D0742557

TISSUE TYPING
AND ORGAN
TRANSPLANTATION

ACADEMIC PRESS RAPID MANUSCRIPT REPRODUCTION

*Proceedings of a Symposium
on Tissue Typing and Organ Transplantation
Held at the University of Minnesota,
Minneapolis, Minnesota
May 14-16, 1970*

TISSUE TYPING AND ORGAN TRANSPLANTATION

Edited by

Edmond J. Yunis

Departments of Laboratory Medicine and Pathology
Division of Immunology
University of Minnesota Medical School
Minneapolis, Minnesota

Richard A. Gatti

Department of Pediatrics
University of Minnesota Hospitals
Minneapolis, Minnesota

D. Bernard Amos

Department of Immunology
Duke University Medical Center
Durham, North Carolina

ACADEMIC PRESS *New York and London* 1973

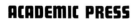

A Subsidiary of Harcourt Brace Jovanovich, Publishers

ACADEMIC PRESS, INC.
111 Fifth Avenue, New York, New York 10003

United Kingdom Edition published by
ACADEMIC PRESS, INC. (LONDON) LTD.
24/28 Oval Road, London NW1

Library of Congress Cataloging in Publication Data

Symposium on Tissue Typing and Organ Transplantation,
    University of Minnesota, 1970.
    Tissue typing and organ transplantation.

    1. Transplantation immunology.–Congresses.
2. Histocompatibility testing–Congresses.
I.   Yunis, Edmond, J., ed.   II.   Gatti, Richard a., ed.
III.   Amos, Dennis Bernard, DATE   ed.   IV.   Title.
[DNLM: 1. Histocompatibility testing.   2. Trans-
plantation immunology. WO 680 Y95t 1973]
RD120.7.S9 1970   617'.95   72–88375
ISBN 0–12–775160–2

CONTENTS

CONTRIBUTORS vii

PREFACE ix

Human Leukocyte Antigens and Antibodies:
An Introduction 1
    Roy L. Walford

Genetics of HL-A Antigens 13
    Jean Dausset

The Prognostic Value of HL-A Typing in Kidney Transplantation . . 49
    J. J. van Rood

The Meaning and Use of the Mixed Leukocyte
Culture Test in Transplantation 71
    Byung H. Park and Robert A. Good

Some Observations on the Mixed-Lymphocyte Culture:
Potential Clinical Uses 93
    Brack G. Hattler, Jr.

Histocompatibility Matching and Donor Selection 117
    D. Bernard Amos and Edmond J. Yunis

Dialysis Today: Its Role and Application 135
    Fred L. Shapiro

Renal Transplantation versus Chronic Dialysis:
Indications and Contraindications 143
    Carl M. Kjellstrand

The Surgeons' View of Tissue Typing in Human Transplantation . . . 159
    John E. Woods

Kidney Transplantation 165
    Richard L. Simmons, Carl M. Kjellstrand,
    and John S. Najarian

CONTENTS

Immune Suppression and the Incidence of Malignancy 281
    Charles F. McKhann

The Biology of Kidney Allograft Transplantation 285
    John E. Foker and John S. Najarian

Pathology in Allograft Recipients 329
    David T. Rowlands, Jr., and Peter M. Burkholder

A Search for Chemical Tags on Transplantation Antigens 357
    R. A. Popp, Mary W. Francis, and Diana M. Popp

The Solubilization and Characterization of the HL-A
Transplantation Antigens 381
    Edward E. Etheredge

Bone Marrow Transplantation: The Minnesota
Experience up to 1970 407
    Hilaire J. Meuwissen

Bone Marrow Transplantation in Combined
Immunodeficiency Disease 413
    W. Douglas Biggar, Byung H. Park, Philip Niosi,*
    Edmond J. Yunis, and Robert A. Good

Bone Marrow Transplantation for Acute Lymphocytic Leukemia . . 437
    Richard A. Gatti, Mark Ballow, and Robert A. Good

Transplantation: A Critical Appraisal 451
    Leonard J. Greenberg, Edmond J. Yunis,
    D. Bernard Amos, and Andreas Rosenberg

SUBJECT INDEX 475

*Deceased

CONTRIBUTORS

D. Bernard Amos, Department of Immunology, Duke University Medical Center, Durham, North Carolina 27710

Mark Ballow, Department of Pediatrics, University of Minnesota Hospitals, Minneapolis, Minnesota 55455

W. Douglas Biggar, Department of Pediatrics, University of Minnesota, Minneapolis, Minnesota 55455

Peter M. Burkholder, Department of Pathology, University of Wisconsin Medical School, Madison, Wisconsin 53706

Jean Dausset, Université de Paris, Hôpital Saint-Louis, 2, Place du Dr. Fournier, 75 Paris, France

Edward E. Etheredge, Department of Surgery, University of Minnesota Health Sciences Center, Minneapolis, Minnesota 55455

John E. Foker, Department of Surgery, University of Minnesota Medical School, Minneapolis, Minnesota 55455

Mary W. Francis, Biology Division, Oak Ridge National Laboratory, Oak Ridge, Tennessee 37830

Richard A. Gatti, Department of Pediatrics, University of Minnesota Hospitals, Minneapolis, Minnesota 55455

Robert A. Good, Sloan-Kettering Institute for Cancer Research, New York, New York 10021

Leonard J. Greenberg, Department of Laboratory Medicine, Division of Immunology, University of Minnesota Medical School, Minneapolis, Minnesota 55455

Brack G. Hattler, Jr., Department of Surgery, Division of Thoracic Surgery, University of Arizona Medical Center, Tucson, Arizona 85721

Carl M. Kjellstrand, Department of Medicine, University of Minnesota, Minneapolis, Minnesota 55455

Charles F. McKhann, Departments of Surgery and Microbiology, University of Minnesota, Minneapolis, Minnesota 55455

Hilaire J. Meuwissen, Department of Pediatrics, Albany Medical College of Union University, Albany, New York 12208

John S. Najarian, Department of Surgery, University of Minnesota Hospitals, Minneapolis, Minnesota 55455

Philip Niosi,* Department of Laboratory Medicine, University of Minnesota, Minneapolis, Minnesota 55455

Byung H. Park, Departments of Pediatrics and Pathology, University of Minnesota Medical School, Minneapolis, Minnesota 55455

Diana M. Popp, Biology Division, Oak Ridge National Laboratory, Oak Ridge, Tennessee 37830

R. A. Popp, Biology Division, Oak Ridge National Laboratory, Oak Ridge, Tennessee, 37830

Andreas Rosenberg, Department of Laboratory Medicine, University of Minnesota Medical School, Minneapolis, Minnesota 55455

David T. Rowlands, Jr., School of Medicine, University of Pennsylvania, Philadelphia, Pennsylvania 19104

Fred L. Shapiro, Medical Director, Community Dialysis Center, Hennepin County General Hospital, and University of Minnesota, Minneapolis, Minnesota 55455

Richard L. Simmons, Department of Surgery, University of Minnesota Hospitals, Minneapolis, Minnesota 55455

J. J. van Rood, Department of Immunohematology, University Hospital, Leiden, The Netherlands

Roy L. Walford, Department of Pathology, UCLA School of Medicine, Los Angeles, California 90024

John E. Woods, Department of Surgery, Mayo Clinic, Rochester, Minnesota 55901

Edmond J. Yunis, Departments of Laboratory Medicine and Pathology, Division of Immunology, University of Minnesota Medical School, Minneapolis, Minnesota 55455

*Deceased

PREFACE

In this book we have tried to provide the student of immunology, medicine, and surgery with an introduction to transplantation biology. Progress in this field has been so rapid that any attempt at a comprehensive treatment of the subject not only presents a formidable task but also appears deficient in many areas immediately after publication. In an effort to minimize such deficiencies we have continously updated various chapters.

The material in this text is roughly divided into two parts: The first part deals with the theoretical and technical aspects of assessing genetic disparity and the chemistry of transplantation antigens; the second part is devoted to surgical and clinical problems of kidney and bone marrow transplantation. The final chapter of this book is a critical appraisal of the whole field of transplantation today which we hope will provide the student with some food for thought and possibly seduce a few individuals into active participation.

We wish to acknowledge the secretarial assistance of Nancy Swanson and Margery Knutson. The editors also wish to thank Dr. Leonard J. Greenberg for editorial assistance.

Edmond J. Yunis
Richard A. Gatti
D. Bernard Amos

TISSUE TYPING AND ORGAN TRANSPLANTATION

HUMAN LEUKOCYTE ANTIGENS AND ANTIBODIES: AN INTRODUCTION

Roy L. Walford

Department of Pathology
UCLA School of Medicine
Los Angeles, California

The delineation of the human leukocyte antigenic systems, particularly the HL-A system, has assumed increasing importance in the last few years. The discipline has arrived at that stage of maturity where its discoveries spill over into and are useful in other fields, for example in blood banking, organ transplantation, and an understanding of the differential susceptibility to disease states, to name only the more obvious practical areas. This maturity was preceded by a long developmental period concerned largely with attaining a methodology reliable enough that the immunogenetic makeup of the highly polymorphic, major histocompatibility system in man, the HL-A system, could be approximated.

Antisera for tissue typing come from three sources. Sera from multiply transfused patients was the original source of leukoagglutinins, and transfusion leads equally well to the production of lymphocytotoxic antibodies. As a rough rule, about half the patients who receive 10 to 20 blood transfusions develop leukocyte-reactive antibodies. Antisera raised by the stimulus of HL-A-unmatched transfused blood is generally quite multispecific.

The second historical source was the sera of postpartum women. As in this case the antibodies are a response to immunization by fetal antigens, and half the fetal genes are of maternal origin, the antiserum produced tends to be less multispecific

1

than that following transfusion. While one antigen, now called HL-A2 or Mac, was roughly defined in 1958 by use of posttransfusional antisera, it was the use of the more simplified postpartum antisera and computer methods that led to the first definition of diallelic systems, including 4a and 4b plus HL-A1 and HL-A2. Complete references are given elsewhere (1,4).

The use of computer methods applied to the reactions of multispecific antisera to define a single, specific antigen can be illustrated by reference to Fig. 1. Using a large cell panel (such as 100 cells) and 2 X 2 tables subjected to Chi-square analysis (Fig. 2), those antisera that are strongly related to one another, i.e., have at least one antibody in common, can be picked out. Then any donor whose cells react with all these highly related antisera can be assumed to possess that antigen which is reactive with the common antibody. In Fig. 1, donor cells 4, 5, 6, and 7 would possess antigen 2, as defined by this analysis.

While the expanded application of the above method has allowed for great advances in defining the leukocyte antigenic systems, the HL-A system is ultimately too complex for dissection with other than monospecific antisera. A few such can indeed be found if large numbers (hundreds) of postpartum sera are screened. An additional method of obtaining monospecific antisera has been the use of planned immunization of volunteer or professional recipients. The subject for potential immunization is typed for HL-A and from a large, similarly typed panel a donor who is identical to the recipient for all but one HL-A antigen is selected. Intradermal or intravenous immunization of the recipient with leukocytes isolated from the selected donor is then carried out.

Three tests for determining HL-A antibodies have been widely employed. The first, historically, was the leukoagglutination test with either the defibrination or EDTA techniques. Except for certain factors ~~that~~ cannot be so definitively measured by other

2

techniques (e.g., 4a and 4b) or even measured at all (the Five system, and 9a, which are wholly indepen- dent of HL-A), leukoagglutination is not much used anymore. The method most popular at present is the lymphocytotoxicity technique, and secondly the platelet complement-fixation test (3). The great majority of HL-A factors are well expressed on platelets.

The general serologic structure or pattern of the HL-A system can now be set forth (Table 1). Because of rapidity of advance in the field, each laboratory tends to develop its own nomenclature. Ten or twelve different nomenclatures have been in use for the HL-A system. In 1968 the WHO Leukocyte Nomenclature Committee met for the first time and began to codify the different systems. Individual nomenclatures are still in use but when a number of different laboratories all have equivalent antisera detecting a new specificy, an HL-A designation is given. The numbers used for different specificities at the 1970 Histocompatibility Testing Workshop (3), where these have not yet been superseded by official HL-A designations, have received semiofficial sanc- tion by usage.

The HL-A system as presently visualized can be divided into two segregant series or loci (Table 1). Within each segregant series the specificities are mutually exclusive: if for example HL-A1 is asso- ciated with the chromosome, none of the other speci- ficities of that series can be. Since each person has two HL-A chromosomes, each has two specificities from the first and two from the second series. Supposedly, no person will express more than four specificities. Many will express fewer, either because of the existence of null factors, or because antiserum to the undetected specificity is not available. The full genotype of an individual might properly be written as, for example, HL-A(1,5/3,13) because each of the two chromosomes will have one specificity from the first and one from the second segregant series.

3

The two segregant series show a considerable
degree of genetic disequilibrium. This means, for
example, that HL-A8 of the second series, when present, is not randomly distributed with respect to the
specificities of the first series. HL-A8 tends to
occur most often with HL-A1. HL-A2 tends likewise
to have HL-A12 with it on the same chromosome. The
situation is similar to that of factors C and D of
the Rh system, to cite another example of genetic
disequilibrium.

Cross-reacting antibodies appear to be common in
the HL-A system and are in part responsible for the
rather appalling complexity of most random posttransfusional or postpartum antisera. Some specimens of anti-Ba* react also with some cells possess-
ing the HL-A2 antigen, of anti-HL-A11 with HL-A1 and
3, and so forth. These assemblages have been termed
"cross-reactive groups." It is uncertain at present
whether the original 4a and 4b of van Rood are very
large cross-reactive groups encompassing most of the
known HL-A factors, represent core substances, or
are in fact separate from both the first and second
segregant series. 4a and 4b appear to show better
correlation with renal homograft survival than the
individual, officially designated HL-A specificities.

The chief areas in which leukocyte typing may
have medical significance are listed in Table 2.
Not all of these will be discussed. With regard to
transfusions, the HL-A antigens are represented both
on white blood cells and platelets as well as other
cells. With recent findings that platelets will
survive in a viable condition for at least 3 days if
kept at room temperature (2), the use of platelet
transfusion in thrombocytopenic or thrombocytopathic
states becomes much more practical than it has been,
for platelets can be made available for component
therapy as part of routine blood banking. However,
it is necessary to transfuse with HL-A compatible
platelets to achieve maximal results and avoid
sensitization. One can select platelet donors either
from a large, typed pool or from among HL-A typed

family members.

HL-A typing will clearly be employed in pater-
nity testing in the future. However, it has not yet
had its first case in court. Terasaki and I have
appeared in one potential case, but the judge would
not accept the testimony, and sent us back to our
own benches. Because the HL-A system is so complex,
a very large number of genetic combinations are possible, and the chance of excluding a falsely labeled
father via HL-A alone is better than for ABO, Rh,
and MNS combined. An example of a family analysis,
in this case a family one of whose children had
acute leukemia, is given in Fig. 3.

In such an analysis, the father, mother, and
children are phenotyped with available HL-A antisera
and the results recorded as (+) or (-) in the manner
shown (Fig. 3). In the example, the father is (+)
for both HL-A2 and 9. As these both belong to the
first series, the rule of mutual exclusivity dic-
tates that they are not on the same chromosome.
Therefore, arbitrarily let HL-A2 be on α chromosome
labeled "a" and 9 on chromosome "b". HL-A2 is not
present on the mother but is on both children, so
both children have "a". W17 is present on the father
but not on mother or children; therefore, W17 resides
on "b" along with HL-A9. Chromosome "a" appears null
at the second series with the listed antisera. The
father's genotype is HL-A(2,?/9,W17). No man who
is not HL-A2(+) and with a null second-series "a"
chromosome could have fathered these children.

HL-A typing has much to offer the expanding
field of anthropology. HL-A differences between
racial groups seem very substantial, and the system
represents a nice, differentiating serologic tool.
The HL-A1 specificity, for example, while present in
monkeys, in man is only found in Caucasians, and not
in the other races so far tested. The next International Histocompatibility Workshop will focus upon
the subject of anthropology and will document HL-A
types from about three dozen different populations
of the world. We ourselves, for example, have chosen

to examine pre-Inca tribes of Peru and Bolivia, with a partial view towards Heyerdahl's well-known thesis that the original Polynesians came by sea from these or related early civilizations. The workshop will also be of inestimable value in helping elucidate the many immunogenetic uncertainties still remaining about the HL-A system.

The most interesting new development in HL-A is the correlation of certain specificities with certain disease states and/or with immune response capacity to specific antigens or possibly to infectious agents. This subject has been reviewed elsewhere in detail (5). Previous attempts to find such disease correlations for the ABO and other standard blood group systems have, with a few exceptions, not amounted to much. It seems unlikely that this will happen with HL-A, because the analogous histocompatibility system, H-2 in the mouse, is proven beyond any doubt to show strong correlations with disease states, viral susceptibilities, and other facets of reticuloendothelial activity. A few diseases for which good evidence of HL-A relationships exists are shown in Table 2, together with those specificities that appear significantly elevated. The 4c, which is elevated in Hodgkin's disease, in fact represents a cross-reactive group, the components of which are HL-A5, R∗, CM∗, and W15 (5). We expect that further work on HL-A and related systems may lead to important advances in our knowledge of the genetic component of disease, and particularly in those instances of so-called "multifactorial" genetic susceptibility or resistance.

Acknowledgement

A portion of the author's work has been supported by the Blood Bank of San Bernardino-Riverside Counties.

References

1. Kissmeyer-Nielsen, F., and Thorsby, E. Human transplantation antigens. Transplant. Rev. 4, 1-176 (1970).
2. Murphy, S., and Gardner, F.H. Platelet preservation. Effect of storage temperature on maintenance of platelet viability - deleterious effect of refrigerated storage. N. Engl. J. Med. 280, 1094-1098 (1969).
3. Svejgaard, A. Isoantigenic systems of human blood platelets. A survey. Ser. Haematol. 2, No. 3 (1969).
4. Walford, R.L. The isoantigenic systems of human leukocytes: Medical and biological significance. Ser. Haematol. 2, No. 2 (1969).
5. Walford, R.L., Waters, H., and Smith, G.S. Histocompatibility systems and disease states, with particular reference to cancer. Transplant. Rev. (1972).

Table 1

The Best Delineated Antigenic Factors of the HL-A System

| First segregant series or locus (the LA locus) | | | Second segregant series or locus (the 4 locus) | | |
Officially named	1970 Workshop number	Other designations	Officially named	1970 Workshop number	Other designations
HL-A1		LA1	HL-A5		Da-5
HL-A2(Mac)		LA2,Mac	HL-A7		7c
HL-A3		LA3	HL-A8		7d
HL-A9		Lc-11	HL-A12		T12,Da-4
HL-A10		Da-17	HL-A13		HN
HL-A11		ILN*			
	W19	{Thompson,La-W / Ao-28,Li		W5	R*,4c*
	W28	Ba*,Da-15,Lc-17 / Lc-26		W15	LND,Te-55
				W10	BB
				W27	FJH
				W22	AA,Bt-22
				W14	Maki,Te-54
					CM*
					TE-57

8

Table 2

Main Areas of Applicability of HL-A Typing

1.	Transfusion	
	The buffy-coat reaction	
	Platelet transfusions	
2.	Organ transplantation	
3.	Paternity studies	
4.	Anthropology	
5.	Disease correlations	
	Hodgkin's disease	4c
	Acute leukemia in children	HL-A2,12
	Non-Hodgkin's lymphomas	HL-A12
	Systemic lupus erythematosus	W15 (=LND)
	Chronic glomerulonephritis	HL-A2

Antiserum

Donor Cells	A		B		C	
1	+	} 1	−		−	
2	+	{	−		+	} 5
3	+	} 3	−		+	
4	+		+		+	
5	+	} 2	+	} 2	+	} 2
6	+		+		+	
7	+		+		+	
8	−		+	} 4	+	
9	−		+		+	} 6
10	−		−		+	

Fig. 1. Hypothetical model showing reactivity of leukocytes of ten donors with antisera: (A) contains three different antibodies (1, 3, and 2), (B) contains two antibodies (2 and 4), and (C) contains three antibodies (5, 2, and 6). Only cells containing antigen 2 would react with all three antisera.

```
                 Reactions
                   with
                  serum 2
                    +  -
Reactions    +   a  b   a=number positive with both sera
                        b=number positive with #1 and
with                       negative with 2
                        c=number negative with #1 and
                           positive with 2
serum 1      -   c  d   d=number negative with both
```

Then $\chi^2 = \dfrac{(ad-bc)^2 N}{(a+b)(c+d)(a+c)(b+d)}$, and $p < .05$ for $\chi^2 > 3.8$

Fig. 2. The Chi-square test to show that two antisera are related, and therefore, as a first approximation, may be assumed to have one antibody in common.

Segregant Series

		First						Second				
Family of Segregant		HL-A 1	HL-A 2	HL-A 3	HL-A 9	HL-A 10	HL-A 11	HL-A 5	HL-A 7	HL-A 8	HL-A 12	HL-A 13	w17
Father	a	−	+	−	+	−	−	−	−	−	−	−	+
	b												
Mother	c	+	−	−	+	−	−	−	−	+	+	−	−
	d												
Leukemic child	a	−	+	−	+	−	−	−	−	−	+	−	−
	d												
Healthy child	a	+	+	−	−	−	−	−	−	+	−	−	−
	c												

Fig. 3.   Immunogenetic analysis of a family. Phenotypic data are given as (+) or (−) under each specificity for each family member. Genotypes can then be derived by simple inspection, assuming the validity of the two segregant series hypothesis plus the rule of mutual exclusivity (allelism) for each series.

11

GENETICS OF HL-A ANTIGENS

J. Dausset

Hopital Saint Louis
2, Place du Dr. Fournier
75 Paris, France

The subject of this presentation will be the genetics of the main histocompatibility system in man, i.e., the HL-A system. I shall therefore consider the theoretical and practical aspects of the choice of a suitable donor and also try to discuss the physiological role of this system, which is maintained in its diversity not in order to irritate the surgeons, but for another and probably more important purpose.

The HL-A system appears to be the most complex genetic system ever known in man. It is the equivalent of the H-2 system in mouse and of other main histocompatibility systems known to exist in all other species studied.

All the work in man was possible because of the precise and patient research made in animals and particularly in mice by Gorer and Snell (49). The link between mice and men was affected by Amos (1a) when, by means of leucoagglutination, he discovered that the H-2 antigens are also present in leucocytes.

The HL-A system has been progressively defined by the joint efforts of several teams all over the world. After our demonstration, in 1958, of the first leucocyte antigen Mac (16), van Rood found the contrasting distribution of two other antigenic entities 4a and 4b (55), and Payne and Bodmer (42) described an allelic pair of antigens LA1 and LA2 (the latter being, in fact, the antigen Mac). Since then, the contributions of other teams, namely

13

Shulman, Amos, Walford, Terasaki, Ceppellini, Lale-
zari, Batchelor, Kissmeyer-Nielsen, Thorsby, and
others, have amassed a large amount of data and have
accelerated the definition of tissue antigens. The
role played by the workshops, so well organized by
Amos, van Rood, Ceppellini, and Terasaki, must be
emphasized (3, 15, 44, 52).

In the history of human blood groups, the role
played by the associations found between antigens
during population studies was extremely important.
For example, the antigens C, D, and E of the Rhesus
system are, at least in the Caucasian population,
frequently associated. Antigens M and S in the MNS
system are also frequently associated.

The same kind of work has been carried out for
leukocyte antigens and, on the basis of the correlations observed in population studies, with Ivanyi
in 1965, we came to the conclusion that all these
antigens belonged to a single system that we proposed
to call Hu-1 (24). Now this system is international-
ly known as the HL-A system.

The present situation of the HL-A system,
slightly modified after the Fourth Conference in
Histocompatibility held in Los Angeles, is illustrated in Fig. 1. One of the chromosomes of the
autosomal pair (still unknown) that bears the HL-A
system is represented. There are two well-defined
loci. Personally, we have no evidence of the existence of a third locus, although some data in this
line have been presented (45).

The various products of the first locus are
listed below. The first segregant series includes
genes HL-A1,A2,A3,A9,A10,A11, and Da-15 (Ba*), and
Da-22 and -25. Other specificities, such as Li and
LAW, also belong to this series. All of them are
mutually exclusive, i.e., only a single of these
genes can be present on the chromosome. The second
segregant series includes genes HL-A5,A7,A8,A12,A13,
Da(6), Da(9), Da-18 (Maki), Da-20 (R*), Da-23 (Te15),
Da-24, BB, FJH, Te-17, Te-18, and probably other
specificities such as SL* and 407*. They are also

mutually exclusive.

Consequently, every man possesses four HL-A sites, two on each of his homologous chromosomes. Therefore, in the present state of our knowledge, he cannot possess more than four antigens; however, the number of combinations is extremely large even for these four sites only.

The frequencies of the various antigens in the Caucasian population is given in Table 1. The most frequent antigen is the Mac or HL-A2 (0.45), whereas the frequency of the other antigens vary from 0.03 to 0.29.

You have accepted the idea of the existence of two segregant series; yet, I must show you some evidence to justify this assertion.

The first evidence is from population studies: In all the populations that have been studied up to now, no individuals having more than two antigens of the first series and two antigens of the second series have been found.

Study by the double-back-cross method of this segregating series in 186 families shows that a parent having two genes of this first series never transmits them together to his children. In other words, the two genes always segregate as alleles (22) (Table 2).

Figs. 2 and 3 illustrate the distribution of these genes in our panel of Caucasian individuals. The complexity is still greater than for the first series; however, no individual possesses more than two of these genes.

Informative families in double-back-cross again show that there is no child being either negative or positive for two antigens of the second series (20, 22). I must say that, among the 300 families studied during the last workshop, many other informative families were observed who showed the same results, thus confirming the two loci or subloci theory (21, 28, 34, 48). The proximity of the two loci on the same chromosome is proved by the usual absence of crossing over between the two loci. In the greatest

majority of cases, the genes of the two loci are
transmitted en bloc. This gene combination is called
"haplotype," that is, half the genotype. For
instance this en bloc transmission of the two genes
is illustrated in the family shown in Fig. 4. The
father possesses the haplotypes HL-A1, 12 on one of
his chromosomes and HL-A3, 7 on the other. The
mother's haplotypes are HL-A2, 5 and Da-15, HL-A8.
Only four types of children are possible, for, in the
absence of crossing over between the two loci, only
four combinations of these four haplotypes can occur.
In this family, only three types of children have
been found.

This is the rule, but a few crossings over have
already been observed, by Ward et al. (57), and by
Kissmeyer-Nielsen et al. (33). We observed an other
example (22).

The family illustrated in Fig. 5 shows an
indisputable crossing over with exchange of genetic
material. Four of the children have received the
parental blocks as expected, but one child has
received from his mother the gene of the first locus
present on one chromosome, Da-15, and the gene of the
second locus present on the other chromosome, HL-A12.

It is not yet possible to establish the rate of
recombinations between the two loci with certainty,
but it seems to be relatively high, perhaps about
0.5%. On the whole, six families with crossing over
have been observed in the world (57).

In our laboratory, 186 families were studied.
We could determine 24 HL-A antigens plus two postulated for 67 others. With the newly discovered
antigens, only 2% of the genes of the first locus
and 6% of the genes of the second locus are still
unknown (Table 1).

Table 3 shows the repartition of the 268
observed haplotypes in the 67 families studied for
HL-A antigens. It is to be noted that there are some
haplotypes that are clearly more frequent than the
others. For instance, HL-A1,8 was observed 20 times
in 170 individuals. HL-A2,12 is also a frequent

combination (15 times), and HL-A3,7 was met 10 times.

This shows that there is what is called a "linkage disequilibrium" between the two loci, which do not behave as if they were perfectly independent of each other. For instance, the association HL-A1,8 is more frequent than one would expect from mere hazard. Maybe this observation is due to a selective advantage for some of these haplotypes, or perhaps it merely reflects that there is not enough crossing over occurring during evolution between the two loci.

The simple combinations of 26 genes on the pair of homologous chromosomes can involve a considerable number of phenotypes, haplotypes, and genotypes. It can be expected that there will be 7672 different phenotypes, 187 different haplotypes, and 17,578 different genotypes.

It must be emphasized that all the antigens have not yet been detected. Consequently, these figures will certainly increase. They already illustrate the fantastic polymorphism of these tissue antigens.

A geneticist will at once ask whether the system studied is in equilibrium, i.e., whether the same percentage of genes will be found again from one generation to the other. This direct study has not yet been made. However, we have studied the segregation of the genes in the families in whom one of the parents was heterozygous for a given gene.

In these matings, $+ - x - -$, we have found a fairly equal number of children who do and who do not have the antigen, which is a good indication for the absence of a rough disequilibrium (Table 4). However, this calculation has been made only on fertile men and therefore does not exclude the possibility of the existence of a gene, analogous to the T locus in mice, closely linked to H2, that would induce sterility.

Finally, we have demonstrated that the HL-A system is independent of many other biological markers: erythrocytes, platelets, serous systems, and erythrocyte enzyme systems (Table 5). We must add that no close linkage with many known normal or

pathological genes has been found as yet (1)
(Table 6).

Thus, in spite of the extreme polymorphism of
this genetic system, it is possible to reach a
logical arrangement that perfectly follows the Men-
delian laws. It has taken a long time and it has
necessitated hard work to demonstrate this genetical
logic. The difficulty was mainly due to a very
peculiar feature of the HL-A gene products.
    The HL-A region is probably composed of at least
two closely linked loci, with 0.5% recombination
fraction. Each locus is a functional unit with
several possibilities for mutations. The direct or
indirect product of this functional unit would be a
molecule with several antigenic determinants or
factors. The allelic products of the same locus
would differ by one or several modifications of these
factors.
    The serological complexity of the HL-A system
is probably due to at least two phenomena: (a) antigenic factors (still hypothetical) and (b) cross
reactions between the different products of a same
locus (well-established fact).
    In a given population, it seems that some
antigenic factors are so frequently associated that
it is impossible to dissociate them when the absorption is carried out with cells from the same population. However, one may expect that in other populations there are individuals lacking one or several of
these factors. The dissociation would then be possible (24).
    Thanks to the discovery, independently made by
Colombani (13, 14, 19) in our laboratory and Svejgaard (50) in Denmark, it is known that the greatest
part of the serological complexity is due to the
extreme frequency of cross reactions between the
antigenic products of the same locus.
    No cross reaction has been observed between

products of the two loci as yet. This might indicate that they have different gene ancestors.

It must be assumed that the common part between allelic products is large enough to allow cross reactions between them. Cross reactions explain the development of "broad" antibodies reacting with several allelic products, thus included in broad specificities.

They explain also the development of what we propose to call "narrow" antibodies, which react with one specificity but are absorbed without reaction by another, leading to the ANAP phenomenon (Agglutination negative, absorption positive) described by van Rood (55) (Fig. 6).

The first example of cross reaction was observed between HL-A2 and Da-15 or Ba* (19). Later on the anti-Da-2 broad antibody was shown to react with both HL-A2 and Da-15, which are two alleles of the first segregant series.

Cross reactions between products of the second series are even more striking. In 1965 an antigen, Da-6, was described, but in 1969 we discovered that Da-6 could be broken into three specificities, all being alleles of the second locus: HL-A5, Da-19, and Da-20 (R*) (14). In 1970, Da-19 was itself broken into two other specificities, Da-23 (LND) and Da-24, which are completely included in Da-19 (14) (Fig. 7).

These cross reactions are of the utmost practical importance, for otherwise it probably would be impossible to find a compatible donor, the number of combinations being much too large.

We shall come back to this point, which is extremely important from the practical angle.

The chemical analysis of the HL-A antigens are now in progress in several laboratories (29, 39, 46). We are working on this problem in collaboration with Davies (29).

The striking analogy of H-2 and HL-A soluble antigens has been already underlined by several authors. It has been shown that HL-A soluble antigens are glycoproteins with 92% proteins and 8% neutral sugar. Their molecular weight is 50,000 to 60,000. According to Mann's and Nathenson's work (39), it seems that the two loci build different molecules that could be separated by ion chromatography and acrylamid gel electrophoresis. This is an argument in favor of the concept of two functional units on the chromosomes.

More clear-cut chemical data are needed before we can express any definite opinion about the relationships between genes and final products. However, we may at least give our present concept of the HL-A system (Fig. 8).

It is quite possible that the parts of the locus governing the main determinants, which behave as alleles in the Caucasian population, are in fact pseudoalleles, and it would not be surprising at all to find two of these main determinants governed in the cis position by the same chromosome in another population.

Now I should like to say a few words about the localization of these substances. They are components of the cellular membrane of most tissues. It has been possible to visualize their presence.

Anti-HL-A antigens have been labeled with ferritin by Kourilsky et al. (36). This electron-microscopic section of lymphocytes shows that, as for the H-2 model, HL-A antigens are gathered in distinct areas. They are not uniformly distributed on the surface. The biological significance of this fact is still unknown.

The localization on the different tissues of the body has also been studied, but this time by absorption experiments. Antigen HL-A2 (Mac) is present in huge quantity in spleen, and in decreasing quantities in liver, lungs, kidney, heart, intestine, and aorta. However, from these preliminary data, it is not possible to conclude that heart, for example, is more easily transplantable than liver or spleen (6).

The localization of HL-A antigens on spermatozoa

was studied by cytotoxicity technique. The haploid expression of HL-A genes on spermatozoa was probably demonstrated.

Table 7 gives an example of this study. The genotype of the donor's spermatozoa was HL-A1,8/ HL-A2,5. Each of the antibodies against these specificities, when used individually, gave a percentage of cytotoxicity of around 50%. When we mixed the antibodies against the product of the two genes in the position (anti-HL-A2 + anti-HL-A8, or anti-HL-A2 + anti-HL-A5) the percentage of killed spermatozoa remained around 50%. However, when the mixture of antibodies was against product in the trans or allelic position, for example anti-HL-A1 + anti-HL-A2, the percentage of killed spermatozoa rose up to 72 to 81%. The same experiment was made with another donor. Here again, the mixture of antibodies against products of genes in the cis position gave less than 50% of killed spermatozoa. The mixture against antigens in trans or allelic position gave from 67 to 78% of killed spermatozoa. A specific anti-HL-A2 against the spermatozoa of individuals who were homozygous for HL-A2 gave a percentage of killed spermatozoa around 80% (30).

The finding of a probable haploid expression in spermatozoa makes available the first mammalian material of this kind. We have also found the same haploid expression of H-2 in mice spermatozoa. If this haploid expression is confirmed, the direct determination of the haplotypes and genotypes of the HL-A system in males will be possible. It will also be possible to study directly the rate of recombination and the rate of mutations. One can also contemplate the possibility of gametic selection based on the use of cytotoxic antibodies recognizing HL-A or other antigens. One might even speculate on the prevention of hereditary diseases governed by linked loci through artificial insemination with one population of spermatozoa.

The other biological implications of the knowledge of the HL-A system are numerous.

It is certainly one of the best markers available because of its extreme polymorphism. Preliminary data indicate that it will be very useful in anthropology. For example, oriental populations are practically devoid of antigens HL-A1 and -A8. Other antigens, for instance Da-15 or Ba* are much more frequent in Negroes than in Caucasions. It is probable that some antigens exclusive to some populations will be found.

It seems to be of utmost importance to establish the world HL-A map before the disappearance of isolated populations. This will be the subject of the next workshop in histocompatibility.

Attention, however, is now focused on two other points: the role of HL-A in transplantation and the role of HL-A in the defense of body integrity and in the susceptibility to diseases.

Regarding transplantation almost everything has been said. Though the role of HL-A in transplantation is widely accepted, there remains a certain degree of scepticism, mostly among surgeons, mainly because of the difficulty of correlating the fate of grafts between unrelated individuals with typing. Obviously, the best results were observed with grafts between related individuals. For example, in skin grafts performed between sibs by Amos (2), or by Ceppellini (10), the longest survivals (21 days) were observed when the two sibs had received the two same HL-A haplotypes from their parents. When they had only one haplotype in common, the survival was 14 days, and when they differed for the two haplotypes, the survival was only 13.1 days.

This observation was confirmed by results of mixed lymphocyte cultures. Bach and Amos (5) could predict the existence of a single main system in man when they observed no stimulation between the lymphocytes of 25% of the sibs studied, that is to say, those who were HL-A identical.

We made the analysis of 156 kidney transplantations performed in Paris. Obviously, the best ones were those performed between HL-A identical sibs.

All the 24 cases are still in perfect condition (23). These data are converging proofs that the HL-A system is the main histocompatibility system in man and that the other histocompatibility systems are weak, having no activity in mixed lymphocyte culture (MLC) tests, or under immunodepression. However there are other systems, undoubtedly, since skin grafts are rejected even between HL-A identical sibs.

The situation is not as good in HL-A haplo-identical situation; that is to say, when one haplo-type is shared by donor and recipient (grafts per-formed between HL-A haploidentical sibs or between child and parent). Here, the possible presence of incompatibilities governed by the haplotype that is not shared is sufficient to shorten the survival time of either skin or kidney grafts. In our statistics, success is 86%.

The results are less good in HL-A different situations, between unrelated individuals, when donors and recipients differ on the two HL-A chromo-somes. Here only 56% of survivals are observed. The fact that the results are directly related to the number of HL-A haplotypes genetically common to donors and recipients is striking (23, 39).

It is now urgent to determine whether some HL-A antigens are more immunological than others. For this purpose, Felix Rapaport and I have carried out an experiment with skin grafts performed from child-ren to fathers (26, 27). The father was grafted with two skins coming from two children, each of them having received one of the two different maternal haplotypes C or D, and 238 grafts were made. We observed that the skins were often rejected in a bimodal fashion. For example, the skins bearing the C haplotype were rejected in 10 days, and those bearing the D haplotype in 13 to 14 days. This also indicates that the HL-A system is the main transplan-tation system, for even when they are identical for the HL-A system, sibs may receive different sets for the other H systems.

The mean survival time of the skin allografts

for the HL-A compatible grafts was 15.10 days, in
contrast with 12.1 days for the incompatible grafts
(p <0.01).

Seventy-eight grafts were performed in the
donor-recipient situation where there were no unknown
relationships at either of the two HL-A loci and the
subjects were also compatible for ABO and C, D, E,
and Rhesus antigens. The survival time varied in
inverse proportion to the number of incompatibilities. The longest survivals (16.66 days) were seen
in the absence of incompatibility and the shortest
(12.43 days) in the presence of two incompatibilities. The most interesting observation is the mean
survival time of grafts for which there is a compatibility by cross reactions, when donor and recipient
possess two different but cross-reacting antigens.
When there is two such compatibilities by cross
reaction, the survival time is 14.83 days. When
there is one such compatibility by cross reaction,
the survival time is 13.44 days.

Thus compatibility by cross reaction appears to
be better than incompatibility, but not as good as
identity: It is intermediate. It seems to us that
this observation is of extreme importance for the
future of transplantation. As a matter of fact, the
number of alleles at the two loci is increasing to
such an extent that it will soon be impossible to
find a compatible donor for all antigens.

Our skin grafts from children to fathers have
also led to the conclusion that no HL-A antigen
seems to be very much stronger than the others. They
have approximately the same strength.

These data and those of other authors make
possible an attempt at delineating the rules of human
transplantation. Of course, the ABO barrier must be
avoided. Donors and recipients must be ABO compatible following the usual transfusion laws (11, 25).
Among other systems, the P erythrocyte system and the
Lp lipoprotein system were incriminated (7). However, in our skin grafts, no such relationship was
observed.

Regarding the HL-A antigens, I strongly believe that donor-recipient relationships at the four HL-A sites are sufficient to explain most of the results. The best situation occurs when there are four identities or compatibilities between donor and recipient, that is to say when the donor has no antigen absent in the recipient. The worst situation occurs in the presence of four incompatibilities. In the absence of complete identity, the next best situation is where there are three identities (or compatibilities) and one only incompatibility. Such a match may be accepted now, in the present state of the technique, in the case of patients needing urgent treatment.

If we consider antigen A and B of the ABO system as well as ten known and one postulated antigens at the first locus, and 16 known and one postulated antigen at the second locus, 32,000 individuals will be necessary to locate one HL-A-identical unrelated donor, if strict HL-A identity for bone marrow transplantation is to be achieved. If we keep to four compatible sites, as may be feasible for kidney transplantation, the number decreases to 2300. However, if, as we suggested (26), we include the presence of cross-reacting antigens, we may only need 3026 instead of 32,000 individuals to locate an "identical" donor, and only 414 instead of 2300 individuals to locate a compatible donor. This number even decreases if, as may be possible in kidney transplantation, we allow the presence of one donor-recipient incompatibility. The size of a reasonable waiting list seems to be around 500. This is, at least for kidney, a goal that it is possible to reach rather quickly, thanks to a good cooperative program in European nations. France-Transplant and Scandia-Transplant already work according to the criteria delineated here.

The second important implication of the HL-A system in human biology is its possible role in the defense of the body. We must admit that the exact fundamental physiological function, if any, of the main histocompatibility system that exists in all species has not been understood as yet. It is possible that it plays a fundamental role in the defense of the body integrity.

In 1959, Thomas (53), and later Burnet (9), proposed that the subtle diversity determined by histocompatibility antigens on cellular membranes would serve as a guardian of the body integrity, eliminating somatic mutations, or cells bearing tumor- or virus-induced antigens.

In this regard, it is interesting to note that a large proportion of recirculating lymphocytes can, at least in vitro, react without apparent immunization against all the histocompatibility antigens of their own species. In fact, the mixed lymphocyte culture test (MLC) is positive even without immunization. Histocompatibility antigens are the only ones that behave this way. This fact has not yet been explained.

It is possible that this apparent state of pre-immunization is merely due to cross reactions between histocompatibility antigens and microorganisms. Immunization would be formed during the first months of life, even in utero. Fetal thymocytes are capable of reacting with foreign histocompatibility antigens (7) but fetal spleen cells are not reactive and progressively become reactive during the first days of life in the newborn (4, 8).

There are already some indications of relationships between mammal main histocompatibility systems and bacteria: By immunization of guinea pigs, rabbits, rats, and mice with heat-killed hemolytic streptococci of group A or staphylocci, Rapaport (43) induced a strong transplantation immunity against the skin of about 80% of unrelated homologous donors, demonstrating a cross reaction between bacterial antigens and tissue antigens. Also, Terasaki recently found that a cross reaction exists between HL-A antigens and M1 protein of streptococci (31).

This correlates with another observation made by Terasaki (40), who found more patients with

26

haplotype HL-A2,X (X for an unknown gene at the second locus) in glomerulonephritis, which is probably related to streptococci infection.

There are also some indications of relationships between the main histocompatibility systems and susceptibility to oncogenic virus.

It is well known that some correlations have been found between the H-2 system and susceptibility to Gross', Tennant's, and Friend's leukomegenic virus, and probably also to Bittner's mammary tumor virus (37, 51). In humans, some recent findings also point in this direction (17): In ten cases of acute lymphoblastic leukemia, Walford (56) observed six cases with HL-A12 haplotypes, which is much higher than the expected figure. Thorsby (54) also published some data in this line. Although we have not observed this frequency in the 133 acute leukemia cases studied in Paris (35), we think that research in this line deserves to be pursued.

It would be of the utmost interest to try to correlate HL-A typing with either high frequency or absence of some malignant diseases in certain well-defined populations. For example, the nasopharyngo-carcinoma is very frequent in South China; however, there is no chronic lymphocytic leukemia in Asiatic populations, in which, as we know, the HL-A1 and A8 antigens are practically absent.

The simplest hypothesis is the molecular mimicry hypothesis. Because the immunological tolerance to

a general rule, it is likely that nces of genetic control in which to respond to a particular anti- ecause it cross reacts with his is shared determinant belongs to a system, a correlation between susceptibility to this agent Obviously, most of the micro-

have many determinants that obscure the picture. Only a few experimental data can be quoted in favor of this hypothesis. The fact that several mammalian species developed a transplantation

immunity after a bacterial immunization (43) indicates clearly that strain determinants exist and
should not be underestimated. The observation by
Nandi (41) that the Bittner virus infects only those
strains that are compatible at the H-2 locus points
also in the same direction and suggest that the virus
is coated with some part of the cell membrane of the
preceding host. Indeed, it is known that RNA
viruses, when budding at the surface of the cell,
carry along in their envelope some structure of the
host cell membrane, possibly bearing the histocompatibility antigens. Such a hypothesis, although not
eliminated, seems unlikely in view of the recent
information brought to electronmicroscopic studies
with labeled antihistocompatibility antigens antibodies.

The strongest argument against the molecular
mimicry hypothesis is the fact that, at least in the
case of the Gross virus and the Friend virus, FS, the
resistance is dominant. The F^1 hybrids from a mating
between a resistant and a susceptible strains
possesses all the antigens of the two parental inbred
lines and, in particular, the postulated shared
antigen of the susceptible one. Therefore, they
should be susceptible and not resistant.

The second hypothesis is built on solid
experimental ground. It postulates the existence
of a gene, closely linked or identical with the
histocompatibility system, that controls the specific
immune response (immune response genes or Ir genes)
(38). The immune response is dominant and therefore
the F^1 hybrids are expected to be resistant, as they
are. The intervention of such Ir genes, demonstrated
in mice as well as in guinea pigs, has been accepted
for synthetic and nonsynthetic antigens but not yet
for a bacterial or viral antigens. However, it is
very likely that this control is a general physiological mechanism of the histocompatibility genes
themselves. It is not possible now to distinguish
between these two possibilities. However, the Jerne
(32) hypothesis, which postulates that each

28

individual is normally able to react immunologically against all the histocompatibility antigens of his own species that he does not possess, has the great merit of providing the missing link between histocompatibility antigens and immune responses.

In conclusion, the role of the genetic background in the susceptibility to diseases, which has been known for a long time but is still obscure, could find a tentative explanation in the intervention of immunological mechanisms linked to the histocompatibility systems, either by a negative association (antigens borrowed from or cross reacting with the tissue antigens) or a positive association (immune response genes). Histocompatibility antigens could be the true guardians, not only against the metabolic errors called mutations, but also against the penetration of foreign particles and against tumors or virus-induced antigens. The intervention of the histocompatibility systems in the defense of the organism can explain the extreme complexity, almost the individuality, of the antigenic combinations of the HL-A system, which would be the result of the mutations and selections that have operated principally after each epidemic over the centuries. Better knowledge of the relationships between viral or bacterial antigens, tumor antigens, and histocompatibility antigens may prove a fundamental key of life equilibrium.

REFERENCES

1. Allen, F.H., and Dausset, J. Unpublished observation
1a. Amos, D.B. The agglutination of mouse leucocytes by iso-immune sera. Brit. J. Exp. Pathol. 34, 464 (1953).
2. Amos, D.B., Hattler, B.G., MacQueen, J.M., Cohen, I., and Seigler, H.M. An interpretation and application of cytotoxicity typing. In "Advances in Transplantation" (J. Dausset, J. Hamburger, and G. Mathe, eds.), p. 203. Williams and

Wilkins, Baltimore, Maryland, 1967.

3. Amos, D.B., and van Rood, J.J., eds. "Histocompatibility Testing 1965." Munksgaard, Copenhagen, 1965.

4. Auebach, R., and Globerson, A. In vitro induction of the graft-versus-host reaction. Exp. Cell Res. 42, 31 (1966).

5. Bach, F.H., and Amos, D.B. Hu-1 The major histocompatibility locus in man. Science 156, 1506 (1967).

6. Berah, M., Hors, J., and Dausset, J. Concentration of transplantation antigens in human organs. Lancet 2, 106 (1968).

7. Berg, R., Ceppellini, R., Curtoni, E.S., Mattiuz, P.L., and Bearn, A.G. The genetic antigenic polymorphism of human serum. β-lipoprotein and survival of skin-grafts In "Advances in Transplantation" (J. Dausset, J. Hamburger, and G. Mathé, eds.), p. 253. Williams & Wilkins, Baltimore, Maryland, 1967.

8. Bortin, M.M., Rimm, A.A., and Saltzstein, E.C. Ontogenesis of immune capability of murine bone marrow cells and spleen cells against transplantation antigens. J. Immunol. 103, 683 (1969).

9. Burnet, M. Role of the thymus and related organs in immunity. Brit. Med. J. 2, 807 (1969).

10. Ceppellini, R. The genetic basis of transplantation. In "Human Transplantation" (F.T. Rapaport and J. Dausset, eds.) p. 21. Grune & Stratton, New York, 1968.

11. Ceppellini, R., Curtoni, E.S., Mattiuz, P.L., Leigheb, G., Visetti, M., and Colombi, A. Survival of test skin grafts in man: Effect of genetic relationship and of blood group incompatibility. Ann. N.Y. Acad. Sci. 129, 421 (1966).

12. Ceppellini, R., Curtoni, E.S., Mattiuz, P.L., Miggiano, V., Scudeller, G., and Serra, A. Genetics of leukocyte antigens. A family study

of segregation and linkage. In "Histocompati-
bility Testing 1967" (E.S. Curtoni, P.L.
Mattiuz, and R.M. Tosi, eds.), p. 149.
Munksgaard, Copenhagen, 1967.

13. Colombani, J., Colombani, M., and Dausset, J.
Cross-reactions in the HL-A system with special
reference to the Da6 cross-reacting group.
Description of Da22, 23, 24, HL-A antigens
defined by platelet complement fixation. In
"Histocompatibility Testing 1970" (P.I. Terasaki, ed.), p. 79. Munksgaard, Copenhagen,
1970.

14. Colombani, M., Colombani, J., Dastot, H., Meyer,
S., Tongio, M.M., and Dausset, J. Définition de
deux nouveaux antigènes du système HL-A: Da19
et Da20. Réactions croisées entre les antigènes
Da19, Da20, HL-A5 et Da6. Rev. Fr. Etud. Clin.
Biol. 14, 995 (1969).

15. Curtoni, E.S., Mattiuz, P.L., and Tosi, R.M.,
eds. "Histocompatibility Testing 1967.
Munksgaard, Copenhagen, 1967.

16. Dausset, J. Iso-leuco-anticorps. Act.
Haematol. 20, 156 (1958).

17. Dausset, J. Les systèmes d'histocompatibilité
et la susceptibilité au cancer. Presse Med.
76, 1397 (1968).

18. Dausset, J. The genetics of transplantation
antigens. Transplant. Proc. 3, 8-16 (1971).

19. Dausset, J., Colombani, J., Colombani, M.,
Legrand, L., and Feingold, N. Un nouvel antigène du système HL-A (Hu-1): l'antigène 15,
allèle possible des antigènes 1, 11, 12. Nouv.
Rev. Fr. Hematol. 8, 393 (1968).

20. Dausset, J., Colombani, J., Colombani, M.,
Legrand, L., and Feingold, N. Génétique du
système HL-A. Fréquence génique, haplotypique
et génotypique observée dans 113 familles.
Nouv. Rev. Fr. Hematol. 9, 749 (1969).

21. Dausset, J., Colombani, J., Legrand, L., and
Feingold, N. Le deuxième sub-locus du système
HL-A. Nouv. Rev. Fr. Hematol. 8, 841 (1968).

22. Dausset, J., Colombani, J., Legrand, L., and Fellous, M. Genetics of the HL-A system. Population and family studies. Deduction of 480 haplotypes. In "Histocompatibility Testing 1970" (P.I. Terasaki, ed.), p. 53. Munksgaard, Copenhagen, 1970.

23. Dausset, J., Hors, J., and Bigot, J. Etude génotypique de l'histocompatibilité HL-A dans 91 greffes de rein. Presse Med. 77, 1699 (1969).

24. Dausset, J., Ivanyi, P., and Ivanyi, D. Tissue alloantigens in human identification of a complex system (Hu-1) In "Histocompatibility Testing 1965" (D.B. Amos and J.J. van Rood, eds.), p. 51. Munksgaard, Copenhagen, 1965.

25. Dausset, J., and Rapaport, F.T. Role of ABO erythrocyte groups in human histocompatibility reactions. Nature (London) 209, 209 (1966).

26. Dausset, J., and Rapaport, F.T. Histocompatibility studies in haploidentical genetic combinations. Transplant. Proc. 1, 649 (1969).

27. Dausset, J., Rapaport, F.T., Legrand, L., Colombani, J., and Marcelli-Barge, A. Skin allograft survival in 238 human subjects. Role of specific relationships at the four gene sites of the first and second HL-A loci. In "Histocompatibility Testing 1970" (P.I. Terasaki, ed.) p. 381. Munksgaard, Copenhagen, 1970.

28. Dausset, J., Walford, R.L., Colombani, J., Legrand, L., Feingold, N., and Rapaport, F.T. The HL-A sub-loci and their importance in transplantation. Transplant. Proc. 1, 331 (1969).

29. Davies, D.A.L., Manstone, A.J., Viza, D.C., Colombani, J., and Dausset, J. Human transplantation antigens: the HL-A (Hu-1) system and its homology with the mouse H_2 system. Transplantation 6, 571 (1968).

30. Fellous, M., and Dausset, J. Probable haploid expression of HL-A antigens on human spermatozoon. Nature (London) 225, 191 (1970).

31. Hirata, A.A., Armstrong, A.S., Kay, J.W.D., and Terasaki, P.I. Cross-reactions between human transplantation antigens and streptococcal M proteins. In "Histocompatibility Testing 1970" (P.I. Terasaki, ed.), p. 475. Munksgaard, Copenhagen, 1970.

32. Jerne, N.K. Generation of antibody diversity and self tolerance in a new theory. In "Immune Surveillance" (R.T. Smith and L. Landy, eds.), p. 343. Academic Press, New York, 1971.

33. Kissmeyer-Nielsen, F., Svejgaard, A., Ahrons, S., and Staub-Nielsen, L. Crossing over within the HL-A system. Nature (London) 224, 75 (1969).

34. Kissmeyer-Nielsen, F., Svejgaard, A., and Hauge, Genetics of the human HL-A transplantation system. Nature (London) 219,1116 (1968).

35. Kourilsky, F.M., Dausset, J., Feingold, N., Dupuy, J.M., and Bernard, J. Leukocyte groups and acute leukemia. J. Nat. Cancer Inst. 41, 81-87 (1968).

36. Kourilsky, F.M., Silvestre, D., Levy, J.P., Dausset, J., Niccolai, M.G., and Senik, A. Immunoferritin study of the distribution of HL-A antigens on human blood cells. J. Immunol. 106, 454 (1971).

37. Lilly, F., Boyse, E.A., and Old, L.J. Genetic basis of susceptibility to viral leukoemogenesis. Lancet 2, 1207 (1964).

38. McDevitt, H.M., and Benacerraf, B. Genetic control of specific immune responses. Advan. Immunol. 2, 31-74 (1969).

39. Mann, D.L., and Nathenson, S.G. Comparison of soluble human and mouse transplantation antigens. Proc. Nat. Acad. Sci. U.S. 64, 1380 (1969).

40. Mickey, M.R., Kreisler, M., and Terasaki, P.I. Leukocyte antigens and disease. II. Alterations in frequencies of HL-A haplotypes associated with chronic glomerulonephritis In "Histocompatibility Testing 1970" (P.I. Terasaki, ed.),

p. 237. Munksgaard, Copenhagen, 1970.

41. Nandi, S. The H-2 locus and susceptibility to Bittner virus borne by red blood cell in mice. Proc. Nat. Acad. Sci. U.S. 58, 485 (1967).

42. Payne, R., Tripp, M., Weiglie, J., Bodmer, W., and Bodmer, J. A new leucocyte isoantigen system in man. Cold Spring Harbor Sympos. Quant. Biol. 29, 265 (1964).

43. Rapaport, F.T. Homograft sensitivity induction by group A streptococci. Science 145, 409 (1964).

44. Russell, R.S., and Winn, H.J., eds. "Histocompatibility Testing," Publ. No. 1229. Nat. Acad. Sci. Nat. Res. Counc., Washington, D.C., 1965.

45. Sandberg, L., Thorsby, E., Kissmeyer-Nielsen, F. F., and Lindholm, A. Evidence of a third sublocus within the HL-A chromosomal region In "Histocompatibility Testing 1970" (P.I. Terasaki, ed.), p. 165. Munksgaard, Copenhagen, 1970.

46. Sanderson, A.R., and Batchelor, J.R. Transplantation antigens from human spleens. Nature (London)219, 184 (1968).

47. Simonsen, M., Engelbreth-Holm, J., Jensen, E., and Poulsen, H. A study of the graft-versus-host reaction in transplantation to embryos, F_1 hybrids, and irradiated animals. Ann. N.Y. Acad. Sci. 73, 834 (1958).

48. Singal, D.P., Mickey, M.R., Mittal, K.K., and Terasaki, P.I. Serotyping for homotransplantation. XVII. Preliminary studies of HL-A subunits and alleles. Transplantation 6, 904 (1968).

49. Snell, G.D. The H_2 locus of the mouse: observations and speculations concerning its comparative genetics and its polymorphism. Folia Biol. (Prague) 14, 335 (1968).

50. Svejgaard, A., and Kissmeyer-Nielsen, F. Cross-reactive human HL-A isoantibodies. Nature (London) 219, 868 (1968).

51. Tennant, J.R., and Snell, G.D. The H_2 locus
     and viral leukemogenesis as studied in congenic
     strains in mice. J. Nat. Cancer Inst. 41, 597
     (1968).
52. Terasaki, P.I., ed. "Histocompatibility Testing
     1970." Munksgaard, Copenhagen, 1970.
53. Thomas, L.

TABLE 1

THE HL-A SYSTEM

Workshop No.	Ph	G	First Locus	Ph	G	Second Locus	Workshop No.
	.224	.130	HL-A 1 ⎫	.295	.161	HL-A 12 ⎫	
	.240	.128	HL-A 3 ⎬ Da-12			TT (EL ?) ⎬	W18
	.094	.048	HL-A 11 ⎭	.036	.018	HL-A 13 ⎫	
						407* (G + .0006) ⎬	
W28	.451	.259	HL-A 2 ⎫ (Ba*, Te-40)	.179	.091	Te 58	
	.078	.040	Da-15 ⎭	.143	.074	HL-A 5 ⎫	W5
	.247	.132	HL-A 9 { HL-A 9'', Da 27 (G = .092); HL-A 9''	.149	.078	Da-20 (R*, Te 50) ⎬	
				.035	.018	Da(6) ⎫ Da 6	
	.117	.060	HL-A 10 { HL-A 10', Da 28 (G = .036); HL-A 10', Da 29 (G = .024)	.084	.043	Da 23 (LND, Te 55) ⎬ Da 19	W15
				.078	.040	Da 24	
	.078	.040	Da 22 (Te 53?, GE33)	.062	.032	ET (G .01); Te 57 (Mapi, Orlina) (G .01); Fe 31/8 (G .01) ⎬	W17
W19	.104	.053	Da 25 (Te-66?) { Da 25', Da 26 (G = .022); Da 25''	.224	.119	HL-A 7	
				.090	.046	BB (Te-60)	W10
	.166	.083	Te 59 (Li, LAW, Thompson ?)	.056	.029	FJH (Te-52) ⎬ 6b(Da 9)	W27
				.072	.034	Da(9) ⎭	
		.027	X'	.055	.028	AA, Bt-22 (Te 51)	W22
				.156	.081	HL-A 8	
				.084	.043	Da 18 (Maki, Te 54)	W14
						Te 61 (G = .04)	
						Te 64 (G = .03)	
						X_2	
					.063		

Ph = Phenotype frequency   G = Gene frequency

Ph and G frequencies in columns were recorded in Paris.

36

TABLE 2

INFORMATIVE FAMILIES BY DOUBLE BACKCROSS STUDY

First Locus

1st	2nd	No. of families	Children +	Children −	p¹
HL-A1	HL-A2	6	10	10	a
	HL-A3	2	2	4	
	HL-A9	3	4	9	
	HL-A10	4	2	11	
	HL-A11	1	1	4	
	Da 15	1	2	3	
	Da 22	2	7	3	
	Da 25	2	1	1	
	Te 19	2	4	4	
HL-A2	HL-A3	3	5	3	f
	HL-A9	9	12	13	c
	HL-A10	4	8	6	d
	HL-A11	4	5	6	e
	Da 15	3	5	3	f
	Da 25	3	6	4	e
	Te 19	2	7	4	e
HL-A3	HL-A9	3	4	4	f
	HL-A10	1	1	2	
	HL-A11	3	8	5	d
	Da 25	4	6	3	f
HL-A9	HL-A10	4	5	10	d
	HL-A11	2	4	2	
	Da 15	4	7	10	d
	Da 22	2	1	4	
	Te 19	1	3	3	f
HL-A10	Da 22	1	2	2	d
	Te 19	2	11	4	
HL-A11	Da 22	3	6	5	e
	Da 25	2	4	5	e
Da 15	Da 25	2	3	1	f
	Te 19	1	4	2	
Da 22	Da 25	1	2	1	

Second Locus

1st	2nd	No. of families	Children +	Children −	p¹
HL-A5	HL-A7	4	9	5	
	HL-A8	4	11	10	
	HL-A12	7	18	11	
	HL-A13	1	3	3	
	Da(6)	2	4	3	
	Da 20	3	2	5	
	Da 23	1	2	1	
	AA	1	1	1	
	BB	1	3	3	
	FJH	2	2	4	
	Te 17	2	4	4	f
HL-A7	HL-A8	2	5	4	
	HL-A12	4	9	6	e
	HL-A13	2	4	3	d
	Da 18	2	3	3	f
	Da 20	3	6	3	f
	Da 23	1	3	1	
	Da 24	1	4	2	
HL-A8	HL-A12	6	8	10	d
	Da(9)	1	4	3	
	Da 18	3	3	1	
	Da 23	3	4	7	
	BB	3	3	3	
HL-A12	Da(9)	2	4	4	f
	Da 18	2	7	6	e
	Da 20	4	3	3	f
	Da 23	1	6	8	d
	Da 24	3	5	5	
	Te 18	3	1	1	e
HL-A13	Da 18	1	1	1	
	Da 24	1	1	1	

Second Locus (continued)

1st	2nd	No. of families	Children +	Children −	p¹
Da(6)	Te 18	1	1	1	d
Da(9)	Da 20	1	1	2	
	Da 23	1	3	1	
	Te 18	1	7	7	d
Da 18	Da 20	2	5	1	
	Da 23	1	2	3	
	Te 18	2	3	3	e
Da 20	Da 24	2	3	4	f
	Te 17	1	2	2	
	Te 18	2	5	3	f
Da 24	BB	1	1	1	
AA	Te 17	2	9	3	d
	Te 18	1	1	2	
BB	FJH	2	6	3	e
	Te 18	1	1	1	
FJH	Te 18	2	3	3	

¹ (a) P 10⁻⁶ (b) P 10⁻⁵ (c) P 10⁻⁴ (d) P 10⁻³ (e) P 0.01 (f) P 0.05

37

Table 3

268 Haplotypes Observed in 67 Families Studied for 26 HL-A Antigens

HL-A	5	7	8	12	13	(6)(9)	18	20	23	24	AA	BB	FJH	Te-17	Te-18	X₂
Da																
1		6	17	3		1		1		1		1	1	4		5
2	9	3	4	11				6	5	5	2	4	2		5	4
3	1	11				1 1	3	5	1	1	2	2		1	2	5
9	5	7	2	7		1	2	1	2	1	1		2		1	
10		2	2			1	1	2	1		1	1	1		2	
11	1	2		2	1	1	2	3	1	1	1	2	2		1	5
15	1	1		1			2		1				1			1
22	1			8			1		1							1
25		1			3					1	1				2	
Te19	2			4			2	2				3			3	1
X₁	2		2	2	1	1	1	1				2	1		1	5

Table 4

Segregation of HL-A Specificities in
+ - X - - Matings

	Children Positive	Children Negative
HL-A1	93	113
HL-A2	154	147
HL-A3	42	35
HL-A9	102	103
Da-15	64	51
Da-17	64	39
Da-21	22	26
Da-22	23	17
Da-22	17	23
Da-4	115	121
HL-A5	75	66
Da-20	31	35
Da-23	23	11
Da-24	12	10
HL-A7	97	102
Da(9)	26	26
HL-A8	17	10
HN	5	3

Table 5

Independence of the HL-A System
with Biological Markers

Erythrocyte Systems

ABO	P
Rhesus	JK
MNSs	Secretor
Kell	
Duffy	
Lewis	

Platelet System

Ko

Serous System

Gm	Lp
Gc	Ag
Inv	Hp
Isf	

Erythrocyte Enzyme

Acide phosphatase A, B, C

Phosphoglucomutase 2

Table 6

HL-A System[1]

No close linkage with:

 ABO, Rh, MN, Duffy, Kidd, Kell, ABH,

  and Lewis secretor

 Gm, Inv, Gc, Ag, Lp

 Ko

 Acid phosphatase, phosphoglucomutase

No loose linkage with:

 ABO, Rh, MN

 Gm

[1] Prepared in collaboration with F. Allen.

TABLE 7

MIXTURE OF ANTIBODIES AGAINST AND

ANTIGENS IN CIS, ALLELIC OR TRANS POSITION

Genotype of the donor's spermatozoa		HL–A 1 8 — ■ □ ■ —
		HL–A 2 5 — ■ □ ■ —

		% of cytotoxicity
Each antibody alone		48 to 59
Mixture in CIS	HL–A 1 + 8	35
	HL–A 2 + 5	42
Mixture in allelic or TRANS	HL–A 1 + 2	73
	HL–A 5 + 8	68
	HL–A 1 + 5	67
	HL–A 2 + 8	78

GENETICAL AND SEROLOGICAL CONCEPT OF THE HL-A SYSTEM
(Autosomal chromosome bearing the HL–A locus)

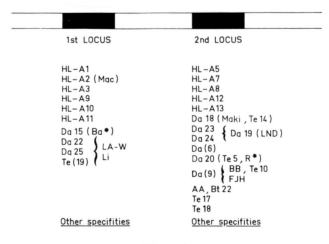

1st LOCUS	2nd LOCUS
HL–A1	HL–A5
HL–A2 (Mac)	HL–A7
HL–A3	HL–A8
HL–A9	HL–A12
HL–A10	HL–A13
HL–A11	Da 18 (Maki , Te 14)
Da 15 (Ba*)	Da 23 Da 24 } Da 19 (LND)
Da 22 Da 25 } LA-W	Da (6)
Te (19) (Li	Da 20 (Te 5 , R*)
	Da (9) { BB , Te 10 FJH
	AA , Bt 22
	Te 17
	Te 18
Other specifities	Other specifities

Fig. 1

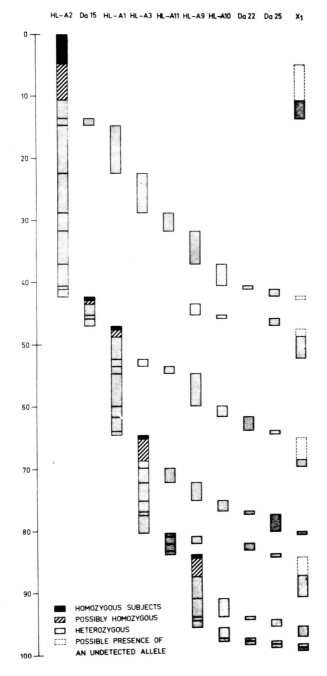

Fig. 2

43

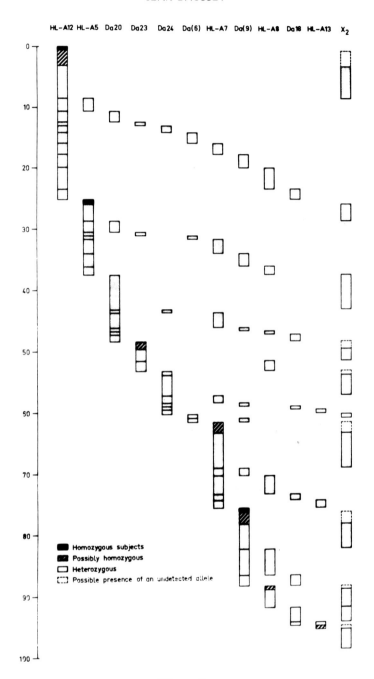

Fig. 3

44

FAMILY B...

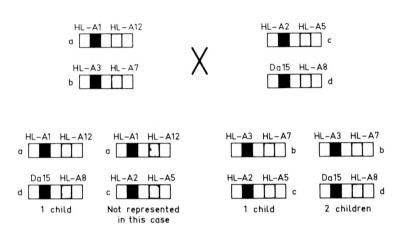

Fig. 4

A FAMILY WITH CROSSING-OVER BETWEEN THE 1st AND 2nd LOCUS

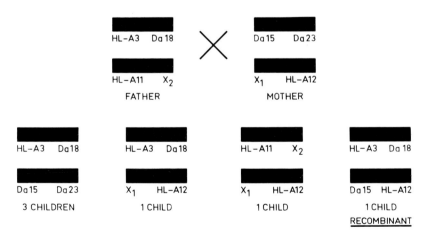

Fig. 5

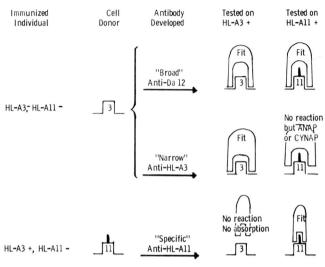

Fig. 6

Da 6 CROSS-REACTING GROUP

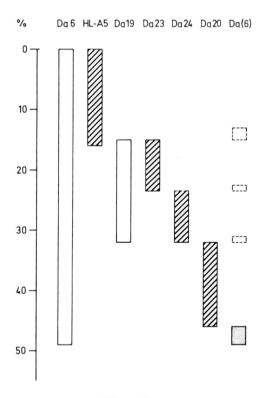

Fig. 7

POSSIBLE INTERPRETATION OF THE HL-A SYSTEM

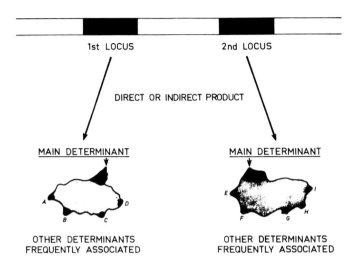

Fig. 8

THE PROGNOSTIC VALUE OF HL-A TYPING
IN KIDNEY TRANSPLANTATION

J. J. van Rood

Department of Immunohematology
University Medical Center
Leiden, the Netherlands

Present evidence suggests that the HL-A system is governed by two loci, LA and 4 (11). Each locus can carry the information for a large number of allelomorphic antigens, more than ten for the LA locus and more than 20 for the 4 locus. Crossing over between the two loci occurs with a frequency of 0.5 to 1% (7, 23, 25).

Each chromosome thus provides genetic information for two histocompatibility antigens. This is called a "haplotype." Because LA and 4 are on an autosomal chromosome, each individual carries four antigens on the surface of his cells. When all four antigens can be recognized separately, this is called a "full house." This is presently possible in about 40% of the general population. In the remainder, either one locus or both carry information for the same antigen or carry information for an antigen that cannot as yet be recognized serologically. These unrecognized allelomorphic genes have a frequency of about 4%, in our laboratory, or in other words, over 95% of the possible alleles in both series can be recognized serologically (29). Many of the anti-HL-A sera will react with two or more so-called cross-reacting antigens, e.g., our anti-8a serum will react with both HL-A2 and W28 (Ba*). Cells carrying either HL-A2 or W28 alone are able to absorb all anti-8a activity out of the serum. Even when these cross-reacting antigens are not taken into account, the

complexity of the HL-A system is enormous, as is
well illustrated by the number of haplotypes: 10 x
20 = 200, which can give rise to 200 x 200/2 =
20,000 genotypes. The number of phenotypes is lower
but is still well above 5000.

Between siblings, HL-A matching is accomplished
by determining which two of the four alternative
haplotypes have been inherited from the parents. The
recognized HL-A antigens are thus utilized as markers
for following the segregation of individual chromosomes. This also obviates the necessity of identify-
ing all of the histocompatibility antigens on each
chromosome. When a potential donor-recipient pair
of siblings shows evidence of having the same two
chromosomes, they are considered a true histocompatibility match. The chances of such a match occurring
in a family are one in four. Kidney transplants
exchanged between such HL-A identical siblings have
a significantly better survival than do grafts from
siblings who differ by one or two chromosomes (22,
28). Obviously, parents can never be a two-haplotype
match with their children since one haplotype must
derive from the other parent.

The situation becomes far more complex when
donor and recipient are unrelated. The number of
different genotypes is almost forbiddingly large and
one could well wonder whether matching for HL-A
outside the sib-sib situation is at all possible.
That it is indeed possible is due to the occurrence
of phenotypes with a relatively high frequency. Over
25% of the population of our part of the world has a
phenotype with a frequency of or over 0.4%. It is
possible to obtain for the majority of them, through
the help of international organ exchange organizations, a kidney that is identical for all four HL-A
antigens, serologically comparable to HL-A identical
siblings (29). When all four antigens of an unrelated donor can be identified, there is little problem as long as the recipient has the same antigens.
Any antigen present in the donor and absent in the
recipient is counted as an incompatibility.

Difficulties start when the donor has less than four
antigens that can be recognized. This is the case in
about 60% of our donor typings. Without family
studies, which are almost always impossible with
cadaveric donors, one is unable to differentiate
whether either the potential donor or recipient are
homozygous for a specific antigen. This creates an
important information gap, because homozygosity in
the donor for an antigen that is also present in the
host represents a histocompatible situation, whereas
the presence of an unidentified antigen at that site
represents incompatibility.

In many publications on this subject this difficulty is not sufficiently taken into account.
Most authors have counted only the recognized incompatibilities, disregarding both the chance of homozygosity in the donor or the possibility that some
antigens have not yet been recognized. As long as it
is not possible to recognize homozygosity in vitro
(without family studies), we believe that it is best
to regard all such instances as possible mismatches.

Table 1 depicts the match of over 200 donor-
recipient pairs who received a kidney in Eurotransplant. In the center column only the mismatched
antigens that can be recognized serologically are
counted. The majority of the donor-recipient pairs
are mismatched for no or at most one antigen, suggesting a very good match. An almost complete reversal occurs if the as yet unrecognized but potential
mismatches are counted (right-hand column). There
are no completely matched donor-recipient pairs and
only a few pairs mismatched for one antigen.
Although this analysis counts more incompatibilities
than there will be in reality (some of the donors
will be homozygous), in our opinion, it is nearer to
the truth than an analysis in which only the recognized incompatibilities are counted.

It is clear from the above that one of the
important aims for the immediate future should be
the development of methods for recognizing homozygosity without having to resort to family studies.

51

The few attempts made in this direction so far
appear not to be reliable and practical enough to be
of use in routine situations. Theoretically, the
mixed leukocyte culture (MLC) test could be of great
interest but it will show stimulation in most HL-A
identical unrelated combinations and will have to be
modified before it will be useful in this situation
(4).

Table 1 illustrates another difficulty. To
truly assess the importance of HL-A matching in
determining prognosis of renal transplants, the
results of two groups of patients - one, well
matched, the other, poorly matched - need to be compared. Results of a poorly matched group are available in this material; however, a well-matched group
(i.e., no mismatches) for comparison is not included.
It is no wonder then that in many of the published
series no significant correlation of HL-A matching
with prognosis could be found (17).

Of 327 kidney grafts that had been followed for
a minimum of 3 months and in which all four antigens
in the donor had been recognized, 100% are still
functioning, whereas of the grafts mismatched for
four antigens, only 67% are functioning. Table 2
shows the results of this analysis for kidneys transplanted in Europe. The difference between the two
groups (0 and 4 mismatches) is of borderline significance (P = 0.03). Of the grafts mismatched for one,
two, and three antigens, approximately 80% functioned
after 3 months. When cross-reactive antigens are
taken into account as compatibilities, significance
rises to P <0.006. The data show thus that HL-A
compatibility significantly improves kidney graft
prognosis at 3 and 6 months. Statistical significance cannot yet be shown at 12 months.

Since the group of full house identical grafts
is small, a definitive assessment must await data
from a larger series of patients. Whereas present
evidence strongly suggests that HL-A matching is able
to improve graft prognosis, it does not constitute
final proof for this. Lack of a significant correla-

tion at 12 months might be due mainly to the small
number of cases not only in the group with no mismatches but also with four mismatches. It should be
stressed that the data shown in Table 2 are a com-
pilation of data of six different organ exchange
groups, each of which includes information from as
many as 50 different centers. The material is thus
extremely heterogenous. This might in itself present
severe handicaps because not only experience but also
immunosuppressive regimen and case evaluation will
vary. This might also be the reason why in some of
the single center series, e.g., the Gothenburg
series, a more impressive correlation was found (13).
To decide whether a kidney graft fails from rejection, recurrent disease, and/or a technical error
(either surgical or through problems in immunosuppressive therapy) can be extremely difficult if not
impossible. The failures in this series should be
analyzed as outlined by the Central Registry of
Matches (29). Special attention should also be given
to the possibility that, although on initial analysis
there seemed to exist no mismatches between donor and
recipient in the zero mismatched group, such differences on further study can be shown to exist. One
could question whether the small percentage of
patients which received a full house identical graft
is really worth the cost of the international organ
exchange organizations. It should not be forgotten,
however, that all of these organizations are young
and that their effectiveness is still improving.
It seems realistic to expect that in the coming year
the percentage of full house identical matches will
increase to near 25% (27). Furthermore, only nine
of 160 patients received a graft mismatched for four
antigens. This is a significant improvement if
compared to the situation where grafts are exchanged
at random; then, about 25% of the grafts will be
mismatched for four antigens (27). Because this
group appears to do worse, at least at 3 months,
such transplants should be avoided in the future.
    We can conclude from this that there is a

statistically significant correlation at 3 and 6
months that is not yet seen at 12 months. It will
thus be necessary to continue our analysis. On the
basis of the results obtained so far, it appears
worthwhile to continue international efforts such as
Eurotransplant.

HL-A identical unrelated donor-recipient pairs
do not do as well as HL-A identical siblings. This
was already apparent from other studies. For
instance, Eijsvoogel et al.(4) have shown that only
an occasional HL-A full-house identical unrelated
donor-recipient pair do not stimulate in the MLC
test, while HL-A identical sibling combinations
almost never stimulate.

Skin grafts exchanged between such HL-A identical unrelated donor-recipient combinations, whether
they were stimulatory or nonstimulatory in the MLC
test, showed at best only a few days prolongation
of graft survival if compared with randomly selected
grafts (14). For these interesting observations a
number of explanations can be offered. (a) Antigenic heterozygosity: Although donor and recipient
appear to carry the same antigens, these antigens in
reality are not always the same and should then be
regarded as cross-reacting antigens. The fact that
the MLC test is, in some instances at least, negative makes it unlikely that this can be the only
explantation. (b) Skin graft survival is influenced
by at least two other loci apart from HL-A. One is
independent of MLC reactivity; the other is associated with such activity and could be called the
MLC locus. Festenstein has provided evidence for
this MLC locus in the mouse (5). It is of interest
that in the mouse this locus appears to be independent from H-2, whereas in man MLC reactivity (and
skin graft survival) is closely linked to HL-A in
siblings. It seems that in man the data so far
obtained could be best explained by a highly polymorphic locus closely linked to HL-A, which would
be in contrast to the situation in the mouse. That
HL-A identical siblings can be found who stimulate

in the MLC test, as reported by Yunis et al. (31,32),
would be in agreement with this assumption. It
will be of extreme importance to recognize the products of this locus also serologically. It might
well be that to this end techniques other than cytotoxicity will have to be applied.

Why is it that some grafts mismatched for three
or four antigens are rejected in a few months whereas
others survive for many years (27)? The answer to
this question is not only of theoretical interest but
also of enormous practical importance. If we could
know in advance which grafts mismatched for three or
four antigens would continue to do well for many
years, the running of organizations like Eurotransplant would be greatly simplified. Unfortunately, a
definite answer cannot yet be given, but it is
already clear that at least two factors play a major
role: (a) the host factors that determine the
immunological response or, more precisely, the homograft reaction and (b) the effect of previous blood
transfusions. We will first discuss them separately
and then try to show how they might interact.

Host factors in the immunological response are
currently a topic of growing interest. The brilliant
work by the group of Sela (20) on artificial antigens, which were shown by Benacerraf and others to
be antigenic in some strains of mice or guinea pigs
but far less so in others, and the studies by
McDevitt and others, showing that the genetic information that determines the capacity to react to these
antigens is linked to the major histocompatibility
locus in these strains, are exciting to every immuno-
logist (15). This locus was called the IR locus or
IR-1 locus in the mouse.
Evidence that this binomial reaction response

(i.e., some mouse strains will react, others will
not) is observed not only for artificial antigens but
also for naturally occurring ones, such as BSA and
antitoxin, underlines the biological significance of
these observations (15).

So far, for man, such correlations have not been
reported, but there are many antigenic stimuli known
that easily induce an antibody response in some
people whereas in others little or no response occurs
occurs. To cite just a few examples: (a) 40% of
Rhesus-negative people will never form Rhesus antibodies if infused with Rhesus-positive blood (18);
(b) 5% of normal individuals will not react to
dinitrochlorobenzene (DNCB) sensitization (Elkerbout,
personal communication); (c) some people will not
react to vaccinia or purified protein derivative
(PPD) vaccination. Studies are underway to determine
whether the ability to react to these antigens is
linked to HL-A.

Already quite a number of studies have appeared
reporting an association between the occurrence of
certain diseases and the presence of an HL-A antigen;
for example, W5 and Hodgkin's disease (1, 6, 26),
W15 and systemic lupus erythematosus (12), and HL-A2
and glomerulonephritis (16). Interestingly enough
these are all diseases that could be caused by viral
or bacterial infections. One could speculate that
they are the result of misguided antibody responses
against these infective agents, but little is known
on this point.

Are these observations relevant for the prognosis of kidney allografts? That host factors play
a role in homograft rejection in man has been shown
by Ceppellini and co-workers (3). They found that
skin grafts from two different donors, when transplanted on the same recipient, showed less difference
in survival time than when skin from one donor was
transplanted onto two different recipients. The
data were significant (P <0.001) and strongly suggest
that the difference is due to nonspecific immunological reactivity of the recipient. Matching for HL-A

was not performed in these experiments and thus the extent to which histocompatibility differences contributed to those observed differences is not known.

That such a host factor(s) might also be of importance for kidney allograft survival in patients receiving immunosuppressive agents is suggested by studies of Tinbergen (24). WAG rats received kidney grafts from BN rats while receiving immunosuppression with Imuran and Prednisone. Although these experiments were carried out under rigorously controlled conditions between two inbred lines of rats, graft survival times varied from 12 to 238 days. When no immunosuppression was given, graft survival varied from 8 to 55 days. These experiments were carried out in a pathogen-free environment. In each experiment the differences for the major histocompatibility locus H-1 or Ag-B was the same. Because the rats were completely inbred (i.e., skin isografts were not rejected), it is unlikely that mismatches at minor histocompatibllity loci would account for the observed variation. In our opinion, the most likely explanation is that the rats were inbred for the histocompatibility loci, but not for their immune response to homograft rejection, suggesting that if this response is governed by one locus, this locus is not closely linked to Ag-B, the major histocompatibility locus in the rat.

Is the capacity to react strongly or weakly in the homograft reaction determined by an as yet unknown IR locus or is some other mechanism operative? Here again we are not able to provide a definite answer. Arguments can be given for both points of view. An alternative to an IR locus could be an acquired variability in the capacity to form circulating antibodies and/or cellular immunity. That such variation in disease states exists is well known. Apart from the inherited immunodeficiencies, there are many possible acquired forms, such as those found in malignancies and uremic patients, that demonstrate a clear-cut and significant decrease in

phytohemagglutinin (PHA) responsiveness. In these
instances, there is a diminished capacity to form
immunity not against the antigen but against all
antigens. The immune potential of the patient is
diminished. It seems a priori highly likely that
this immune potential will also show a biological
variation in the normal population. Some people will
be good antibody formers against almost any antigen
and others will be poor responders. The same probably occurs in cellular immunity. This biological
variation could be the result of the sum of the
effect of an IR locus and/or acquired factors. A
kidney allograft in an individual with a poor capacity to develop cellular immunity will probably have
a much better prognosis than a kidney graft in some-
one with a strong cellular immunity.

Some highly suggestive evidence in this regard
is reported by Wilson and Kirkpatrick (30). Twenty-
four candidates for a kidney allograft were tested
for seven antigens (phytohemagglutinin (PPD), histoplasmin, Candida, etc.) for delayed cutaneous hypersensitivity. Thirteen patients were unresponsive to
all antigens: in 11, reactivity against one or more
antigens was demonstrable. They write, "The mean
time of onset of the rejection reaction in the 13
unresponsive patients was 14.8 days. By contrast,
the onset of the reaction in the group of 11 reactive
patients occurred on an average of 4.3 days after
transplantation." No data are presented relating the
reactivity in delayed cutaneous hypersensitivity to
long-term prognosis. On the basis of the considerations and observations presented above, it seems a
matter of the highest urgency to get further documentation on this point.

Blood transfusion is a unique antigenic stimulus
because the HL-A antigens are carried on lymphocytes,
granulocytes, platelets, and reticulocytes and can
immunize the recipient against transplantation antigens present in a kidney graft he will later receive.
If a kidney is transplanted over a positive cross-
match, i.e., the serum of the recipient will react

with the lymphocytes of the donor, that kidney will
be hyperacutely rejected in most instances (12,19).
In instances where rejection occurs despite a negative crossmatch the techniques used to detect leukocyte antibodies may not be sufficiently sensitive.
It is even more difficult to explain how a kidney
could continue to do well in a recipient whose serum
contains an antibody that reacts with the donor
lymphocytes (9). In such cases, a dissociation
exists between humoral immunity against the graft
and graft rejection. Table 3 summarizes our thoughts
on this issue. We would postulate that in the majority of cases antibodies in the recipient that react
against the donor lymphocytes will coincide with, but
are not primarily responsible for, hyperacute graft
rejection (category I). The rejection would not be
primarily due to the direct action of the circulating
antibodies (although they probably do play some role)
but instead to simultaneously activated cellular
immunity or homograft reactivity against the graft.
This activated cellular immunity would be primarily
responsible for the acute graft rejection. In those
instances where the graft remains functioning despite
a positive crossmatch homograft, sensitivity was not
activated (category II). Here, a state of enhancement might exist. In a third situation, hyperactive
rejection in patients with a negative crossmatch
could be due to insensitivity of the serological
techniques but also to an activated homograft sensitivity in the absence of humoral immunity (category
III). It should be stressed that these are as yet
only postulates.

From what has been said above it is clear that
any blood transfusion may induce a variety of immunologic responses. It can activate the dormant immunocompetent cells committed to HL-A. If the immunological potential of the recipient is deficient for
cellular immunity, but adequate for the formation of
circulating antibodies, this could be a blessing in
disguise: The circulating antibodies actually could
enhance the graft. It is evident that as long as we

are not better informed on the immune potential of our patients, giving blood transfusions and hoping for the best is playing Russian roulette with the prognosis of the graft at stake.

We feel that it is therefore imperative that blood intended for potential renal transplant recipients be obtained from donors who are either HL-A identical or compatible. That this is feasible is shown in Table 4, which shows the number of HL-A identical donors found in a group of 1685 people typed for 30 patients on dialysis in Leiden. An average of 8.4 HL-A identical donors per patient were identified among 1685 individuals. For all but three, three or more HL-A identical donors could be found. We believe that it is especially here that great improvements can be made in the prognosis of transplanted organs.

Considering all of the above, what should be our future policy? At least for the present, HL-A matching plays an important role in determining the prognosis of kidney transplants: a 6 month prognosis of 100% for an optimal match in contrast to a 76% prognosis for a mismatched kidney and an even more impressive contrast in, for instance, the Gothenburg series.

The availability of a good match for a given patient will to a large extent depend upon the frequency of the patient's HL-A phenotype in the general population. The most significant uncontrollable factor at present is the influence of the immunological potential of the patient on the graft. It seems highly likely that some patients will have a strong immune potential and others a weak one. In further analysis of this factor, differentiation should be made between cell-mediated and circulating antibody responses to immunologic challenge.

Strong immune potential for cellular immunity in a recipient can be influenced by immunosuppressive therapy. Antilymphocyte globulin (ALG) with its selective action on cellular immunity might be especially suitable for this. Sheil et al. (21) showed, in a well-controlled study, that there is a significant improvement in cadaveric kidney allograft survival if ALG is given. On the other hand, these data should be interpreted with caution because a similar success rate for cadaveric kidney allograft survival has been reported without the use of ALG (8).

On the basis of all these considerations, we will not attempt to outline a protocol for future treatment of renal transplant patients. We expect that if the immune potential is studied, it will be possible to divide the patients into four categories: (a) Immunological potential for cellular immunity is high and HL-A phenotype is of a high frequency. These patients should receive only HL-A identical blood. Only kidneys that are completely matched are acceptable. ALG treatment should be considered. (b) Immune potential for cellular immunity is low, but HL-A phenotype frequency high. This is the group with the best prognosis. If possible, compatible blood should be given and transplant delayed until a well-matched kidney is available. ALG is probably not necessary. (c) Cellular immunity is strong and the HL-A phenotype is infrequent. This group of patients will be the most difficult to manage. HL-A compatible blood transfusions should be given at any cost. The sooner the patient is transplanted, probably the better. These patients should receive ALG. (d) Weak capacity for cellular immunity and a rare HL-A phenotype. These patients will probably have a reasonable prognosis, independent of matching. If matched blood is available, it should be given. As chances are slight for a full house identical match, a kidney mismatched for one or two antigens should be accepted. ALG treatment can probably be withheld.

In summary, the prognosis of a kidney allograft is dependent upon a number of interacting factors.

At the moment the most important ones seem to be matching for HL-A, the immune potential of the recipient, previous blood transfusions, and immuno-suppressive regimens. Intelligent interpretation of the information on these points will almost certainly improve kidney allograft prognosis and will uncover other new and exciting areas to explore.

ACKNOWLEDGEMENT

In part supported by the National Institutes of Health (contract PH 43-65-992), the Dutch Organization for Pure Research (FUNGO), the Dutch Organization for Applied Research (TNO), the J.A. Cohen Institute for Radiology and Radiation Protection, and the Whitehall Foundation. Portions of this manuscript appear in the "Proceedings of the First International Congress of Immunology" (Academic Press).

REFERENCES

1. Amiel, J.L. In "Histocompatibility Testing 1967" (E.S. Curtoni, P.L. Mattiuz, and R.M. Tosi, eds.), p. 79. Munksgaard, Copenhagen, 1967.
2. Bodmer, W., and McDevitt, H.O. Transplant Proc. (1972). (in press).
3. Ceppellini, R., Curtoni, E.S., Mattiuz, P.I., Leigheb, G., Visetti, M., and Colombi, A. Ann. N.Y. Acad. Sci. 129, 421 (1966).
4. Eijsvoogel, V.P., Schellekens, P.T.A., Breur-Vriesendorp, B., Konig, L., Koch, C.T., van Leeuwen, A., and van Rood, J.J. Transplant. Proc. 3, 85 (1971).
5. Festenstein, H. Personal communication (1971).
6. Forbes, J.F., and Morris, P.J. Lancet 2, 349 (1970).
7. Gatti, R.A., Meuwissen, H.J., Terasaki, P.I., and Good, R.A. Tissue Antigens 1, No. 5, 239 (1971).
8. Go, I.H., Hintzen, A., van Rood, J.J., Struyven-

berg, A., Terpstra, J.L., Veegens, C., Vink, M., and de Graeff, J.J. To be published. (1972).
9. Heale, W.F., Morris, P.J., Bennett, R.C., Mortensen, P.J., and Ting, A. Med. J. Aust. 2, 382 (1969).
10. Joint International Statement. Transplant Proc. (1971). (in press).
11. Joint Report of the Fourth International Histocompatibility Workshop. In "Histocompatibility Testing 1970" (P.I. Terasaki, ed.), p. 17. Munksgaard, Copenhagen, 1970.
12. Kissmeyer-Nielsen, F., Olsen, S., Posborg Petersen, V., and Fjeldborg, O. Lancet 2, 662 (1966).
13. Kissmeyer-Nielsen, F., Staub Nielsen, L., Lindholm, A., Sandberg, L., Svejgaard, A., and Thorsby, E. In "Histocompatibility Testing 1970" (P.I. Terasaki, Ed.), p. 105. Munksgaard, Copenhagen, 1970.
14. Koch, C.T., Frederiks, E., Eijsvoogel, V.P., and van Rood, J.J. Submitted for publication (1972).
15. McDevitt, H.O., and Benacerraf, B. Advan. Immunol. 11, 31 (1969).
16. Mickey, M.R., Kreisler, M., and Terasaki, P.I. In "Histocompatibility Testing 1970" (P.I. Terasaki, ed.), p. 237. Munksgaard, Copenhagen, 1970.
17. Mickey, M.R., Kreisler, M., Albert, E.D., Tanaka, N., and Terasaki, P.I. Tissue Antigens 1, No. 2, 81 (1971).
18. Mollison, P.L., Frame, M., and Ross, M.E. Brit. J. Haematol. 19, No. 2, 257 (1970).
19. Patel, R., and Terasaki, P.I. N. Engl. J. Med. 280, 735 (1969).
20. Sela, M. Advan. Immunol. 5, 29 (1969).
21. Sheil, A.G.R., Kelly, G.E., Storey, B.G., May, J., Kalowski, S., Mears, D., Rogers, J.H., Johnson, J.R., Charlesworth, J., and Stewart, J.H. Lancet 1, 359 (1971).
22. Singal, D.P., Mickey, M.R., and Terasaki, P.I.

Transplantation 7, 216 (1969).
23. Svejgaard, A., Bratlie, A., Hedin, P.J., Hogman, C., Jersild, C., Kissmeyer-Nielsen, F., Lindblom, B., Lindholm, A., Low, B., Messeter, L., Moller, E., Sandberg, L., Staub-Nielsen, L., and Thorsby, E. Tissue Antigens 1, No. 2, 81 (1971).
24. Tinbergen, W.J. Thesis, Leiden University, Waltman, Delft, The Netherlands (1971).
25. van Leeuwen, A., and van Rood, J.J. Unpublished observations (1971).
26. van Rood, J.J., and van Leeuwen, A. Transplant. Proc. 3, 1283 (1971).
27. van Rood, J.J., Freudenberg, J., van Leeuwen, A., Schippers, M.A., II, Zweerus, R., and Terpstra, J.L. Transplant. Proc. 3, 933 (1971).
28. van Rood, J.J., van Leeuwen, A., and Brunning, J.W. J. Clin. Pathol. 20, 504 (1967).
29. van Rood, J.J., van Leeuwen, A., Freudenberg, J., and Rubinstein, P. Transplant. Proc. (1972). (in press).
30. Wilson, W.E.C., and Kirkpatrick, C.H. In "Experience in Renal Transplantation" (T.E. Starzl, ed.), p. 239. Saunders, Philadelphia, Pennsylvania, 1964.
31. Yunis, E.J., and Amos, D.B. Proc. Nat. Acad. Sci. U.S. 68, No. 12, 3031 (1971).
32. Yunis, E.J., Plate, J.M., Ward, F.E., Seigler, H.F., and Amos, D.B. Transplant. Proc. 3, 1 (1971).

TABLE 1

Matching in Eurotransplant

Number of antigens mismatched	Identified antigens alone[2]	Identified antigens plus possible ones
0	108	0
1	109	18
2	29	74
3	8	109
4	2	55

[1] From van Rood et al. (29).

[2] Number of donor-recipient pairs.

Table 2a

Pooled International Survival Results of 160 First-Set Renal
Allografts Obtained from HL-A Full-House Cadaver Donors[1]

	Incompatibilities assessed without HL-A cross reactions		
Number of donor-recipient HL-A incompatibilities	Number of grafts surviving at:		
	3 months	6 months	12 months
0	15/15 = 100%	12/12 = 100%	8/9 = 89%
1	35/103= 83%	55/73 = 75%	23/32 = 72%
2	35/46 = 76%	20/26 = 77%	13/18 = 72%
3	10/11 =	6/8 = 75%	5/7 =100%
4	6/9 = 67%	3/3 = 100%	3/3 =100%
Statistical comparison between the group with no and the sum of the groups with 1, 2, 3, and 4 incompatibilities	$P<0.03$	$P<0.03$	n.s.

[1] These data were compiled by Batchelor, Dausset, Festenstein, Govaerts, Harris, Hors, Jeannet, Kissmeyer-Nielsen, Thorsby, and van Rood.

Table 2b

Pooled International Survival Results of 160 First-Set Renal Allografts Obtained from HL-A Full-House Cadaver Donors[1]

Number of donor-recipient HL-A incompatibilities	Incompatibilities assessed with HL-A cross reactions[2] Number of grafts surviving at:		
	3 months	6 months	12 months
0	25/25 = 100%	19/19 = 100%	9/13 = 69%
1	84/103= 82%	55/73 = 75%	27/33 = 82%
2	29/40 = 73%	16/22 = 73%	11/16 = 69%
3	8/8 = 100%	4/6 = 67%	3/5 = 60%
4	5/8 = 63%	2/2 = 100%	2/2 = 100%
Statistical comparison between the group with no and the sum of the groups with 1, 2, 3, and 4 incompatibilities	P<0.006	P<0.006	P<0.006 n.s.

[1] These data were compiled by Batchelor, Dausset, Festenstein, Govaerts, Harris, Hors, Jeannet, Kissmeyer-Nielsen, Thorsby, and van Rood.
[2] The following crossreacting antigens were considered: HL-A2 and W28 (Ba*), HL-A3 and HL-A11, HL-A5, and W5 (R*), HL-A7 and W27 (FJH).

TABLE 3

Dissociation Between Cellular and Humoral
Immunity in Homograft Rejection

Category	Humoral immunity	Cellular immunity	Cross match	Homograft reaction
I	Present	Increased	pos.	Hyperacute rejection
II	Present	Not increased	pos.	Normal graft survival; enhancement?
III	Absent	Increased	neg.	Hyperacute rejection

TABLE 4

The Number of HL-A Identical Donors
Found for Individual Patients in Leiden

Patient's Eurotransplant number	Patient's phenotype		Number of HL-A identical donors
	LA	4	
1133	1,3	7,8	37
0673	1,2	8,12	20
0473	3	7,7b	19
1419	2,3	7	18
0335	1,3	7	3
0911	1	12	2
0555	2	7,13	1
0387	Ba*	5,12	0

THE MEANING AND USE OF THE MIXED LEUKOCYTE
CULTURE TEST IN TRANSPLANTATION

B. H. Park and R. A. Good

Department of Pediatrics, Pathology and Microbiology
University of Minnesota
Minneapolis, Minnesota

INTRODUCTION

In 1946, Medawar (1) showed that the intradermal injection of leukocytes from rabbit D into rabbit R induced a state of sensitivity to subsequent
grafts of D's skin to R. This indicated that leukocytes, skin, and other organs shared at least some
important transplantation antigens. It was later
observed that tolerance of skin allografts could be
induced in very young rodents by inoculation with
living leukocytes from other individuals of the same
genetic origin, indicating that leukocytes must
express all the transplantation antigens of skin and
other tissues. These findings and the ease with
which leukocytes could be obtained made leukocyte
typing the most important approach to histocompatibility testing.

By serological analysis, more than 30 different
leukocyte antigens have been recognized; most of them
belong to the HL-A (human leukocytes-antigen) system.
Analysis of HL-A antigens through family studies has
revealed that many antigens that had no apparent
association in a random population were, in fact,
linked to markers known to be determined by the HL-A
locus. A further advantage of family studies is
that the haplotypes of parents can be deduced from
the HL-A types of the children.

The clinical importance of HL-A typing was clearly shown by skin grafts exchanged between siblings with identical HL-A types. Grafts between HL-A identical siblings survived significantly longer than did grafts between HL-A unidentical siblings. However, the inadequacy of HL-A typing in predicting the outcome of grafting was readily apparent when it was shown that grafts between HL-A identical but unrelated persons survived for much shorter periods than grafts between HL-A identical siblings. This finding indicated that there must have been as yet unidentified HL-A antigens that exerted influence on the outcome of grafts. The influence of these undetermined leukocyte antigens was presumed to be shown in vitro by the mixed leukocytes culture (MLC) test. Thus, the mixed leukocyte culture test gained popularity over other methods of histocompatibility testing, e.g., inverse skin grafting, the normal lymphocyte transfer test, the third man test, and the irradiated hamster test.

IN VITRO TRANSFORMATION OF LYMPHOCYTES

Asgood and Brook (2), in 1955, were the first to describe the technique for culturing human leukocytes from peripheral blood and bone marrow. Hungerford (3), in 1959, adapted this technique to his study of human chromosome analysis. Nowell (4) discovered in 1960 that blast transformation and mitosis in the culture of normal human leukocytes were actually caused by the mitogenic effect of phytohemagglutinin (PHA), which had been used to isolate leukocytes. PHA, an extract of the kidney bean Phaseolus vulgaris, had been known to be a potent hemagglutinating agent that was frequently used as a means of enhancing sedimentation of red blood cells, thereby easily separating leukocytes from the whole blood (5). Schrek and Stefani suggested that lymphocyte transformation by PHA was an immunological phenomenon (6) on the basis of their experiments on skin testing (delayed type) and transformation of lymphocytes by

72

PHA in man, rat, and guinea pig. This view of an immulogic nature of in vitro lymphocyte transformation was supported by the findings of others, who showed that a similar transformation of lymphocytes could be induced by specific antigens. Pearmain (7) was the first to show that lymphocytes from patients with positive tuberculin tests transformed in the presence of tuberculin in vitro. Similar findings were reported by many others using a wide variety of antigens from bacteria, fungi, viruses, pollens, drugs, synthetic amino acid polymers, and, finally, transplantation antigens (8, 9). Thus, the immunologic nature of lymphocyte transformation was established. Although much subsequent evidence makes it clear that the response to mitogens like PHA does not in itself reflect adaptive immunological response, the relation of this quasiimmunological process to the immunologic stimuli may still reflect some fundamental aspect of its nature that induces the lymphocytes to proliferate by an appropriate stimulus at the membrane.

MIXED LEUKOCYTE CULTURES

By 1963, it was clear that a large number of antigens, in addition to PHA, were capable of activating lymphocytes sensitive to the antigens and of inducing transformation and proliferation in vitro. It was also known that lymphocytes carry on their surface a number of important transplantation antigens. This background, together with the incidental observation made by Schrek and Donnelly in 1961 (10) that mitosis was noted in the mixed culture of leukocytes (without PHA present) from two patients with hemochromatosis, led Bain et al. (11, 12) to carry out further detailed study of mixed leukocyte cultures in normal healthy persons, including twins (identical and unidentical). The results clearly indicated that the reaction (transformation and synthesis of new DNA) by lymphocytes in the mixed leukocyte cultures are related to genetic differences

73

and the allograft immunity of the two individuals
from whom the leukocytes were obtained. It was further shown that no prior sensitization of the cells
of donors to the antigens of the other was necessary
for the MLC reaction.

Because the degree of interaction of the lymphocytes from various donors appears to be related to
the genetic disparity in allogeneic systems of the
two individuals, the mixed leukocyte culture (MLC)
or mixed leukocyte reaction (MLR) has inevitably
received a good deal of attention as a potential
basis for histocompatibility testing (13-18). When
the leukocytes from two individuals react against
each other in a test tube, it is difficult, if not
impossible, to determine the degree of response of
each population. Therefore, it is necessary to have
the leukocytes from one individual in a static state
in terms of their proliferating activity while the
capacity to stimulate leukocytes from the other individual is being expressed. For the purpose of
attaining this unidirectional stimulation, various
means, e.g., leukocyte extracts, disrupted leukocytes
(19), frozen cells, nitrogen mustard treatment, and
irradiation (20), were tried but did not give reproducible results. In 1966, Bach and Voynow (21)
described their technique of one-way stimulation in
mixed leukocyte cultures. Stimulating cells were
incubated with mitomycin-C at the concentration of
25 mg/ml for 20 min. at 37°C to prevent the replication of DNA while such mitomycin-treated lymphocytes
continued to be capable of stimulating normal lymphocytes of an allogeneic individual. The procedure is
relatively simple and the results highly reproducible.
This method has become a preferred method for the
one-way mixed leukocyte culture test.

The standardization of culture conditions has
been a problem in the study of mixed leukocyte cultures. The number and concentration of cells in the
culture, the role of macrophage and polymorphonuclear
leukocytes, the means of measuring the degree of
reaction (i.e., the morphologic observation of

transformed cells, the measurement of uptake of radioactive precursor of DNA), the type and shape of
the culture tube, the kind of culture medium, the
concentration of radioactive precursor, the period
of culture, and the time of pulse are major factors
known to influence the results of MLC tests (22).
Recently, Sengar and Terasaki (23) reported a semi-
micro method of MLC test. By this method, quantitation of the response is possible with reasonable
reproducibility. A similar method was described by
Hartzman et al. (24). In this method, most of the
variables were standardized and the entire procedure
was reduced to a microscale. We have adapted this
method with slight modification and the results have
been quite consistent.

HL-A TYPING AS A MEANS OF HISTOCOMPATIBILITY TESTING

Because it has been shown that the lymphocytes
carry most of (if not all) the transplantation
antigens in man (25, 26), a proper and precise typing
of human lymphocytes would naturally provide a useful
means of selecting donor and recipient in the transplantation of cells, tissue, and organs.

Dausset (27) was the first to demonstrate by
serological means the existence of leukocyte isoantigens in man, which he designated as leukocyte group
Mac. That these antigens are genetically controlled
was shown in twin (28, 29) and family studies (30-
32). However, the exact characterization of leukocyte groups was hampered by the lack of a standard
serological procedure and the lack of monospecific
sera. van Rood and van Leeuwen, in 1963 (33),
refined the method of the leukoagglutinin test and
employed monospecific sera obtained from pregnant
women in this analysis. By the use of a cross-
absorption technique monospecificity was insured.
The data were analyzed statistically by computer
according to Fisher's 2 x 2 table. The results
clearly disclosed the existence of a genetic locus in
man determining leukocyte isoantigens. This locus

was designated as 4, with two possible alleles, 4a or 4b. The gene frequency for the alleles was estimated to be 0.38 and 0.62, respectively.

Earlier attempts to correlate the identified leukocyte antigens with skin graft survival (32, 34), however, showed only marginal difference, although skin graft induced specific antileukocyte antibodies in the recipient (35, 36). This lack of good correlation was largely caused by the inadequacy of the technique for serotyping leukocytes at the time. Terasaki and McClelland, in 1964 (37), developed a method for assaying lymphocytotoxins on a microscale in order to circumvent the many difficulties of the leukoagglutinin test. They found this micromethod reproducible, rapid, and extremely sensitive and thus of practical use in human lymphocyte typing. By the use of this method, Terasaki et al. (38) characterized 154 samples of native human lymphotoxic antisera with respect to their strength, frequency, and grouping and their relevance to kidney transplantation. The discriminatory capacity of a large panel of unabsorbed sera was sufficient to distinguish the lymphocytes of nine pairs of duplicates from the lymphocytes of 273 random persons. Two-thirds of the 154 antisera could be classified as belonging to seven major groups. Two of the groups were shown to be associated with the LA-1 and LA-2 groups previously established by Payne et al. (39) using a leukoagglutinin method. The cytotoxic reaction did not completely parallel the reaction of all leukoagglutinating sera. When the seven groups of leukocytes were compared in 49 recipients of successful kidney transplants, it was found, contrary to expectation, that only marginal correlation existed between the groups of lymphocytes in recipients and donors. van Rood et al., in 1965 (40), reported five new leukocyte antigens based on the study of 147 sera and pointed out that there is good correlation between leukoagglutinin and lymphocytotoxin in the grouping of human leukocytes. The correlation between the normal lymphocyte transfer test (NLT), skin graft survival, and the compatibility of leukocytes was reported to be rather poor.

Exchange of typing sera among laboratories from different parts of the world and the holding of several international workshops on histocompatibility testing (41-44) resulted in further definition of the antisera and antigens and arrival at a standard nomenclature for human lymphocytes. The antigens were recognized as a major genetically determined system which was called HL-A (45, 46).

Despite the refinement of serologic determinations and more precise definition of a large number of antigens, the correlation of HL-A system with the survival of skin grafts between unrelated individuals has been rather poor (47-49). However, the survival time of skin graft between related persons, especially between siblings, has been shown to be well correlated with the HL-A type of leukocytes (50, 51). Dausset et al. (52) performed 238 skin grafts between HL-A haploidentical individuals and concluded that the HL-A system plays a dominant role in transplantation over the other histocompatibility system excluding the ABO system, and that there is a direct correlation between the survival time of skin grafts and HL-A compatibility. Mickey et al. (53) reviewed the results of 1200 kidney transplantations and arrived at the conclusion that the HL-A system is useful in predicting the outcome of kidney grafts among relatives but does not provide significant correlation in unrelated persons. A similar conclusion was reached by Hors et al. (54) on the basis of 179 renal transplants.

The extreme polymorphism of the HL-A system, with more than 30 alleles (55), and the influence of as yet unidentified leukocyte antigens are believed to account in a major way for the poor correlation between the grafts of unrelated persons and leukocyte antigens.

THE MIXED LEUKOCYTE CULTURE TEST AS A
MEANS OF HISTOCOMPATIBILITY MATCHING

In the mixed leukocyte culture (MLC) test, the sum total of antigenic disparity between two individuals is measured without defining the kind and the number of antigens involved. A genetic analysis of the MLC test suggested that a single genetic locus with a minimum of 20 alleles is involved (56, 57). This conclusion was based on the facts that 28.2% of 291 sibling pairs was nonstimulatory in the MLC test and that 80 instances of parent-child pairs and more than 600 unrelated pairs were found to be always stimulating. It was further proposed that the locus controlling MLC reactivity is the same locus that determines the majority of the leukocyte antigens, i.e., the major histocompatibility locus in man.

Iványi et al. (58) studied 104 MLC tests with respect to ten leukocyte antigens, and concluded that the reactivity of leukocytes in the MLC test was correlated with leukocyte antigens 1, 2, 3, and 7, but that there was no correlation between the vigor of MLC response and the number of differences among these antigens. Albertini and Bach (59), in a family study, showed that the cells of siblings differing from the responding sibling by both alleles at HL-A stimulated more than did cells of siblings differing by one allele in every instance. In other words, a direct correlation between the vigor of response in the MLC test and the antigenic disparity of leukocytes in siblings was found. Findings were reported by Debray-Sachs et al. (60) on the basis of 140 pairs of MLC tests. Schellekens et al. (61) carried out an extensive study of HL-A antigens and the MLC test and concluded (a) that the degree of reaction in the MLC test is completely dependent upon HL-A incompatibility, (b) that the difference of two alleles resulted in two times more stimulation than did a difference of one allele, and (c) that three of HL-A identical unrelated pairs showed strong stimulation despite the HL-A identity. Thus, it became clear that the good correlation between the MLC test and HL-A type was found only among relatives but that no correlation existed between the two unrelated individuals. The strong stimulation in the MLC test between unrelated individuals with identical HL-A types was believed to be caused by the disparity of as yet undetected antigens in the leukocytes. Therefore, the MLC test is useful in measuring the overall disparity of known and unknown antigens of leukocytes and provides a practical means of matching histocompatibility between donor and recipient that will probably remain standard and can be detected by serological means (62).

Russel et al. (63), in 1966, reported a good correlation between MLC testing and skin graft survival in man. This was confirmed by Bach and Kisken (64). The study of 35 kidney transplants by Bach et al. (65) showed that there was a highly significant correlation between the degree of MLC reaction and the function of the grafted kidney and that the MLC test had predictive value in distinguishing between successful cases and cases of failure.

A NEW ASPECT OF THE GENETIC CONTROL OF HL-A SYSTEM, MLC REACTION, AND TRANSPLANTATION IMMUNITY

The concept that a single genetic locus controls both the HL-A system and the MLC reaction, and that this locus is the major histocompatibility locus of man, may have to be modified in the light of recent findings.

In a 1968 report by Amos and Bach (57), an instance of HL-A mismatched sibling pair that was nonstimulatory in the MLC test was recognized. The possibility that this represented a recombination within the genetic material was considered. A clear example of recombinant mismatch of HL-A was observed in a family in which the recombinant sibling, mismatched at an antigen of the LA series, was used as a marrow transplant donor (66). The HL-A mismatched sibling not only failed to be stimulated in the MLC test but gave a very mild graft versus host (GVH) reaction upon marrow transplantation. This finding suggested to us that HL-A and MLC, as well as HL-A mismatch and severe GVH reaction, could be dissociated.

Yunis et al. (67) reported on two families in which HL-A identical siblings were stimulated in the MLC test. Further, they found one unusual family in which two pairs of siblings showed HL-A match, one with the other. In one sibling pair, the HL-A match was associated with an absence of response in the MLC test. In the other sibling pair, the HL-A match was associated with vigorous MLC response. Furthermore, the leukocytes of one of the second pair stimulated vigorously the leukocytes of both members of the first pair in MLC test, whereas the leukocytes of the second member of the second pair failed to stimulate the leukocytes of either member of the first pair. These findings, coupled with further evidence from Yunis and Amos (71) of vigorous stimulation between a parent and child who were HL-A identical and our own observation of haplotype mismatched siblings who did not stimulate in the MLC test, make it certain that HL-A and MLC systems can segregate independently.

Yunis and Amos proposed several hypotheses to explain these findings: (a) possibility of the inheritance of different, strong, or cumulative non-HL-A antigens that are not closely linked to HL-A and are not detectable by current serologic test; (b) the possibility that some of these antigens are more effective in the MLC reaction and nonetheless undetectable serologically as such, so that recombination involving these determinants would go unnoticed; (c) or the possibility that the HL-A locus is linked to but separated from the MLC locus. Koch et al. (68) reported that two of nine HL-A identical unrelated individuals failed to stimulate in the MLC test, but a skin graft between them was rejected as fast as that of an unrelated donor. They suggested that in addition to the possibility of the influence of as yet undetected HL-A antigens, there might be at least

two other loci apart from HL-A locus, one for MLC
reactivity and one for graft survival. Dupont et al.
(69) studied the one-way MLC test on seven siblings,
one of whom represented a recombinant between the LA
and the 4 series of the HL-A system. Their findings
suggested that the MLC reactivity is elicited by, or
correlated with, the antigens of the 4 series rather
than the LA series. They proposed a third locus that
may control the MLC reaction, closely linked to the
locus that controls the 4 series. Sengar et al. (70)
studied eight pairs of unrelated HL-A identical individuals and five parent-child HL-A identical pairs
and concluded that, with the improved serotyping, the
MLC stimulation of cells that were thought to be HL-A
identical by earlier criteria may in fact be caused
by new antigens, possibly of a third HL-A segregant
series. Yunis and Amos (71), on the basis of their
studies of the MLC test in two families and six
individuals with identical HL-A types, then proposed
that the rejection time of skin and organ transplants
is dependent upon immunization of the recipient
against the products of two, or possibly three, separate but closely linked genetic systems, i.e., the
HL-A system, the MLC reaction system, and the hypersensitivity delayed reaction system (HDR). This
hypothesis of an independent MLC locus is further
strengthened by the report of HL-A unidentical, unrelated pair who did not stimulate each other in the
MLC test (72, 73).

THE IMPORTANCE OF THE MLC TEST
IN BONE MARROW TRANSPLANTATION

That histocompatibility matching is a crucial
factor in the success of bone marrow transplantation
has been clearly shown both in animals (74-76) and in
man (77). With the advancement of tissue typing and
matching techniques, it is now possible to reconsti-
tute immunologic function in patients with combined
immune deficiency disease. Bone marrow transplantation has been regularly successful when the donor

and recipient are identical in their HL-A genotype and are siblings. However, in spite of HL-A identity and MLC matching in sibling pairs, a varying degree of severity of the graft versus host reaction has been regularly observed during the clinical course of bone marrow transplantation. This indicates strongly that there must be another as yet unidentified factor influencing the graft versus host reaction in bone transplantation. Bone marrow grafting between HL-A unidentical individuals, including siblings, results in either rejection of the graft or fatal GVH reaction. When the HL-A identity is doubtful in siblings, nonreaction in the MLC test establishes the HL-A identity of the siblings with the rare exception mentioned above.

Recently we attempted to correlate the severity of the GVH reaction in bone-marrow transplanted patients with the third party MLC test in the donor and recipient (78). In the third party MLC test, the degree of difference in capacity of the cells from the donor and the recipient to stimulate an unrelated person's cells in the MLC test was measured. The difference is expressed in terms of a disparity index. It was found that there appeared to be direct correlation between the disparity index and the severity of graft versus host reaction. It is suggested that study of the disparity index may be useful in selecting better matched donors among siblings with HL-A identical genotypes and that this index may be useful in predicting the severity of graft versus host reaction after bone marrow transplantation. This finding may be an important factor in calculating the optimum number of bone marrow cells for successful grafting and reconstitution of immunologic function.

SUMMARY

Human leukocytes carry most of their transplantation antigens on their surfaces. Serotyping, ultimately using microcytotoxic assay, established the HL-A system in man to which more than 30 of the leukocyte antigens so far identified belong. By family study of these antigens, the haplotype of each individual can be deduced.

The HL-A type of leukocytes and the survival of grafts are shown to be well correlated among family members, but not between unrelated pairs. A similar correlation was found between the HL-A type of leukocytes and the reaction of the MLC test; i.e., (a) HL-A identical sibling pairs do not generally stimulate each other; (b) the degree of reaction in the MLC test is directly proportional to the degree of difference in HL-A types of the members of the family; (c) HL-A unidentical pairs regularly stimulate each other; (d) HL-A identical unrelated individuals regularly stimulate each other. The MLC test is useful in conjunction with HL-A typing for histocompatibility matching, but the two do not correlate well in unrelated individuals. The MLC test is a most useful means of matching donor and recipient in bone marrow transplantation. The disparity index of the third party MLC test may be useful in predicting the severity of the graft versus host reaction. The concept that a single locus controls the HL-A system and the MLC reaction needs to be modified in the light of recent reports (a) that in rare instances, HL-A identical siblings were found to be stimulative in MLC; (b) that HL-A unidentical siblings failed to stimulate in certain cases; (c) that HL-A unidentical unrelated individuals can be nonstimulatory in the MLC test but that the rejection of skin grafts occurs as fast as in an unrelated MLC reactive pair. This evidence indicates that the genetic loci for the HL-A antigens, MLC reaction, and transplantation immunity may be separate but closely linked and perhaps influenced by one another. However, the influence of as yet unidentified leukocyte antigens may be responsible for the apparent disparities in some of these reactions. The complexity of the chromosomal region associated with the HL-A system needs further study to define the immunogenetics of transplantation in man in more operational terms.

ACKNOWLEDGEMENTS

Aided by grants from The National Foundation-March of Dimes, The John A. Hartford Foundation, Inc., the US Public Health Service (AI-08677 and AI-00798), the American Cancer Society, and the Arthritis Foundation, Minnesota Chapter.

REFERENCES

1. Medawar, P.B. Relationship between the antigens of blood and skin. Nature (London) 1, 161-162 (1946).
2. Asgood, E.E., and Brooke, J.H. Continuous tissue culture of leukocytes from human leukemic bloods by application of "gradient" principles. Blood 10, 1010-1022 (1955).
3. Hungerford, D.A., Donnelly, A.J., Nowell, P.C., and Beck, S. The chromosome constitution of human phenotypic intersex. Amer. J. Hum. Genet. 11, 215-236 (1959).
4. Nowell, P.C. Phytohemagglutinin; an inhibitor of mitosis in cultures of normal human leukocytes. Cancer Res. 20, 462-466 (1960).
5. Li, J.G., and Asgood, E.E. A method for the rapid separation of leukocytes and nucleated erythrocytes from blood or marrow with a phytohemagglutinin from red bean (Phaseolus vulgaris). Blood 4, 670-675 (1949).
6. Schrek, R., and Stefani, S.S. Lymphocytic and intradermal reactions to phytohemagglutinin. Fed. Proc., Fed. Amer. Soc. Exp. Biol. 22, 428 (1963).
7. Permain, G., Lycette, R.R., and Fitzgerald, P.H. Tuberculin-induced mitosis in peripheral blood leukocytes. Lancet 1, 637-638 (1963).
8. Ling, N.R. "Lymphocytes Stimulation," pp.147-174. North-Holland Publ., Amsterdam, 1968.
9. Valentine, F.T. The transformation and proliferation of lymphocytes in vitro In "Cell Mediated Immunity. In Vitro Correlates," J.P.

Revillard, Ed.), pp. 6-50. Karger, Basel, 1971.

10. Schrek, R., and Donnelly, W.J. Difference between lymphocytes of leukemic and non-leukemic patients with respect to morphologic features, motility, and sensitivity to guinea pig serum. Blood 18, 561-571 (1961).

11. Bain, B., Vas, M., and Lowenstein, L. A reaction between leukocytes in mixed peripheral blood cultures. Fed. Proc., Fed. Amer. Soc. Exp. Biol. 22, 428 (1963).

12. Bain, B., Vas, M.R., and Lowenstein, L. The development of large immature mononuclear cells in mixed leukocytes cultures. Blood 23, 108-116 (1964).

13. Hirschhorn, K., Bach, F., Kolodny, R.L., Firschein, I.L., and Hashem, N. Immune response and mitosis of human peripheral blood lymphocytes in vitro. Science 142, 1185-1187 (1963).

14. Jackson, J.F., and Hardy, J.D. Lymphocyte transformation as an in vitro histocompatibility test. Lancet 1, 453-455 (1965).

15. Elves, M.W., Isräels, M.C.G., and Booth, J. Lymphocyte transformation in culture of mixed leukocytes; a possible test of histocompatibility. Lancet 1, 1184-1186 (1965).

16. McClaurin, B.P. Homograft interactions in the test-tube. Lancet 2, 816-821.(1965).

17. Marshall, W.H., Rigo, S.J., and Melman, S. Lymphocyte transformation and mitosis in vitro initiated by homologous macrophages; an improved method for histocompatibility testing. Lancet 1, 730-732 (1966).

18. Bach, F., and Hirschhorn, K. Lymphocyte interaction; a potential histocompatibility test in vitro. Science 143, 813-814 (1964).

19. Bain, B., and Lowenstein, L. Genetic studies on the mixed leukocyte reaction. Science 145, 1315-1316 (1964).

20. Ceppellini, R., Franceschini, P., Miggiano, V.C., and Tridenti, G. Directional activation of mixed lymphocytes cultures. In "Histocom-

patibility Testing 1965" (D.B. Amos and J.J. van Rood, eds.), pp. 223–228. Munksgaard, Copenhagen, 1965.

21. Bach, F.H., and Voynow, N.K. One way stimulation in mixed leukocyte culture. Science 153, 545–547 (1966).

22. Ling, N.R. "Lymphocytes Stimulation," pp. 117–145. North-Holland Publ., Amsterdam, 1971.

23. Sengar, D.P.S., and Terasaki, P.I. A semi-micro mixed leukocyte culture test. Transplantation 11, 260–267 (1971).

24. Hartzman, R.J., Segall, M., Bach, M.L., and Bach, F.H. Histocompatibility matching. VI. Miniaturization of the mixed leukocyte culture test; a preliminary report. Transplantation 11, 268–273 (1971).

25. Friedman, E.A., Retan, J.W., Marshall, D.C., Henry, L., and Merrill, J.P. Accelerated skin graft rejection in humans pre-immunized with homologous peripheral leukocytes. J. Clin. Invest. 40, 2162–2170 (1961).

26. Rapaport, F.T., Laurence, H.S., Thomas, L., Converse, J.M., Tillett, W.S., and Mulholland, J.H. Cross reaction to skin homograft in man. J. Clin. Invest. 41, 2166–2172 (1962).

27. Dausset, J. Iso-leuko-anticorps. Acta Haematol. 20, 156–166 (1958).

28. Dausset, J. and Brecy, H. Identical nature of the leukocyte antigens detectable in mono-zygotic twins by means of immune iso-leuk-agglutinins. Nature (London) 180, 1430–1431 (1957).

29. Lalegari, P., and Spaet, T.H. Studies on the genetics of leukocyte antigens. Blood 14, 748–758 (1959).

30. Payne, R., and Rolfs, M.R. Fetomaternal leukocyte incompatibility. J. Clin. Invest. 37, 1756–1763 (1958).

31. Payne, R., and Hackel, E. Inheritance of human leukocyte antigens. Amer. J. Hum. Genet. 13, 306–315 (1961).

32. van Rood, J.J., van Leeuwen, A., and Basch, L.J. Leukocyte antigens and transplantation immunity. Proc. Congr. Eur. Soc. Haematol., 8th, 1961 p. 199 (1962).

33. van Rood, J.J., and van Leeuwen, A. Leukocyte grouping, a method and its application. J. Clin. Invest. 42, 1382-1390 (1963).

34. Colombani, J., Dausset, J., and Préaux, J. Homogreffe de peau chez l'homme en relation avec les iso-antigènes leukocytaires. Nouv. Rev. Fr. Hematol. 3, 499-505 (1963).

35. Walford, R.L., Carter, P.K., and Anderson, R.E. Leukocyte antibodies following skin homografting in the human. Transplant. Bull. 29, 16-18 (1962).

36. Colombani, J., Colombani, M., and Dausset, J. Leukocyte antigens and skin homograft in man. Demonstration of humoral antibodies after homografting by the antiglobulin consumption test. Ann. N.Y. Acad. Sci. 120, 307-321 (1964).

37. Terasaki, P.I., and McClelland, J.D. Microdroplet assay of human serum cytotoxins. Nature (London) 204, 998-1000 (1964).

38. Terasaki, P.I., Mickey, P.I., Vredevoe, D.L., and Goyette, D.R. Serotyping for homotransplantation. IV. Grouping and evaluation of lymphotoxic sera. Vox Sang. 11, 350-376 (1965).

39. Payne, R., Tripp, M., Weigle, J., Bodmer, W., and Bodmer, J. A new leukocyte isoantigen system in man. Cold Spring Harbor Symp. Quant. Biol. 29, 285-295 (1964).

40. van Rood, J.J., van Leeuwen, A., Schipper, A.M. J., Vooys, W.H., Fredriks, E., Balner, H., and Eerniss, G. Leukocyte groups, the normal lymphocyte transfer test, and homograft sensitivity. In "Histocompatibility Testing 1965" (D.B. Amos and J.J. van Rood, eds.), pp. 37-50. Munksgaard, Copenhagen, 1965.

41. "Histocompatibility Testing (1964). Nat. Acad. Sci. - Nat. Res. Counc.,Washington, D.C., 1965.

42. Amos, D.B., and van Rood, J.J., eds. "Histo-

compatibility Testing 1965." Munksgaard, Copenhagen, 1965.

43. Curtoni, E.S., Mattiuz, P.L., and Tosi, R.M., eds. "Histocompatibility testing 1967." Munksgaard, Copenhagen, 1967.

44. Terasaki, P.I., ed. "Histocompatibility Testing 1970." Munksgaard, Copenhagen, 1970.

45. Amos, D.B. Human histocompatibility laws HL-A. Science 159, 659-660 (1968).

46. Allen, F., Amos, D.B., et al. Joint report of fourth international histocompatibility workshop. In "Histocompatibility Testing 1970" (P.I. Terasaki, ed.), pp. 2-47. Munksgaard, Copenhagen, 1970.

47. Hatler, B.G., Hutchin, P., Zmijewski, C.M., Amos, D.B., and Stickel, D.L. Human leukocyte typing in selection of compatible donors. Surg. Forum 17, 243-244 (1966).

48. van Rood, J.J., van Leeuwen, A., Schipper, A.M.J., Ceppellini, R., and Mattiuz, P.L. Leukocyte groups and their relation to homotransplantation. Ann. N.Y. Acad. Sci. 129, 467-489 (1966).

49. Walford, R.L., Colombani, J., and Dausset, J. Retrospective leukocyte typing of unrelated human donor-recipient pairs in relation to skin allograft survival times; a study of welldefined specificities. Transplantation 7, 188-193 (1969).

50. Amos, D.B., Hatler, B.G., MacQueen, J.M., Cohen, I., and Seigler, M.F. An interpretation and application of cytotoxicity typing. In "Advances in Transplantation" (J. Dausset, J. Hamburger, and G. Mathé, eds.), p. 203. Williams & Wilkins, Baltimore, Maryland, 1967.

51. Ceppellini, R., Mattiuz, P.L., Schudeller, G., and Visetti, M. Experimental transplantation in man. I. The role of the HL-A system in different genetic combinations. Transplant. Proc. 1, 385-389 (1969).

52. Dausset, J., Rapaport, F.T., Legrand, L.,

Colombani, J., and Marcelli-Barge, A. Skin allograft survival in 238 human subjects. In "Histocompatability Testing 1970," (P.I. Terasaki, ed.), pp. 381-397. Munksgaard, Copenhagen, 1970.
53. Mickey, M.R., Krusler, M., Albert, E.D., Tanaka, N., and Terasaki, P.I. Analysis of HL-A incompatibility in human transplants. Tissue Antigens 1, 57-67 (1971).
54. Hors, J., Feingold, N., Fradelizi, D., and Dausset, J. Critical evaluation of histocompatibility in 179 renal transplants. Lancet 1, 609-612 (1971).
55. Ceppellini, R., Curtoni, E.S., Mattiuz, P.L., Miggiano, V.M., Scudeller, G., and Serra, A. Genetics of leukocyte antigens; a family study of segregation and linkage. In "Histocompatibility Testing 1967" (E.S. Curtoni, P.L. Mattiuz, and R.M. Tosi, eds.), pp. 149-187. Munksgaard, Copenhagen, 1967.
56. Bach, F.H., and Amos, D.E. Hu-I: Major histocompatibility locus in man. Science 156, 1506-1508 (1967).
57. Amos, D.B., and Bach, F.H. Phenotypic expression of the major histocompatibility locus in man (HL-A): Leukocyte antigens and mixed leukocyte culture reactivity. J. Exp. Med. 128, 623-637 (1968).
58. Iványi, D., Rychlikova, M., Sasports, M., Iványi, P., and Dausset, P. Leukocyte antigens and the mixed lymphocyte culture reaction. Vox Sang. 12, 186-198 (1967).
59. Albertini, R.J., and Bach, F.H. Quantitative assay of antigenic disparity at HL-A - the major histocompatibility locus in man. J. Exp. Med. 128, 639-651 (1968).
60. Debray-Sachs, M., Dormont, J., Bach, J.F., Descamps, B., Dausset, J., and Hamburger, J. Leukocyte typing versus transformation in mixed lymphocyte culture. Lancet 2, 318-320 (1968).
61. Schellekens, P.Th.A., Vriesendorp, B., Eijs-

voogel, V.P., Van Leeuwen, A., van Rood, J.J. Miggiano, V., and Ceppellini, R. Lymphocyte transformation in vitro. II. Mixed leukocyte culture in relation to leukocyte antigens. Clin. Exp. Immunol. 6, 241-254 (1970).

62. Bach, F.H. Transplantation: Pairing of donor and recipient. Science 168, 1170-1179 (1970).

63. Russel, P.S., Nelson, D.S., and Johnson, G.J. Matching tests for histocompatability in man. Ann. N.Y. Acad. Sci. 129, 368-385 (1966).

64. Bach, F.H., and Kisken, W.A. Predictive value of results of mixed leukocyte cultures for skin allograft survival in man. Transplantation 5, 1046-1052 (1967).

65. Bach, J.F., Debray-Sachs, M., Crosnier, J., Kreis, H., and Dermont, J. Correlation between mixed lymphocyte culture performed before renal transplantation and kidney function. Clin. Exp. Immunol. 6, 821-827 (1970).

66. Gatti, R.A., Meuwissen, H.J., Allen, H.D., Hong, R., and Good, R.A. Immunological reconstitution of sex-linked lymphopenic immunological deficiency. Lancet 2, 1366-1369 (1968).

67. Yunis, E.J., Plate, J.M., Ward, F.E., Seigler, H.F., and Amos, D.B. Anomolous MLR responsiveness among siblings. Transplant. Proc. 3, 118-120 (1971).

68. Koch, C.T.,Eijsvoogel, V.P., Frederiks, E. and van Rood, J.J. Mixed-lymphocyte-culture and skin graft data in unrelated HK-A identical individuals. Lancet 2, 1334-1336 (1971).

69. Dupont, B., Nielsen, L.S., and Svejgaard, A. Relative importance of four and LA loci in determining mixed-lymphocyte reaction. Lancet 2, 1336-1340 (1971).

70. Sengar, D.P.S., Mickey, M.R., Myhre, B.A., Chen, H.H., and Terasaki, P.I. Mixed leukocyte culture response in HL-A "identical individuals." Transfusion (Philadelphia) 11, 251-257 (1971).

71. Yunis, E.J., and Amos, D.B. Three closely linked genetic systems relevant to transplanta-

tion. <u>Proc. Nat. Acad. Sci. U.S.</u> <u>68</u>, 3031–
3035 (1971).

72. Pentycross, C.R., Klouda, P.T., and Lawler, S.D.
The HL-A system and the mixed lymphocyte culture reaction. <u>Lancet 1</u>, 95 (1972).

73. Dupont, B. Personal communication (19).

74. Uphoff, D.E., and Law, L.W. An evaluation of
some genetic factors influencing irradiation
protection by bone marrow. <u>J. Nat. Cancer
Inst.</u> <u>22</u>, 229–240 (1959).

75. Simonsen, M. Graft-versus-host reactions.
Their natural history and applicability as tools
of research. <u>Progr. Allergy</u> <u>6</u>, 349–467 (1962).

76. Yunis, E.J., Hilgard, H.R., and Martinez, C.
Studies on immunologic reaction of thymectomized mice. <u>J. Exp. Med.</u> <u>121</u>, 607–632 (1965).

77. Good, R.A. Progress toward a cellular engin-
eering. <u>J. Amer. Med. Ass.</u> <u>214</u>, 1289–1300
(1970).

78. Park, B.H., and Good, R.A. Third party MLC
test: A new method of histocompatibility testing. <u>Proc. Nat. Acad. Sci. U.S.</u> <u>69</u>, 1490
(1972).

SOME OBSERVATIONS ON THE MIXED-LYMPHOCYTE
CULTURE - POTENTIAL CLINICAL USES

Brack G. Hattler, Jr.

Department of Surgery
Division of Thoracic Surgery
University of Arizona Medical Center
Tucson, Arizona

INTRODUCTION

Schrek and Donnelly (1), in 1961, were the first
to observe a number of large cells with prominent
nuclei and nucleoli in a culture consisting of a mixture of bloods from two patients with hemachromato-
sis. This report went largely unnoticed until 1963,
when Bain et al. (2,3) described a proliferative
interaction that resulted when blood leukocytes from
immunogenetically disparate but normal donors were
mixed and placed into culture. Shortly thereafter,
Bach and Hirschhorn (4) reported a similar observation. Here, a small percentage of cells underwent
morphological transformation into lymphoblasts. The
number of cells transformed could be estimated by
microscopic inspection; however, counting was frequently difficult because of intermediate cell forms.
Greater reliability in the determination of cell
transformation was achieved by measuring the incorporation of radioactive metabolic precursors into
newly formed nucleic acid. In unmixed control cultures, few cells were found to transform or to incor-
porate ^{3}H-thymidine.
    The following year, Bain and Lowenstein (5)
reported the critical finding that mixed cultures of
cells from identical twins did not respond and that
those of closely related individuals responded only

93

slightly. These studies were done, however, using a two-way test system in which it was impossible to control for possible technical errors that might have led to false-negative results. Using a one-way method of stimulation, Bach and Amos (6,7) were able to confirm Bain's findings and to show that approximately 28% of sibling mixtures failed to stimulate. These observations suggested that the response observed in cultures was genetically controlled and therefore an expression of antigeneic similarity or dissimilarity of lymphocyte populations in vitro.

Numerous experiments with animal cells not only confirmed the original observations made with human blood lymphocytes but also established the immuno-genetic basis of the phenomenon. Thus, the interaction of mixed leukocytes was shown to be a response on the part of small lymphocytes from normal animals, i.e., unsensitized by recognized criteria. The mixed-lymphocyte culture (MLC) response could be elicited not only with blood lymphocytes, but with equal effectiveness with lymphoid cells from spleen and lymph nodes. Using spleen cells, Dutton (8) demonstrated with various inbred strains of mice that a correlation between the magnitude of the MLC response and the degree of histoincompatibility could be made only with respect to differences at the H2 locus. This observation suggested that the MLC measured mainly incompatibilities at the major H locus of the species. Silvers et al. (9) confirmed these observations with genetically defined populations of rats in which ^{3}H-thymidine uptake in MLC was observed only when donors differed at the major (Ag-B) histocompatibility locus. Wilson (10,11), using rat lymphocyte mixtures of parental strain and F1 hybrid origin, concisely showed that the reaction was unidirectional, with only parent lymphocytes responding to the stimulus of F1 antigens. Sex chromosome markers provided direct evidence for this contention.

As a unidirectional reaction, many of the qualities of the MLC have provided a rational basis

for its employment as an in vitro model for the allograft reaction (12). Its reactivity is controlled by
the major H histocompatibility system in every
species in which the MLC has been studied (6,9,12).
Most recently, in the human, Bach and Amos (6,7)
have shown a close correlation between MLC reactivity
and the HL-A locus. The same major locus detected by
suitable isoimmune antisera appears to be identical
or closely linked to genetic material, determining
MLC reactivity. These observations have extended
preliminary findings that show a correlation in two-
way MLC stimulation with incompatibilities for certain white cell antigens (13).

Although a large body of data supports the concept that the major histocompatibility locus in various species determines MLC reactivity, two findings
applicable to the HL-A locus in the human argue
against this concept. First, HL-A identical siblings have been reported who do stimulate in mixed-
lymphocyte reactions. Second, only a small fraction
(less than 1%) of identical nonrelated individuals do
not stimulate in a mixed-lymphocyte interaction.
This has been interpreted by Amos and Yunis (14,15)
as indicating that the MLC locus, although closely
linked to HL-A, may be separable from it by crossing
over. They have, in fact, suggested a three-point
genetic map in which the MLC locus lies adjacent to
and outside of the genetic material determining the
four (second) segregant series of antigens within the
HL-A system.

These findings, however, do not detract from
the use of the MLC as an in vitro test simulating the
allograft response. Abundant data support the
conclusion that the MLC may be a faithful reproduction of the allograft reaction proceeding from the
inductive phase to the effector mechanisms. The
evidence for this has been recently reviewed by
Wilson (16). Whether a separate MLC locus exists or
not, the vast majority of evidence points to the very
close correlation between proliferation in the mixed-
lymphocyte culture and the histocompatibility

differences between responding and stimulating lymphocytes. The very fact that lymphocytes are the cells responding in vitro and that their proliferative response can take place without any prior history of sensitization places this reaction in a unique position. In contrast, proliferation to the delayed hypersensitivity antigens in vitro requires that the lymphocyte donor be sensitized to the appropriate antigen. Wilson (16) has identified the responding cell in MLC as thymus derived. Lymphocytes from neonatally thymectomized animals are markedly hampered in their MLC response and responding cells from tolerant animals do not react to antigens governed by the major histocompatibility locus of the animal utilized in the production of tolerance but do undergo proliferation to indifferent (control) cells (17).

It is not intended here to review most of the recent evidence supporting the parallel between the primary allograft reaction and MLC reactivity. Much of this work has appeared in recent composite publications. Papers that are central to this discussion are cited. Certain aspects of work under study in our laboratory are stressed, although we realize that such an approach omits by necessity the contributions of many to this subject. We are seeking a working model, one that will guide further experiments, rather than a complete description of what has been done.

Cellular Contributions to Mixed-Lymphocyte Culture Reactivity.

One of the main drawbacks to the use of the mixed-lymphocyte culture as an assay for following allograft reactivity has been its general lack of reproducibility. This is not surprising when one attempts to assimilate in vitro observations on the role of macrophages, T-B cell interactions, recruiting or augmenting factors, and the in vitro responses to soluble antigens and various mitogens.

96

Apart from the response to mitogens, stimulation of lymphocytes by allogeneic cells results in the activation of a large (1-3%) population of lymphocytes (18 - 20). One suggestion has been that specificity is essentially the end result of the way in which presentation of determinants occurs (21). A necessary correlation of such a contention must, however, encompass a high frequency of cross-reactivity with responding cells displaying more than a unipotent potential to antigen stimulation (22).

Of the various factors that may effect the mixed-lymphocyte culture, those that have been most thoroughly studied relate to the culture conditions themselves. Possibly of equal importance are the requirements for various cellular components, some specific and others lacking specificity, and the relative contributions of subpopulations of lymphocytes to the total reaction. Indeed, it appears reasonable to assume that for any given response to an antigen there is a crucial step that involves antigen interaction with a critical cell population (22,23).

The necessity for an adherent or macrophage cell has recently been stressed. Although this requirement is small in comparison to the total number of cells present, a lack of these cells results in an attenuated mixed-lymphocyte culture response. In contrast, the reactivity recorded to certain mitogens can be demonstrated in the absence of macrophages. Interestingly, Bach et al. (24) have shown that the macrophage requirement for MLC reactivity lacks specificity and may be substituted for by supernatants derived from macrophage cultures that have never come in contact with the antigen.

In contrast to the reports of others, we have found, as has Bach, that the presence of polymorphonuclear cells in certain concentrations markedly inhibits the response in mixed-lymphocyte culture (25,26). The ability to separate pure granulocytes (>95%) and lymphocytes free of granulocyte contamination allows us to explore this relationship. To

lymphocytes prepared from peripheral blood by Ficoll-
Isopaque density gradient centrifugation, relative
proportions of granulocytes are added. These cells
are readily available by sedimentation of heparinized
peripheral blood in plasmagel, followed by layering
of the buffy coat on a discontinuous gradient consisting of bovine serum albumin (BSA) (density, 1.083)
below a layer of Ficoll-Isopaque. After centrifuging
at 200G for 20 min, the lymphocytes are collected at
the (Ficoll-Isopaque)-blood interphase and the
granulocytes at the BSA-(Ficoll-Isopaque) interphase.
The majority of red cells pass through to the bottom
of the tube and those contaminating the granulocytes
are lyzed following treatment with Tris-ammonium
chloride. As the percentage of granulocytes is
increased, the mixed-lymphocyte culture response progressively diminishes (Table I). This effect is nonspecific and is equally evident when granulocytes
from either responder, stimulator, or an indifferent
third person are added to the mixed-lymphocyte interaction. As can be seen in Table I, comparing values
in which total cell numbers are kept constant, inhibition is not a function of cell concentration.

The etiology of the granulocyte effect is not
apparent yet but may reside in an enzyme (thymidine
phosphorylase) present in granulocytes and known to
facilitate thymidine breakdown to substances that are
not incorporated into DNA (27-29). It is not surprising, therefore, that with the elimination of
granulocytes many workers note an improved reproducibility with mixed-lymphocyte culturing (26-30).

Human peripheral blood lymphocytes are very
heterogeneous with regard to life span, origin, and
function. One may speculate, therefore, that apart
from the role that other cells play, some of the day-
to-day variability that can be seen in the culture
response of lymphocytes may be secondary to daily
fluctuations in lymphocyte subpopulations. To this
effect, a series of recent experiments are of interest. Ficoll-Isopaque separated peripheral blood
lymphocytes were resuspended in 17% BSA and layered

on top of a discontinuous BSA gradient. After centrifugation for 30 min at 400G, three distinct and an occasional fourth band could be found at the following interphases: band I, between 17% and 19% BSA; band II, at the 19-21% area; band III, at the 21-23% interphase; and an occasional fourth band between the 23% and 25% bovine serum albumin layers. Good day-to-day reproducibility with cultures of these bands (Table II) was seen and was better than that obtained with Ficoll -Isopaque separated lymphocytes. Cells from layer I not only responded best to PHA and to MLC but also stimulated better. We saw, however, subjects whose cells after BSA gradient separation consistently showed maximum responsiveness in layer three (III). In these instances PHA reactivity also peaked in this band.

Recently, we have performed experiments utilizing the ability of human lymphocytes to form rosettes directly with sheep red blood cells (E cells) as a T-cell marker and receptors for activated complement (EAC cells) as a property of B lymphocytes (31). Peripheral blood lymphocytes separated by Ficoll-Isopaque gradients consistently demonstrate 30-40% E rosettes and 20-30% EAC rosettes. The E cells are concentrated, after further separation on BSA gradients, to 50-70% in those bands showing maximum PHA and MLC responsiveness, whereas EAC cells are only sporadically demonstrated here. It appears that at least two subpopulations of human lymphocytes are being distinguished for when lymphocytes are incubated with both E and EAC; the rosettes counted are the approximate sum of E and EAC complexes as separately determined. In addition, the inability to account for all lymphocytes by E or EAC rosette formation implies that other subpopulations have yet to be identified. To what extent day-to-day shifts in the stratum of lymphocyte subpopulations may effect MLC reproducibility is under investigation and may depend on fluctuations in peripheral blood lymphocyte representation as a function of numerous variables, i.e., antigen exposure at any point in time.

Regardless of the explanation, we have found that the
reproducibility of the MLC is further improved after
BSA gradient separation and the culturing of cells of
similar density on various days.

Some Potential Clinical Uses of the Mixed-Lymphocyte
Culture Other than for Histocompatibility Matching.

   If we accept that various culture conditions may
affect the day-to-day reproducibility of MLC reactivity between the same donor-recipient pair, it becomes
increasingly evident that, when such variables are
carefully controlled, the test becomes a sensitive
assay for following cellular immunity and factors
that may modify it. As such, in the dog undergoing
unmodified renal allograft rejection, several pertinent observations have been made (30,32,33).
During rejection there is a loss of MLC-reactive
lymphocytes from the peripheral blood of recipient
animals. This cellular unresponsiveness, although
demonstrable to a greater degree with stimulation by
irradiated donor cells, may also be seen with cells
of indifferent (normal) dogs and occurs regardless of
whether cultures are performed in recipient or normal
dog plasma. It therefore represents a true loss of
cellular reactivity from the peripheral blood
lymphocyte compartment. Further experimentation
indicates, however, that this change is spurious, for
with the simultaneous culturing of splenic lymphocytes from the same animal reactivity to donor antigens can be found at this level. Therefore, in spite
of loss of MLC-reactive lymphocytes in the peripheral
blood, clones of responding cells remain centrally
situated (Table III).
   Loss of reactivity from the peripheral blood can
be ascribed to entrapment of the MLC responsive cell
in the allografted kidney. We have recently been
able to separate these cells by density gradient
centrifugation from other cells within kidneys
removed at the peak of allograft rejection (32). By
sex karyotyping, these cells have proved to be of

recipient origin. Such lymphocytes contain 5-20% lymphoblasts within their population and do respond to stimulation with irradiated donor cells (Table III). Following rejection and kidney removal, a gradual return of MLC peripheral lymphocyte reactivity is seen over the ensuing 2 to 4 weeks when cultures are set in normal plasma and may be caused by the absence of the allograft and consequently the lack of a "cellular sponge" and/or to seeding of the peripheral blood with lymphocytes from the more centrally situated clones. Thus, in the human, we have also shown that peripheral blood lymphocyte and central (splenic) lymphocyte reactivity do not always parallel each other. Peripheral blood lymphocyte reactivity may be absent in the presence of a prompt and dramatic splenic lymphocyte response (34).

Similar observations have now been made in over 15 consanguinous kidney transplants studied preoperatively by HL-A typing and mixed lymphocyte culture reactivity against their prospective donors and indifferent individuals (35-37). The MLC was followed sequentially after transplantation as well. When HL-A identity was present, and in some cases of nonidentity, MLC reactivity against the donor was absent or minimal pre- and postoperatively, whereas the response against indifferent lymphocytes remained strong (Table IV). In this setting there were no detectable rejection episodes. When preoperative MLC reactivity against both donor and indifferent lymphocytes was strong, postoperatively there was a disappearance of this reactivity with rejection, which occurred more specifically against donor lymphocytes. The decrease in MLC reactivity preceded the clinical detection of rejection episodes. This was followed by a gradual return of reactivity with successful therapy and in spite of increased immunosuppression. Here again, entrapment of MLC-reactive cells within the allograft has been demonstrated (35). Unfortunately, the time interval required for culturing makes this test at present an interesting in vitro observation with little clinical application.

Possibilities for temporally scaling down the reaction time may overcome this objection (38).

In addition to the use of the mixed lymphocyte culture to sequentially monitor changes occurring during allograft rejection, it appears that blocking of lymphocyte activation is at present a sensitive means of detecting antibodies against lymphocytes and one of the few techniques available for detecting antibodies without cytotoxic effects (39-41). Thus, immunoglobulin G appearing several months after transplantation in the serum of three closely matched kidney recipients has been demonstrated to progressively inhibit unidirectional mixed-lymphocyte cultures when donor lymphocytes are used either as responding or stimulating cells (36). The gamma G demonstrated specificity for donor cells, was noncytotoxic by lymphocytotoxicity and, most important, the effect could be reversed by carrying out a two-stage mixed-lymphocyte interaction (Table V). For cultures set using donor responding cells plus indifferent stimulating cells (D + Ix) in recipient (R) plasma - MLC inhibitory, noncytotoxic - no stimulation above autologous control values was seen. If, however, on day 2 the cultures were spun down and R plasma was replaced by normal (I) plasma, stimulation was demonstrated as the culture period resumed. Such inhibition must take place early in the culture period. When R plasma is added after the first 24 hr of culture no inhibition is seen. It therefore appears that, once the cell has been activated, the inhibitory IgG is no longer effective. This is in contrast to those results recorded when a known cytotoxic antibody is used in a parallel series of experiments. Here, there is no reversal of inhibition and the effect can be demonstrated at any time in culture (Table V).

Similar blocking patterns have not been detected in patients in whom rejection has been a problem. The specificity of the MLC inhibitory immunoglobulin for donor cells, its association with an unremarkable postoperative clinical course, and the ability most

recently to elute this antibody from biopsies taken
from these kidneys (36) all point to a possible
immunoregulatory role for this immunoglobulin in the
long-term success of kidney transplants.

Cytotoxic antibody also inhibits MLC reactivity.
Table VI presents data from a recent series of experiments designed to ascertain the sensitivity and
specificity of the assay as a test for antibody in
patients awaiting transplantation. Patient FRO, a
multiparous woman whose serum reacted with over 80%
of a cell panel representing all recognized HL-A
phenotypes, was tested in unidirectional mixed-
lymphocyte cultures with irradiated stimulating cells
from four subjects. Immunoglobulin G separated from
the serum of a normal individual and from FRO's serum
by DEAE column chromatography (identified as one band
on immunoelectrophoresis) was available. FRO's lymphocytes responded to the stimulating cell panel.
No significant differences were evident regardless of
whether normal sera or normal IgG was added to the
basic cultures set in normal plasma. However, when
heat inactivated serum from patient FRO was present,
marked MLC inhibition was discernible. The inhibitory effect, found in the IgG fraction, could be
completely removed for subject SOB's cells by
absorbing FRO's serum or IgG with spleen cells available from patient SOB. Interestingly, there appeared
to be no correlation between conventional lymphocytotoxicity and MLC inhibition. Indeed, for subject
SPA, even though lymphocytotoxicity was removed following absorption of FRO's serum or IgG, the materials were still markedly MLC inhibitory and remained
so even when titered out to a 1 : 64 dilution (not
illustrated). In contrast, for subject HUP, Table
VI, lymphocytotoxicity was not removed for HUP's
cells in spite of repeated absorption of FRO's IgG or
serum. Inhibition of MLC reactivity was still evident.

To what extent the inhibitory effect noted in
MLC is cytotoxic or possibly blocking is yet to be
clarified. Several possibilities exist: (1) Two

different classes of antibodies are present, one
cytotoxic, one blocking in nature. Thus, for patient
SPA's cells, absorption of FRO's serum removes the
cytotoxic component and the blocking factor remains.
In this particular instance, however, (1) appears
unlikely because with mixed lymphocyte cultures of
FRO plus SPA cultured initially in FRO's absorbed
IgG and 1 day later reset in normal plasma (two-
stage reaction) the inhibitory effect was unchanged
(not illustrated). As previously shown, the inhibitory effect on MLC reactivity demonstrated in the
presence of blocking antibodies is reversible. (2)
The antibodies are predominantly cytotoxic. Mixed
lymphocyte culture inhibition, however, provides a
more sensitive assay for their detection. Although
one cannot rule out blocking factors, in the example
cited above it appears that the reaction predominantly detected is cytotoxic. In spite of the fact that
in this instance the sera studied are from chronic
renal failure patients, it is felt that our results
do not necessarily equate with those in vitro inhibitory effects described by others for uremic serum in
which antibody has not been shown to play a role
(42). In contrast, the inhibitory effect described
here can be found in the IgG fraction. We have been
unable to detect any traces of urea nitrogen or
creatinine in these IgG preparations and feel that
it is highly unlikely that after chromatography and
repeated dialysis of the immunoglobulin we are
simply recording the effect of a "uremic toxin" that
has fortuitously migrated and remained with immunoglobulin G. In addition, the specificity illustrated
by the absorption experiments argues against nonspecific toxicity.

We have described, therefore, a few of the areas
in which the mixed-lymphocyte culture interaction may
be used in the clinical and experimental evaluation
of the allograft reaction. Its use depends initially
on the availability of a reproducible assay. Critical questions may then be asked.

ACKNOWLEDGEMENTS

The author wishes to point out that many of the arguments presented in this paper were developed in collaboration with Dr. J. Miller. The expert technical assistance of B. Soehnlen, B. Auchter, and M. Davis are gratefully acknowledged.

REFERENCES

1. Schrek, R., and Donnelly, W.J. Blood 18, 561 (1961).
2. Bain, B., Vas, M.R., and Lowenstein, L. Fed. Proc., Fed. Amer. Soc. Exp. Biol. 22, 428 (1963).
3. Bain, B., Vas, M.R., and Lowenstein, L. Blood 23, 108 (1964).
4. Bach, F.H. and Hirschhorn, K. Science 143, 813 (1964).
5. Bain, B. and Lowenstein, L. Science 145, 1315 (1964).
6. Amos, D.B., and Bach, F.H. J. Exp. Med. 128, 623 (1968).
7. Bach, F.H. and Amos, D.B. Science 156, 1506 (1967).
8. Dutton, R.W. J. Exp. Med. 123, 665 (1966).
9. Silvers, W.K., Wilson, D.B. and Palm, J.E. Science 155, 703 (1967).
10. Wilson, D.B. J. Exp. Med. 126, 625 (1967).
11. Wilson, D.B., Silvers, W.K. and Nowell, P.C. J. Exp. Med. 126, 655 (1967).
12. Bach, F.H., Bock, H., and Graupner, K. Proc. Nat. Acad. Sci. U.S. 62, 377 (1969).
13. Dausset, J. Ivanyi, P. and Ivanyi, D. In "Histocompatibility Testing 1965" (D.B. Amos and J.J. van Rood, eds.), p. 51. Munksgaard, Copenhagen, 1965.
14. Amos, D.B. and Yunis, E.J. Cell. Immunol. 2, 517 (1971). Editorial.
15. Yunis, E.J., and Amos, D.B. Proc. Nat. Acad. Sci. U.S. 68, 3031 (1971).

16. Wilson, D.B. In "Progress In Immunology" (D.B. Amos, ed.), p. 1045. Academic Press, New York, 1972.
17. Wilson, D.B., and Nowell, P.C. J. Exp. Med. 131 131, 391 (1970).
18. Simmons, M.J., and Fowler, R. Nature (London) 209, 588 (1966).
19. Simonsen, M. Cold Spring Harbor Symp. Quant. Biol. 32, 517 (1967).
20. Wilson, D.B., Blyth, J.L., and Nowell, P.C. J. Exp. Med. 128, 1157 (1968).
21. Mitchison, N.A. Symp. Int. Soc. Cell Biol. 7, 29-42 (1968).
22. Zoschke, D.C., and Bach, F.H. Science 170, 1404 (1970).
23. Dutton, R.W., and Mischell, R.I. Cold Spring Harbor Symp. Quant. Biol. 32, 407 (1967).
24. Bach, F.H., Zoschke, D.C., Solliday, S., Day, E., Alter, B., and Bach, M.L. Int. Immunopathol. Symp., 6th, p. 271 (1970).
25. Johnson, M.C., Hattler, B., Currier, C., and Alexander, J. Fed. Proc., Fed. Amer. Soc. Exp. Biol. 30, 467 (1971).
26. Bach, M.L., Bach, F.H., Widmer, M., Oranen, H., and Wolberg, W.H. Transplantation 12, 283 (1971).
27. Merey, P., and Cox, R.P. Experientia 28, 711 (1972).
28. Rubini, J.R. J. Lab. Clin. Med. 68, 566 (1966).
29. Bain, B. Clin. Exp. Immunol. 6, 255 (1970).
30. Miller, J., Hattler, B., Davis, M., and Johnson, M.C. Transplantation 12, 65 (1971).
31. Stjernswerd, J., Jondal, M., Vanky, F., Wigzell, H., and Sealy, R. Lancet 2, 1352 (1972).
32. Hattler, B.G., Jr., Miller, J., and Johnson, M.C. Transplantation 14, 47 (1972).
33. Miller, J., Hattler, B.G., and Johnson, M.C. Transplantation 14, 57 (1972).
34. Hattler, B.G., Jr., and Soehnlen, B.J. Fed. Proc., Fed. Amer. Soc. Exp. Biol. 31, 800 (1972).

35. Hattler, B.G., Jr., and Miller, J. Transplant. Proc. (1972) (in press).
36. Hattler, B.G., Jr., and Miller, J. Transplant. Proc. (1973) (in press).
37. Miller, J., and Hattler, B.G., Jr. Surgery (1972) (in press).
38. Rosenberg, S.A. Fed. Proc., Fed. Amer. Soc. Exp. Biol. 31, 790 (1972).
39. Hattler, B.G., Jr., Karesh, C., and Miller, J. Tissue Antigens 1, 270 (1971).
40. Quadracci, L.J., Hellstrom, I.E., Striker, G.E., Marchioro, T.M., and Hellstrom, K.E. Cell. Immunol. 1, 561 (1970).
41. Ceppellini, R. In "Progress In Immunology" (D.B. Amos, ed.), p. 973. Academic Press, New York, 1972.
42. Newberry, W.M., and Sanford, J.P. J. Clin. Invest. 50, 1262 (1971).

Table I

Effect of Granulocytes on Mixed-Lymphocyte Culture Reactivity[a]

Stimulating cells[b]		Counts per minute
Mononuclears, x 10^5/ml	Granulocytes, x 10^5/ml	x 10^3/culture
3	0	19.4[c]
3	3	17.0
3	6	15.8
3	9	8.1
6	0	25.0
6	3	22.1
6	6	15.3
6	9	10.0
9	0	31.3
9	3	24.1
9	6	17.2
9	9	11.0
0	3	0.4
0	6	0.4
0	9	0.3
0	0	0.7

[a] Three milliliter cultures all set with 6 x 10^5 responding cells per milliliter; 7 day cultures.
[b] Irradiated with 1500 R.
[c] Mean of triplicate cultures; standard error 9.4% or less.

Table II

The Response of Bovine Serum Albumin Separated Subpopulations of Human Peripheral Lymphocytes to Phytohemagglutinin and Mixed-Lymphocyte Culture Stimulation on Different Days[a]

Responding cell	PHA[b]		S_x[c]		S_{I_x}[d]		S_{II_x}[d]		S_{III_x}[d]	
	Day 1	Day 2	Day 1	Day 2	Day 1	Day 2	Day 1	Day 2	Day 1	Day 2
R[c]	3,915	6,	9,	20,857	52,159	51,517	15,617	18,920	22,918	19,855
R_I[d]	32,411	38,393	78,166	85,456	69,911	71,459	55,001	61,311	60,911	69,249
R_II[d]	7,466	7,942	23,673	14,942	63,673	54,515	10,041	6,294	24,119	17,930
R_III	5,111	4,858	31,589	40,580	59,589	64,024	13,918	10,040	28,698	20,755

a Values expressed as the mean counts per minute (cpm) of five cultures. Standard error 6% or less. Cultures 0.2 ml volume. 10^5 lymphocytes responding to 10^5 stimulating and 10^5 responding cells in mixed lymphocyte culture. PHA – 3 day culture. Control for phytohemagglutinin (cells without) culture – 7 day culture period. Autologous controls for mixed lymphocyte cultures less than 450 cpm for all cultures. cultures less than 650 cpm for all cultures.

b Phytohemagglutinin.

c Lymphocytes separated on Ficoll-Isopaque. 95% lymphocytes-monocytes. Subscript (x) denotes 1500 R irradiation for stimulating cells.

d Lymphocytes from Ficoll-Isopaque separation further fractionated on bovine serum albumin gradients, see text. Cells from same subjects used on both days.

Table III

Mixed-Lymphocyte Culture Reactivity
Following Allografting[a]

Responding cells	Counts per Minute/culture
I. Pretransplant	
1	
PB[b]	19,812
S[c]	24,672
II. Days Posttransplant	
3	
PB	14,309
S	20,218
5	
PB	2,391[d]
S	28,678
K[e]	14,742
7	
PB	1,339[f,g]
S	19,458
9	
PB	4,710
S	21,901
11	
PB	6,881
S	20,090

Table III, cont.

14		
PB		15,949
S		17,811

[a] Three milliliter cultures (7 day incubation), set in normal dog plasma; responding cells from recipient dog (peripheral blood or splenic lymphocytes); stimulating cells from kidney donor (peripheral blood cells irradiated with 1500 R).

[b] Peripheral blood lymphocytes.

[c] Splenic lymphocytes.

[d] All autologous control cultures 2500 cpm or less. Values expressed as mean of three cultures. Standard error 10% or less.

[e] Allograft removed at 5 days and lymphocytes extracted from the kidney.

[f] Responses to stimulation by donor lymphocytes depicted. In this experiment and others, however, loss of reactivity to indifferent (normal dog) lymphocytes was also seen.

[g] Although only 7 day culture responses depicted, incubation times of from 2 to 14 days showed no reactivity with peripheral blood lymphocytes.

Table IV

Preoperative Comparison of Haplotype Match,
MLC Response and Clinical Course

Patients	Haplotype	Donor	MLC Response		
			R + Dx	R + Ix	R + Rx
JC	U[a]	Sib[b]	1,056	5,469	555
JW	I[c]	Sib	547	15,960	654
SH	U	P[d]	368	5,499	241
IF	U	P	390	10,069	363
MB	U	Sib	498	11,680	501
PC	U	Sib	901	15,680	649
LF	U	P	14,457	15,808	1,804
SW	U	P	6,021	5,871	361
TS	U	Sib	12,133	10,648	1,668
MA	I	Sib	810	4,581	668
AB	U	P	23,863	34,789	732
SH	U	Sib	10,740	10,108	1,794
AS	U	Sib	21,833	18,941	1,900
DA	U	Sib	2,736	12,460	708
DO	I	Sib	410	40,120	478

[a]One haplotype nonidentical; all these patients
donors possessed no more than one antigen not shared
by recipients.

[b]Sibling.

[c]Haploidentical.

[d]Parent.

Table IV, cont.

Patients	Number of rejection episodes	Day post-transplant	Current status	
			Serum creatinine, mg%	Creatinine clearance ml/min
JC	1	590	0.9	75
JW	0	565	1.8	84
SH	0	535	1.4	100
IF	0	375	1.2	100
MB	0	345	1.5	91
PC	0	295	0.9	80
LF	3	225	2.1	46
SW	2	175	1.7	57
TS	3+	165	1.2	62
MA	0	135	0.9	70
AB	1	125	1.5	60
SH	1	105	1.3	70
AS	2	90	1.3	65
DA	0	60	1.0	80
DO	0	45	1.3	75

Table V

Reversible Inhibition of MLC Reactivity:
Noncytotoxic versus Cytotoxic Antibody[a] (D + Ix)

Serum treatment		MLC results,[b] days after reset					
Day 0	Day 2 (reset)	Noncytotoxic[a] serum			Cytotoxic[c] serum		
		3^d	5^d	7^d	3	5	7
R	I	981	1617	4911	191	208	109
I	R	4197	6833	6042	583	677	404

[a] Cultures prepared with donor responding cells (D) and indifferent stimulating cells (Ix). R serum from a kidney transplant recipient, clinically doing well, 4 months after allografting a kidney from donor (D). R serum MLC inhibitory but nonlymphocytotoxic.

[b] Mean of five cultures (cpm), standard error less than 10%.

[c] Lymphocytotoxic titer of 1/16 against D cells.

[d] Total time in culture 5, 7, and 9 days, respectively.

Table VI

Inhibition of Mixed-Lymphocyte Culture Reactivity as a Test for Antibody[a]

	Normal[b]				Patient FRO[c]				Patient FRO[d]			
	Sera		IgG		Sera		IgG		Sera Absorbed		IgG Absorbed	
	MLC	Cytox.[e]	MLC	Cytox.	MLC	Cytox.	MLC	Cytox.	MLC	Cytox.	MLC	Cytox.
FRO	769± 192	–	641± 102	–	1,231± 200	–	1,080± 92	–	1,461± 312	–	891± 98	–
SAC	42,636±2,081	–	38,911±1,843	–	24,838±3,081	–	6,794±1,118	–				
SPA	43,511±2,624	–	33,981±1,991	–	671± 81	+	967± 113	++	5,811± 581	–	4,001± 666	–
SOB	24,146±1,011	–	18,718± 841	–	4,018± 818	–	5,121±1,483	–	20,911±1,561	–	26,779±2,109	–
HUP	33,227±2,312	–	29,712±1,843	–	1,037± 587	++	1,599± 793	++	2,038± 481	++	3,433± 390	+

[a] Mixed-lymphocyte cultures (MLC) set in normal plasma with patient FRO lymphocytes as responding cells. All cultures 0.2 ml with 1 x 10^5 responding and 1 x 10^5 stimulating cells. Culture period 7 days. Values expressed as mean ± S.E. of five cultures. The numbers in the table all represent numbers of stimulating cells, irradiated with 1500 R, i.e., SPAx, found.

[b] 0.06 ml normal sera or IgG added to culture (3 mg/ml).

[c] 0.06 ml patient FRO sera or IgG (3 mg/ml) added to culture.

[d] 0.06 ml patient FRO sera or IgG (3 mg/ml) added to culture after absorption of serum or IgG with spleen cells from patient SOB.

[e] Lymphocytotoxicity per modified Amos technique:–,>85% viable; +, 60–85% viable; ++, 40–60% viable.

115

HISTOCOMPATIBILITY MATCHING AND DONOR SELECTION

D. B. Amos and E. J. Yunis

Division of Immunology
Duke University Medical Center
Durham, North Carolina

Department of Laboratory Medicine
University of Minnesota Hospitals
Minneapolis, Minnesota

There is disagreement concerning the success of attempts to predict the outcome of renal and other homografts. At one extreme are those who believe that adequate immunosuppression compensates for any except the very strongest degree of histoincompatibility (1,2). At the other extreme are those who believe just as passionately that by selecting the most histocompatible donor it is possible to avoid strong rejection reactions and thus to obtain a well-functioning organ with a minimum requirement for immunosuppression (3-6). Both sides can point to significant successes. Certain transplant series have been conspicuously successful despite the inclusion of many grossly mismatched pairs in them (1). Other series, in which very careful matching has been achieved, can point to the correlation between match or mismatch and graft performance (3,5,7). Many of these arguments are discussed in this monograph or other monographs devoted to renal transplantation.

It is the purpose of this chapter to put some of the factors involved into perspective. To do this it is necessary to define clearly some of the concepts and terms. By "tissue typing" is usually meant the serologic determination of the presence of certain antigenic specificities on the surface membrane of cells of a prospective donor and by "matching" is meant the selection of a recipient whose antigens most nearly resemble those of the donor. Matching includes techniques that may not detect or define the antigens tested for in tissue typing. In MLC matching, lymphocytes from one or more possible donors are incubated with mitomycin-treated or x-irradiated cells of one or more recipients. Compatibility is equated inversely with the degree of stimulation attained (8-10). Skin graft assessment of histocompatibility and matching has been applied to families to supplement the in vitro methods. Grafts are placed between family members (other than the future recipient), previously genotyped for HL-A, in such a way that one or more grafts is incompatible with respect to each HL-A allele or haplotype possessed by the potential donor and absent from the recipient within the family. A skin graft from a child with, say, the paternal A allele and the maternal C placed on an AD sibling gives a measure of the C allele, the A being common to both, and so on (11, 12).

Typing for compatibility has passed through several phases. Before the two loci or two segregant series hypothesis was accepted, matching by tissue typing usually meant grouping donor-recipient pairs in terms of overall phenotypic similarity. Several extensive series reported compatibility in terms of degrees of compatibility as "match grades" A, B, C, or D and claimed a correlation between match grade and graft survival (13,14). However, the correlation, although significant, was far from absolute. After the two loci hypothesis was formulated, compatibility was given in terms of the number of antigens (0-4) shared or as a ratio based on this, called the "net histocompatibility ratio" (15). This, too, was generally discounted as a fallible method although

118

that small proportion of donor-recipient pairs
sharing four antigens appeared to fare better than
those differing by one or more antigens (16,17).
Within a family, the same loose correlation held.
Siblings who shared both haplotypes were the best
donors of allografts. Parent-child combinations and
sibling pairs who differed at one allele might make
ideal donors, or a graft might be violently rejected
(18-20). There was no correlation between incompatibility for any single known HL-A specificity ar
the speed of rejection (21,22).

With respect to MLR (mixed-leukocyte reactions,
pairs who are phenotypically HL-A identical are
mutually stimulatory in most instances (23-28). On
the basis of available data, the absence of stimulation is not correlated with prolonged skin graft
survival (29). Furthermore, in the family study
reported from the Duke group, there was no correlation between skin graft survival in haploidentical
pairs (i.e., pairs sharing only one HL-A haplotype)
and the degree of stimulation in MLR (30). However,
an overall correlation between zero-allele, one-
allele and two allele incompatibility; degree of
stimulation, and graft survival was observed.

Several factors must be taken into consideration
to explain the discrepancy between in vitro attempts
and matching and the outcome of a graft: (1) The
fine detail of the HL-A specificities; (2) technical
problems affecting the results of the MLR or of the
cytotoxocity test generally used to detect HL-A
specificities; (3) recombination within HL-A;
(4) recombination between HL-A and other factors of
the HL-1 histocompatibility complex (31); (5) the
effects of immune response loci; (6) environmental
effects, including prior sensitization to specific
or crossreactive antigens, or to the action of
naturally occurring immunosuppressive agents, such as
certain viruses; and (7) differences in sensitivity
of the individual and of his immune system to immunosuppression.

I.   HL-A

As originally defined, six HL-A specificities could be recognized; these were HL-A1, -A2, -A3, -A4, -A5, -A7 and -A8.   Soon thereafter, HL-A9, -A10, -A11, -A12, and -A13 were added and a number of less well-defined specificities were given W designations: W5, -10, -14, -15, etc.; whereas yet other specificities remained associated with private symbols, Te60, Da23, etc. (Table I).

Concomitant with the recognition of new specificities was the realization that some of the originally described HL-A antigens were complex.   For example, Walford (32) and later Dausset (33), Amos and Yunis (34), and others recognized that HL-A9 was not one antigen but consisted of at least two components.   The same appeared to be true of HL-A1, -A2, -A3, -A4, -A7, -A10, and -A12.   Some of these antigens appeared to be divisible into not just two but into many specificities.   If these specificities of restricted frequency were being described for the first time, they would undoubtedly have been given distinctive HL-A designations.   Because the broad specificities were described first, the real differences between the subcomponent restricted specificities tended to be overlooked.

The crossreactivity between the subspecificities W23 and W24, W25 and W26, etc., appears to be essentially similar to that observed between HL-A1 and -A11, HL-A3 and -A11, HL-A10 and -A11, HL-A5 and W5, and W5 and W18, HL-A2 and HL-A9, and HL-A2 and W28, all of which appear to be very pronounced. Crossreactivity is here based solely upon the basis of serologic crossreactivity direct as in cytotoxicity testing or indirect as in absorption or elution (35,36).   Most anti HL-A11 sera tend to react with cells from at least some HL-A1 or HL-A10 donors; a serum containing anti-W28 can be absorbed with HL-A2 cells to remove anti-W28, whereas a serum containing anti HL-A2 is not readily absorbed by W28 cells, and so on.   To what extent crossreactivity reflects shared amino acid sequences and to what extent an

120

affinity similarity, not based on sequence, is quite unknown. However, the existence of crossreactivity and of many apparent subspecificities is at present obscuring the interpretation of HL-A serology. When donor and recipient are both said to be, for instance, 1-8/2-12 and stimulate in mixed culture, the immediate question is raised, "Which 1, which 12, which 2, or which 8?" There is no easy answer and one can only say, "They appear to be identical with respect to their reactivity with a large battery of sera and their absorptive capacity." In some instances we can add, "and also in their inability to induce an antibody in each other," but none of these descriptions is completely adequate. Only where there is clear genotypic inheritance within a family do we know that the haplotypes are identical and then (with only very rare exceptions) there is no stimulation in MLR.

II.   The Performance of the MLR.

Theoretically, the MLR is an extremely simple test. In practice it is an exceedingly complex reaction. Cells from the same two subjects reacting under apparently identical culture conditions on different occasions provide widely divergent estimates of the degree of stimulation. Cells separated on Ficoll gradient stimulate less strongly than do cells separated on nylon or by gravity (Table II). Others found conflicting results (37). If the cell suspension used includes an excess of granulocytes, the reaction is inhibited; but it also is if there are too few macrophages (38). The identity of the plasma used, the time and temperature between collection of the blood and the setting up of the cultures, the time of incubation before cell mixing, and the equilibrium between the individual and his microbial flora all may have a great influence on the degree of stimulation and hence upon the stimulation index (26).

III. Lymphocyte Stimulation

Lymphocyte stimulation owes nothing to the serologically potent antigens of the first segregant

series. Many studies have now confirmed the earlier
report of Yunis et al. (28,39-43) that stimulation
is associated with incompatibility at the 4 series
and not at the LA series, the 4 apparently corresponding to the K end of H-2 and the LA series to the
D end specificities of the mouse. In other families
we have shown that the locus responsible for MLC
stimulation segregates independently of the loci
controlling HL-A. Therefore, the significance of
HL-A and of the MLR stimulation locus in transplantation is not properly defined (26,28).

From a consideration of MLR, haplotype inheritance, and graft survival times in man and mouse,
Yunis and Amos conclude that HL-A and MLR loci alone
were probably inadequate to explain many facts of
graft survival. They therefore postulate the existence of a fourth locus in the histocompatibility
complex that controls the production of a product
that can elicit delayed hypersensitivity responses
(HDR) but that is either silent or only occasionally
detectable by serological reagents. It is convenient
to refer to the whole histocompatibility complex as
HL-1. It is known that HL-A and MLR-S are highly
polymorphic loci because of the serologic complexity
of HL-A and because of the frequency with which MLR
stimulation is observed in related or unrelated
subjects who are not HL-A identical. The original
estimate by Bach and Amos(8) was of a single locus
with 15 or more alleles; nothing since has been
published to suggest that 15 was an underestimate and
MLR-S would appear to qualify as a very polymorphic
system. However, nothing is known about the degree
of polymorphism of HDR. There is indirect evidence,
as, for example, from a consideration of the trans-
plantability of HL-A mismatched kidneys, to suggest
that HDR is not a highly polymorphic locus and very
indirect evidence to suggest that there are two
separate HDR loci. If this duality of HDR is true,
then the degree of polymorphism of each must be
extremely restricted.

The reasoning that suggests that there are two

HDR loci is as follows. In the mouse, graft rejection has been studied in combinations that include a recombinant between the D and K regions. Incompatibility for the K end is associated with both MLR stimulation and graft rejection. Incompatibility at the D end is associated with a very different form of MLR reactivity (44-47); D end incompatibility is also associated with skin graft rejection that in some combinations is moderately rapid. If graft rejection is really an attribute of a delayed type reaction and H-2 (or HL-A) determines a product that is primarily responsible for immediate hypersensitivity, then there ought logically to be two HDR loci, one at the D end and one at the K. The Shreffler-Klein model for H-2 explains this very easily (48). The primordial H locus is thought to be a single genetic region, closely linked to the SsSlp gene. Reduplication of the H gene is accompanied by inversion, trapping SsSlp between the two H-2 genes. Now, if the HDR locus were adjacent to H-2 and the MLR locus were more remote, the inversion could have separated HDR from MLR; alternatively during reduplication an HDR gene remains associated with the second H-2 gene. It is emphasized that these hypotheses are still extremely tenuous, but they appear to be consistent with many observations in mouse and in man.

In skin graft exchanges between unrelated human subjects, the median survival time is approximately 11 days and the range is generally 6-15 days. However, occasional grafts persist for longer than 15 days and some may persist for over 21 days (3,22, 49). These long surviving grafts, which account for approximately 5% of all grafts, approach the survival times of grafts exchanged between HL-A identical siblings. Some of the donor-recipient pairs are phenotypically HL-A identical, whereas others are clearly different. If graft survival is determined by HDR rather than by HL-A, the observed long survivals can be explained by one HDR locus with six alleles or two HDR loci with only three allelic

forms. In agreement with the long survival of a proportion of skin grafts between unrelated pairs, certain kidneys from unrelated donors have been found to
function well and to give no evidence of rejection,
despite minimal or inadequate immunosuppression.

One classic example was reported in the first
series of Hume et al. (50), in which a kindey from a
Bostonian functioned well in a Peruvian recipient who
received only low doses of steroids as an antiinflam-
matory drug. The distinction between well-accepted
and poorly accepted cadaveric kidneys was most apparent in the earlier transplant series. The exact proportion of kidneys accepted as if they were from HL-A
identical donors was approximately 10% (13). This
would also be more in accord with a relatively simple
HDR locus or loci than with the highly polymorphic
HL-A system.

Additional support for the HDR hypothesis came
from observations with three mutations at H-2. The
first of these was observed by Dr. Carl Cohen during
an experiment in which C57BLxDBA/aF$_1$ hybrid mice were
being challenged with the DBA/a lymphoma L1210. Of
the many hundred mice tested, three F$_1$ hybrids rejected the tumor. Two of these were infertile and were
not further examined. The third gave progeny that
were serologically indistinguishable from the H-2^d of
DBA/2 but that were resistant to L1210 (51). The
second example was reported by Egorov, who found a
mutant indistinguishable from H-2^d (52), except for
possible weak reactivity with H-2.10. Because this
specificity was not fully established and probably
should be withdrawn from the H-2 table, this also
appeared to have been a serologically silent mutant.
The third example was found by Bailey as one mutant
of several thousands tested that gave rapid rejection
of C57BL skin. This mutation was associated with
H-2^b but despite intensive efforts by Snell and
Cherry it was found to be impossible to detect any
antigenic deviation from H-2^b by serological methods.
All three mutants were capable of responding strongly
to tumor or tissue transplants. These mutations

would appear to be at the HDR rather than at the H-2
locus.

The hypotheses that can be advanced to account
for the discrepancy between in vitro tests and graft
behavior seem to be (1) that HL-A as originally
described is the major H antigenic system in man. In
support are reports of improved kidney graft survival in subjects phenotypically HL-A identical.
Against support are the high frequency of MLR stimulation between phenotypically identical pairs; poor
correlation of HL-A type with skin graft survival;
and no apparent difference between kidney graft
survival, whether the pairs are mismatched at one,
two, or three antigens. (2) The HL-A locus is more
complex than has been previously recognized (a)
because there are more than two segregant series of
antigens or (b) because many of the specificities
have been inadequately defined. It is difficult to
obtain clear documentation of (a). Several investigators, including Walford, Terasaki, and Kissmeyer-
Nielsen (53-55), have attempted to document a third
series based on serological reactions but have not
been able to demonstrate such a locus convincingly.
This may justify an intensive study of sera that fail
to give concordant results in family typing. Such
antigens as JN-AJ or Ao54 appear to be candidates for
such a series. Inadequate definition of the HL-A
specificities is being acknowledged. Reference has
already been made to HL-A9, which is a composite of
at least two crossreactive specificities. HL-A10
appears to consist of at least two and possibly as
many as four crossreactive components, based on the
reactions of such sera as those that react with
HL-A11 cells and also with some HL-A10 cells. The
complexity of HL-A12 is readily recognized; many
HL-A12 sera are available that react with only a proportion of HL-A12 cells, and so with many other specificities. These subdivisions become especially
apparent when cells from donors of different populations are tested.

(3) The interpretation of HL-A specificities is

125

incorrect. The whole of the elaborate HL-A super-
structure is founded on cytotoxicity testing. By
agglutination of antiglobulin tests, many additional
reactivities become apparent. Possibly, some of the
antigens now regarded as distinct but crossreacting
are not distinct; therefore, instead of 40 or more
antigens there may be only five or six actual antigens and matching should be based upon these rather
than on the apparent individual specificities that
may reflect minor surface modifications.

(4) The HL-A region includes a series of
different genes. These include genes coding for
HL-A, MLR-S, and HDR (the chromosomal region we have
called HL-1) (31). The different attributes may also
be carried by the same molecular complex if some of
the properties of the molecule are determined by side
chains. The core molecule, recognized by the antigenic marker LYO, may be the carrier for side chains,
which can be peptide, oligosaccharide, or glycopep-
tide, and the HL-A or H-2 genes may then control the
production of transferases rather than the actual
antigens themselves. However, because HDR is
probably lymphocyte restricted, the immune response
to lymphocyte may, as suggested by Elkins (56),
trigger immunity to the transplant.

In summary, methods for predicting histocompatibility are only partially successful. This suggests
that the products of the major histocompatibility
complex HL-1 are being only incompletely identified.
Emphasis on the role of the response to passenger
lymphocytes in the graft and of antigenic specificities linked to HL-A and, therefore, part of HL-1,
which are normally found only on lymphoid cells,
offers a new approach to matching for transplantation
that has as yet been inadequately explored.

ACKNOWLEDGMENTS

Supported in part by PHS grants HL-06314,
AI-18399 and funds from the Department of Laboratory
Medicine, University of Minnesota.

REFERENCES

1. Simmons, R. L., Kjellstrand, C. M., and Najarian, J. In "Tissue Typing and Organ Transplantation" (E. J. Yunis and D. B. Amos, eds.), p. , Academic Press, New York, 1972.

2. Starzl, T. E., Groth, C. G., Terasaki, P. I., Putman, C. W., Brettschneider, L., and Marchion, T. L. Surg. Gynecol. Obstet. 127, 1023 (1968).

3. Amos, D. B., Hattler, B. G., MacQueen, J. M., Cohen, I., and Seigler, H. F. In "Advances in Transplantation" (J. Dausset, J. Hamburger, and G. Mathé, eds.), p. 203, Williams and Wilkins, Baltimore, Maryland, 1967.

4. Stickel, D. L., Seigler, H. F., Amos, D. B., Ward, F. E., Gunnels, J. C., Price, A. R., and Anderson, E. E. Ann. Surg. 172, 160 (1970).

5. Dausset, J., Rapaport, F. T., Legrand, L., Colombani, J., and Marcelli, B. A. In "Histocompatibility Testing 1970" (P. I. Terasaki, ed.), p. 381, Munksgaard, Copenhagen, 1970.

6. Ceppellini, R. In "Human Transplantation" (F. T. Rapaport, and J. Dausset, eds.), p. 21, Grune and Stratton, New York, 1968.

7. Morris, P. J., Ting, A., and Kincaid-Smith, P. In "Histocompatibility Testing 1970" (P. I. Terasaki, ed.), p. 37, Munksgaard, Copenhagen, 1970.

8. Bach, F. H., and Amos, D. B. Science 156, 1506 (1967).

9. Albertini, R. J., and Bach, F. H. J. Exp. Med. 129, 639 (1968).

10. Jeannet, M. Helv. Med. Acta 35, 168 (1970).

11. Amos, D. B., and Stickel, D. L. Advan. Intern. Med. 14, 15 (1968).

12. Amos, D. B. Transplantation 5, 1015 (1967).
13. Terasaki, P. I., Vredevoe, D. L., and Mickey, M. R. Transplantation 5, 1057 (1967).
14. Mickey, M. R., Kreisler, M., Albert, E. D., Tanaka, N., and Terasaki, P. I. Tissue Antigens 1, 57 (1971).
15. Rapaport, R. T., and Dausset, J. Science 167, 1260 (1970).
16. van Rood, J. J. In "Progress in Immunology" (D. B. Amos, ed.), p. 1028, Academic Press, New York, 1972.
17. Dausset, J., and Hors, J. Nature (London) 238, 150 (1972).
18. Amos, D. B., Hattler, B. G., MacQueen, J. M., Cohen, I., and Seigler, H. F. In "Advances in Transplantation" J. Dausset, J. Hamburger, and G. Mathé, eds.), p. 203, Williams and Wilkins, Baltimore, Maryland, 1967.
19. van Rood, J. J., van Leeuwen, A., Schippers, A. M. V., Ceppellini, R., Mattiuz, P. L., and Curtoni, E. S. Ann. N. Y. Acad. Sci. 129, 467 (1966).
20. Dausset, J., Rapaport, F. T., Ivanyi, P., and Colombani, J. In "Histocompatibility Testing 1965" (D. B. Amos and J. J. van Rood, eds.), p. 63, Munksgaard, Copenhagen, 1965.
21. Dausset, J., Rapaport, F., Legrand, L., Colombani, J., and Marcelli-Barge, A. In "Histocompatibility Testing 1970" (D. B. Amos and J. J. van Rood, eds.), p. 63, Munksgaard, Copenhagen, 1970.
22. Ward, F. E., Seigler, F.H., Southworth, J. G., Andrus, C. H., and Amos, D. B. In "Histocompatibility Testing 1970" (P. I. Terasaki, ed.), p. 399, Munksgaard, Copenhagen, 1970.
23. Sorensen, S. F., and Nielsen, L. S. Acta Pathol. Microbiol. Scand. 78B, 719 (1970).
24. Schellekens, P. T. A., and Eijsvoogel, V. P. Clin. Exp. Immunol. 7, 229 (1970).

25. Bach, F. H., Day, E., Bach, M. L., Myhre, B. A., Sengar, D. P. S., and Terasaki, P. I. Tissue Antigens 1, 39 (1971).
26. Sorensen, S. F. "The Mixed Lymphocyte Culture Interaction. Techniques and Immunogenetics." Vald Pedersens Bogtrykkeri A-S, Copenhagen, 1972.
27. Eijsvoogel, V. P., Schellekens, P. R. A., Breur-Briesendorp, B., Koning, L., Koch, C., van Leeuwen, A., and van Rood, J. J. Transplant. Proc. 3, 85 (1971).
28. Yunis, E. J., and Amos, D. B. Proc. Nat. Acad. Sci. (U.S.) 68, 3031 (1971).
29. Koch, C. T., Frederiks, E., Eijsvoogel, V. P., and van Rood, J. J. Lancet 2, 1334 (1971).
30. Seigler, H. F., Ward, F. E., Amos, D. B., and Stickel, D. L. J. Exp. Med. 133, 411 (1971).
31. Amos, D. B., Seigler, H., Simmons, R. L., and Yunis, E. J. Transplantation (1972), (in press).
32. Walford, R. L., Wallace, O., Shambrom, E., and Troup, G. M. Vox. Sang. 15, 338 (1968).
33. Dausset, J. Transplant. Proc. 3, 8 (1971).
34. Amos, D. B., and Yunis, E. J. Unpublished studies.
35. Dorf, M. E., Eguro, S. Y., and Amos, D. B. Transplantation 14, 474 (1972).
36. Yunis, E. J., Dorf, M., and Amos, D. B. Transplantation (1972) (in press).
37. Bain, B., and Pshyk, K. Transplant. Proc. 4, 163 (1972).
38. Bach, M. L., Bach, F. H., Widmer, M., Oranem, H., and Wolberg, W. H. Transplantation 12, 283 (1971).
39. Yunis, E. J., Plate, J. M., Ward, F. E., Seigler, H. F., and Amos, D. B. Transplant. Proc. 3, 118 (1971).
40. Dupont, B., Staub-Nielsen, L., and Svejgaard, A. Lancet 2, 1336 (1971).

41. Plate, J. M., Ward, F. E., and Amos, D. B.
In "Histocompatibility Testing 1970"
(P. I. Terasaki, ed.), p. 531, Munksgaard,
Copenhagen, 1970.
42. Sasportes, M., Lebrun, A., Rapaport, F. T.,
and Dausset, J. Transplant. Proc. 4, 209
(1972).
43. Eijsvoogel, V. P., Koning, L., de Groot-Koog,
L., Huismans, L., van Rood, J. J., van Leeuwen,
A., and du Toit, E. D. Transplant. Proc. 4,
199 (1972).
44. Klein, J. Folia Biol.(Praha) 12, 168 (1966).
45. Dimant, P., and Nonza, K. Folia Biol. (Praha)
17, 410 (1971).
46. Rychlikova, M., Dimant, P., and Ivanyi, P.
Nature (New Biol.), 230, 271 (1971).
47. Plate, J. (personal communication).
48. Shreffler, C. S., David, H. C., Passmore, H. C.,
and Klein, J. Transplant. Proc. 3, 176 (1971).
49. Rapaport, F. T., Lawrence, H. S., Thomas, L.,
Converse, J. M., Tillett, W. S., and Mulholland,
J. H. Ann. N. Y. Acad. Sci. 99, 564 (1962).
50. Hume, D. M., Merrill, J. P., Miller, B. F.,
and Thorn, G. W. J. Clin. Invest. 34, 327
(1955).
51. Cohen, C., and Amos, D. B. (unpublished
observations).
52. Egorov, I. K. Folia Biol. (Praha) 13, 169
(1967).
53. Walford, R. L., Filkelstein, S., Hanna, C., and
Collins, Z. Nature (London) 224, 74 (1969).
54. Sengar, D. P. S., Mickey, M. R., Myhre, B. A.,
Chen, H. H., and Terasaki, P. I. Transfusion
11, 251 (1971).
55. Kissmeyer-Nielsen, F., Svejgaard, A., and
Thorsby, E. Transplant. Proc. 3, 81 (1971).
56. Elkins, W. L. Transplantation 11, 555 (1971).

ACKNOWLEDGMENT

We wish to acknowledge the secretarial assistance
of Nancy Swanson and Margery Knutson.

TABLE Ia

Nomenclature of Antigens of HL-A System (1972)

First HL-A Locus (LA Locus)

Official Name	1970 Workshop No.	Other Designations	1972 Workshop No.
HL-A 1		Ao 19, LA$_1$, To 8, Da 11, Te 1, Lc 1	
HL-A 2		Ao 1, LA$_2$, To 9, Da 1, Te 2, Lc 2, <8a	
HL-A 3		<Ao 40, <To 10, <Da 12, <Te 8, Lc 3, <LA$_3$	
HL-A 9		LA 4, To 12, Da 16, Te 4, Lc 11	
	9.1	9' (Da 27), Lc 12	W23
	9.2	9" (Da 32) BIM	W24
HL-A 10		To 13, Da 17, KN, Te 12	
	10.1	To 31, 10" (Da 29)	W25
	10.2	To 40, 10' (Da 28)	W26
HL-A 11		To 26, Da 21, ILN*, Te 13	
	W19	Li, Thompson	
	19.1	Ao 77, Da 22, Te 63	W29
	19.2	Da 25	
	19.3	Da 25' (Da 26), Lc 21	W30
	19.4	Law, Da 25" (Da 33), Lc 26.1, Te 66	W31
	19.5	Ao 28, To 30	W32
	19.6		
	W28	Da 15, Ba*, Te 28 or 40, Lc 17, <8a	

Supertypic Specificities
HL-A 2 + W28 = 8a
HL-A 3 + 11 = LA$_3$, Da 12, ILN
HL-A 3 + 11 + <1 = Ao 14

TABLE Ib

Second HL-A Locus (4 locus)

Official Name	1970 Work- shop No.	Other Designations	1972 Work- Shop No.
HL-A 5		Ao 12, ‹4c, To 5, Da 5, Te 11	
HL-A 7		Ao 2, ‹7c, Lc 8	
HL-A 8		Ao 56, To 7, Da 8, 7a, Lc 7	
HL-A 12		Ao 12, To 11, Da 4, T12, Te 9, Merrit A	
HL-A 13		To 21, HN, Te 26	
	W5	Ao 13, ‹4c, To 25, Da 20, R*, Te 5 or 50	
	W10	To 23, BB, Te 10 or Te 60	
	W14	To 27, Da 18, Maki, Te 14 or 54	
	W15	Da 23, LND, Te 15 or 55, ‹4c	
		U18, Sa 583, Te 64	W16
	W17	Ao 70, SL-MaPi, MaPi, Orlina, Te 57	
	W18	‹4c, CM*+CM-SL, Te 18 or Te58	
		AJ	
		Da 24, ET, Te 61	W20
	W22	To 28, AA, ‹7c	W21
	W22.1	AA*, Te 22 or Te 51	
	W22.2	AA-AJ	
	W27	To 29, FJH, Te 27 or Te 52	
	subdiv.	FJH-AJ	
	subdiv.	FJH*	

Supertypic Specificities:

4a = HL-A 12 + 13 + HL-A 5 + SL* + W17 + W27
4b = HL-A 7 + HL-A 8 + W5 + W18 + W15 + W10 + W22 + W14
6a = 7b + 7a + W10 + W22
6b = 7c + W10
7c = HL-A 7 + W22 + W27
7b = HL-A 12 + HL-A 13 + HL-A 5 + W5 + W18 + SL* + W17

TABLE II

Depressed Reactivity in Mixed-Leukocyte Cultures after
Separation of Mononuclear Cells on Ficoll-Hypaque[1]

| HL-A type of cells | Lymphocyte separation of stimulating cells | | | | | |
| | Am | | Bm | | Cm | |
	F[2]	S[3]	F	S	F	S
HN (A) HL-A1,2,8,12	75	156	546	1487	329	1680
HK (B) HL-A1,2,8,12	663	5104	148	209	3000	9912
MS (C) HL-A1,2,8,W10	1291	1697	3758	5260	128	150

[1] Cell mixtures consist of 5×10^5 responding and 5×10^5 mitomycin-treated lymphocytes. Cultures terminated after 3 days.

[2] Mixed cultures performed following the method of D. D. Hartzman et al. Transplantation 11: 260 (1971). Ficoll-Hypaque (F) lymphocytes separated by the method of E. Thorsby: In "Histocompatibility Testing 1970" (P.I. Terasaki, ed.), p. 655, Munksgaard, Copenhagen, 1970.

[3] Sedimented cells prepared by incubation of blood at 37°C for 30 min.

DIALYSIS TODAY: ITS ROLE AND APPLICATION

Fred L. Shapiro
Medical Director, Community Dialysis Center
Associate Professor of Medicine

Hennepin County General Hospital
Portland Ave. and So. 5th St.
Minneapolis, Minnesota 55415

University of Minnesota
Minneapolis, Minnesota 55455

The improved success of renal transplantation in the treatment of patients with end-stage renal disease has significantly influenced the role of chronic hemodialysis programs. Some investigators have suggested that dialysis should be used simply as a stepping stone to renal transplantation. As more experience with dialysis has been acquired, the role of dialysis has expanded to fulfill many other functions. This paper will discuss our current concepts of the role of chronic dialysis and some of the basic philosophy we use in its application (1).

One of the most important roles of dialysis is to maintain patients with end-stage renal disease until transplantation can be accomplished. These patients require dialysis in preparation for major surgical procedures and occasionally after transplantation if acute renal insufficiency develops. Dialysis may also be required in the late transplant period should chronic rejection develop. Transplantation and dialysis programs should be integrated so that when patients reject transplants they can be maintained by dialysis. This integrated approach is particularly important in transplantation programs that rely heavily on cadaveric donors. A much higher proportion of cadaveric transplants, as compared to live related donor transplants, fail because of chronic rejection.

A second very important function of chronic dialysis is as definitive therapy for patients unsuitable for transplantation. This group of patients includes several categories such as: (a) Patients with preformed antibodies. These patients have a higher incidence of acute rejection reactions and a decreased rate of graft survival. Unfortunately, the number of patients in this group is continuing to grow because of sensitization due to blood administration, kidney transplantation, and pregnancy. It is hoped that the rate of growth of the size of this group will be lessened with the decreased use of blood transfusions and the use of frozen blood when transfusion is indicated. (b) Patients with neoplastic disease are currently considered poor candidates for transplantation because of the potential carcinogenic effect of the immunosuppressive agents. Many of these patients can achieve successful rehabilitation and a productive life if chronic dialysis is provided for them. We currently are treating patients who have or have had multiple myeloma, hypernephroma, and alveolar ridge carcinoma. (c) Patients who tolerate immunosuppressive therapy poorly and develop such problems as significant leukopenia or thrombocytopenia, recurrent infections, hepatic dysfunctions, or multiple complications of steroid therapy can usually be maintained on chronic dialysis. (d) Another group of patients who do poorly on transplantation are those patients who are physiologically old, particularly patients over the age of 50. We recently compared results achieved in 29 patients over the age of 50 at the time dialysis was instituted with the results in 93 patients who were under 50 at the time dialysis was begun. In every parameter studied, the older group did as well as the younger group. The factors compared included

mortality, cannula survival, blood utilization, in-
patient complication time, and rehabilitation
results. It is our opinion that the patients over
50 years old adjust emotionally to hemodialysis
extremely well. (e) Another category of patients
requiring definitive dialysis is that group in which
the primary disease is likely to recur in a transplanted kidney or may significantly affect their
tolerance of immunosuppressive agents. Diseases in
this category include rapidly progressive glomerulonephritis, some types of systemic lupus erythematosus, diseases associated with antiglomerular basement membrane antibodies, amyloidosis, and diabetes.
Although initial results with cadaveric transplantation in diabetics were somewhat encouraging, most
of these kidneys ultimately failed. Very few transplant centers will now consider cadaveric transplantation for diabetics. We have had experience in
treating over 20 diabetics with chronic dialysis and
some significant palliation can be accomplished.
The results compared to nondiabetic patients, however, are somewhat disappointing, with much higher
mortality rates, poor rehabilitation, and more complications necessitating in-patient hospital care.
(f) There are some patients who just prefer not to
have a transplant. Some of these patients are
reluctant to undergo the major surgery while others
may refuse transplantation on religious grounds,
such as two patients whom we are treating with dialysis who are Jehovah's Witnesses. We feel that the
patient should be provided with the statistics for
the various forms of therapy and that wherever possible he should participate in the decision about
which form of therapy he will receive at a given time
time. There are numerous factors that enter into
this decision, such as family status, finances, complicating medical problems, occupation, residency,
home status.

The third fundamental role for chronic dialysis
programs is as a component of a comprehensive nephrology training program. The dialysis program serves

as a stimulus for referral of patients with chronic
renal failure. The majority of these patients can
be managed initially by conservative techniques,
including diet, fluid and electrolyte control, and
appropriate medications. During this interval, the
patients serve as vivid examples of disturbed renal
pathophysiology and illustrate how these factors can
be controlled by the application of appropriate conservative measures. There is ample opportunity to
train the house staff in the techiques of peritoneal
dialysis and hemodialysis. Another important benefit derived from integrating chronic dialysis into
nephrology programs is that there is an experienced
team of physicians and nurses available to treat
patients with acute renal failure; this increases
the survival rate and lessens the cost of therapy.
The successful treatment of patients with acute renal
failure is probably the most rewarding aspect of the
dialysis programs. Chronic dialysis patients are
prone to develop unusual complications that frequently are multiple and require the application of
sophisticated internal medical principles. Such
patients provide stimulating and challenging learning
experiences to both trainees and staff.

A fourth major role for dialysis programs is
stimulating both clinical and basic research, particularly in the fields of uremia and its complications, in the technique of dialysis, and in the
regional approach to health care delivery. The latter has been of particular interest to us and over
the past 6 years we have developed a comprehensive
regional program for the treatment of patients with
chronic renal failure. The program utilizes conservative medical management for as long as is reasonable, at which time chronic dialysis or kidney transplantation is made available. Our chronic dialysis
program is unique in that dialysis treatments are
performed in several different locations, including
the parent center at Hennepin County General Hospital, the patient's own home, small satellite units
in private hospitals throughout the region, and in

the 20-bed limited-care type of facility in Minneapolis. These several methods of providing dialysis
are integrated with each other and also serve as
maintenance and backup facilities for the renal
transplant program. The parent facility provides
numerous services, which include the acute treatment
of patients with acute and chronic renal failure;
training of personnel; evaluation and selection of
patients; continuous surveillance of medical, rehabilitation, and financial progress; and backup treatments for all significant complications. Currently,
there are 95 patients being treated with chronic
hemodialysis in our program.

During the past several years, we have developed
certain concepts relative to providing care to
patients with end-stage renal disease. The most
important is that to only sustain life is not an
adequate accomplishment. A meaningful existence involving vocational, psychological, social, and econ-
omic rehabilitation is necessary for truly successful
therapy.

In selecting patients for our program, our only
major criterion currently is rehabilitation potential
to some form of meaningful life. Other factors, such
as age, medical status, and finances, are considered
but these influence what kind of therapy will be
provided not whether the patient will receive treatment.

We initiate dialysis when the patient can no
longer continue in his normal vocational activities.
A trial of conservative management usually is effective initially, particularly in patients with
creatinine clearances of over 4 ml/min and urine
volumes exceeding 200 ml/day. If the patient
develops decreased nerve conduction velocity, uremic
symptoms, pericarditis, uncontrolled hypertension or
fluid retention, congestive heart failure, bleeding
disorders, mental aberrations, or excessive weakness,
dialysis therapy is begun. It is very important that
the patients be followed closely in out-patient
clinics during the time they are receiving conserva-

tive therapy to insure that dialysis is begun prior to the development of major complications, many of which may be difficult to control or correct.

Dialysis performed outside the patient's home should retain some of the rehabilitation aspects that the home patient enjoys. The patient should not have to travel excessive distances to receive dialysis, as this would directly affect his rehabilitation. Dialysis should be provided at a time when the patient loses as little of his active living time as is possible. This usually means providing treatment during the evening or night. We are not satisfied with 2 or 3 days a week rehabilitation, and therefore, all of the satellite units and the limited care unit provide dialysis treatments during the evening and night. The dialysis unit should be quiet, pleasant, safe, and conducive to sleeping so that the patient is well rested and able to work regularly without interruption due to dialysis treatment or lack of sleep.

One of the most important practical aspects of maintenance dialysis is to provide enough dialysis treatment. Many of the problems and complications that were considered inherent in patients maintained with dialysis, including neuropathy, anemia, and pericarditis, are now known to be prevented or controlled by providing sufficient duration of dialysis treatment and adequate nutrition. Three treatments weekly usually are required to achieve near normal strength, minimize complications, and allow maximal rehabilitation and physical activities. Another technological advance that has improved the quality of patients' lives has been the use of arteriovenous fistulas instead of external cannulas for access to the bloodstream. Prior to the time we began using fistulas, approximately 50% of the complications requiring in-patient care resulted from cannula-related problems. A successful arteriovenous fistula effectively reduces this problem.

SUMMARY

There are several forms of treatment for patients with chronic renal failure. Transplantation is preferred for the younger patients with primary renal disease. Chronic maintenance dialysis is also an effective treatment when administered properly. Dialysis and transplantation programs should be closely affiliated to provide continuous comprehensive care to patients with end-stage renal disease.

The role of dialysis programs includes providing care for patients awaiting transplantation, as well as for those who are unsuitable for transplantation. Dialysis has become an integral part of nephrology training and research programs. The effective application of rehabilitation-oriented dialysis treatment can result in a meaningful existence for many patients with end-stage renal disease.

REFERENCES

1. Shapiro, F.L. Comprehensive regional approach to the chronic renal failure problem. Perspect. Biol. Med. 13, No. 4, 597 (1970).

RENAL TRANSPLANTATION VERSUS CHRONIC DIALYSIS: INDICATIONS AND CONTRAINDICATIONS

C. M. Kjellstrand

Department of Medicine
University of Minnesota
Minneapolis, Minnesota

Both renal transplantation and chronic dialysis are accepted methods of treating end-stage renal failure. While there is common agreement that the patient with a well-functioning renal transplant is better off than a chronic dialysis patient, opinions differ and quidelines are lacking as to which patient would benefit most from transplantation and which would benefit most from dialysis. We have attempted to answer this question by comparing our transplantation results with the results of experienced dialysis groups.

In order to get more meaningful data, the transplant patient material was divided up into several different subgroups. The first division separates patients with transplants done before and after December 31, 1967. The material was also bisected into those patients who received related kidneys and those who received unrelated kidneys. It was further subdivided into ideal candidates, i.e., patients between 15 and 45 years of age without systemic disease and with a normal urinary tract, and high-risk patients. The latter group included four subgroups in order to isolate certain risk factors: (a) patients below age 15, (b) patients above age 45, (c) patients with diabetes and (d) patients with other problems which are thought to increase the risk of transplantation (other systemic disease, outflow problems, etc.). For each of these different groups

143

comparable dialysis-patient materials were available
with the exception of the subgroup "patients with
other problems."

Table 1 is a summary of the patient material
(121 patients) from 1968 through 1970. There were
83 patients transplanted during 1963-1967: 43
received related transplants, 18 or 42% died; 40
received unrelated kidneys, 75% are dead. The observation period ended June, 1971, and no patient had
been observed for less than 6 months. All patients
transplanted between 1963 and 1967 had been observed
for at least 3½ years. Actuarial survival curves (4)
were then constructed for all groups and compared to
similar curves for patients on chronic dialysis.

Figure 1 shows the survival curves for two
groups of patients transplanted during 1963-1967 and
1968-1970, those who received (a) cadaver or (b)
related kidneys. These curves are compared to the
results of chronic dialysis in Seattle (5). It is
obvious that the results of both cadaver and related
transplantation have improved considerably between
the two periods of time. A similar improvement does
not seem to have taken place in dialysis. Ginn (2a)
noted no difference in survival of patients started
on chronic hemodialysis before or after December 31,
1966. It thus seems reasonable to focus on our
recent results (1968-1970) of transplantation and
compare them to those of dialysis even if the time
periods are not exactly the same. From Fig. 1 it
would seem as if transplantation from a related donor
is the method of choice and that chronic dialysis and
cadaver transplantation now have approximately equal
4 year success. However, if the transplantation
material is divided into ideal candidates and high
risk patients, a different picture emerges (Fig. 2).
From this curve it would seem that transplantation of
kidneys from related persons to either an ideal can-
didate or to a high risk patient and transplantation
of kidneys to ideal candidates are the methods of
choice whereas transplantation of cadaver kidneys
to high risk patients obviously has a much worse

mortality than chronic hemodialysis.

Figures 3 through 6 compare the results of transplantation (1968–1970) to that of dialysis for the subgroup material of high risk patients (except for the group "patients with other problems"). In all groups, transplantation of a kidney from a relative is the method of choice although the difference in mortality is very small from that of chronic dialysis for children below age 15. The results of cadaver transplantation are much worse both for the older and the younger patient. Cadaver transplants to diabetic patients were too few to allow any comparison.

The results of cadaver transplantation to older patients are very dismal with only a 30% 2 year survival. If the number of patients in this group (transplantation with a cadaver to patients older than 45) is subtracted from the results of cadaver transplantation to the high risk patient, Fig. 2, even the results of cadaver transplantation to the high risk patient equal that of dialysis. An obvious criticism that could be leveled against this comparison is that in Fig. 2 the results of dialysis have not been divided up into high risk or ideal candidates; however, no truly high risk group of patients in dialysis has been defined. Both Cohen et al. (1) and Lewis et al. (3) could not find any significant difference in mortality in patients above or below age 50 or above or below age 45 treated with chronic hemodialysis. The Seattle group (5), however, has described a markedly increased mortality in patients above age 56 on chronic hemodialysis.

The patients with other problems are listed in Table 2. Three of these patients died. In one case, P. B., the basic problem, polyarteritis nodosa, was directly responsible for the patient's death with cerebral hemorrhage. In the second case, J. M., gastroduodenal ulcer contributed significantly to death as there was a marked weight loss and inability to maintain good nutrition leading to the episode of infection with pulmonary abscesses that caused the

145

patient's death. In the third case, A. M., with
lupus erythematosus, the basic disease did not contribute to the patient's death of rejection-infec-
tion. In 13 patients there were multiple high risk
factors involved. These patients are listed in
Table 3. In nine of these, old age was one factor,
and in four, young age was one factor. In the previous survival curves these patients have been
included in their age group and not in the curve for
other problems. Of the seven deaths, six occurred in
patients over 45 years. In four, C. P. (gastroduodenal ulcer), Y. H. (pulmonary fibrosis), R. K.
(diverticulosis), and L. S. (bronchiectasis), the
basic problem was directly related to the cause of
death. In one, R. Re., gastroduodenal ulcer contributed to death. In case M. Mc. (diabetes) and
R. R. (Wilms tumor) there was no direct connection
between the other problem and the patient's death.

If the materials listed in Table 2 and Table 3
are analyzed together (Table 4), some problems
deserve particular attention. None of the three
patients with previous heart disease had cardiac
problems during or following transplantation. Of six
patients with previous gastroduodenal ulcers, three
are dead and both patients with previous gross lung
pathology are dead. On the other hand, none of five
patients with previous urinary tract disease have
died after transplantation. One patient of two with
lupus erythematosus is dead, but no problem with the
basic disease was encountered during or after transplantation in either case. Of the remaining seven
patients, four are dead. In two (one diverticulosis
and one polyarteritis) the basic problem was directly
related to the patient's death.

Table 5 summarizes all 21 deaths that occurred
in patients transplanted between 1968 and 1970.
Seven of the 21 deaths (33%) occurred in the group of
12 patients over age 45 who received a cadaver kidney
(only 10% of the total material). In five of the
deaths, L. S., Y. H., P. B., R. K., and C. P., there
was a basic other problem that was directly related

to the patient's demise. In two cases, R. Re. and J. M., another problem contributed significantly to the patient's death. In two (A. K., R. R.), a technical problem was the cause of death. In six (A. M., M. B., C. J., W. R., E. B., D. R.), infection caused death. Two (L. K., L. P.) died after a long period of dialysis and in three (M. Mc., W. A., S. B.) rejection per se caused the patient's demise. D. C. died of dissecting aortic aneurysm.

It is evident that the above interpretations must be viewed with caution. Despite the fact that the group of transplanted patients is very large, 204 patients, subgrouping reduces the size of some groups significantly. On the other hand, we feel this subgrouping is very necessary when trying to derive indications for transplantation versus dialysis. It appears to us that transplantation from a related donor is the treatment of choice for any patient with end-stage renal failure. Interpretation of the results for cadaver transplantation versus chronic dialysis are more difficult: The success rate here is approximately equal with the exception of the patient over age 45 for whom chronic dialysis would appear to be the method of choice. In addition, our results suggest that at this time old age combined with other disease processes besides renal failure must be regarded as a contraindication for cadaver transplantation since no less than five of six such patients have died after transplantation.

REFERENCES

1. Cohen, S.L., Comty, C.M., and Shapiro, F.L. The effect of age on the results of regular hemodialysis treatment. Proc. Eur. Dialysis Transplant Asso. 7, 254-260 (1970).
2. Drukker, W., Haagsma-Schouten, W.A.G., Alberts, C., and Spoek, M.G. Report on regular dialysis treatment in Europe. Proc. Eur. Dialysis Transplant Asso. 7, 3 (1970).
2a. Ginn, H.E. Dialysis, U.S.A. - 1969. Amer. Soc.

2b. Kjellstrand, C. M., Simmons, R. L., Bouselmeier, T. J., and Najarian, J. S. Recipient selection and medical management of renal transplant patients. In "Transplantation" (J.S. Najarian and R.L. Simmons, eds.), p. 418.

3. Lewis, E.J., Foster, D.M., De La Puente, J., and Scurlock, C. Survival data for patients undergoing chronic intermittent hemodialysis. Ann. Intern. Med. 70, 311-315 (1969).

4. Merrell, M., and Shulman, L.E. Determination of prognosis in chronic disease illustrated by systemic lupus erythematosus. J. Chronic Dis. 1, 12-32 (1955).

5. Pendras, J.P., and Pollard, T.L. Eight years' experience.with a community dialysis center: The Northwest Kidney Center. Trans. Amer. Soc. Artif. Intern. Organs 16, 77-84 (1970).

6. Potter, D., Larsen, D., Leumann, E., Perin, D., Simmons, J., Piel, C.F., Holliday, M.A. Treatment of chronic uremia in childhood. II. Hemodialysis. Pediatrics 46, 678-689 (1970).

TABLE 1

Summary of Results of Renal Transplantation at the University
of Minnesota 1968-1970; Observation Time June 30, 1971

	Total	Mortality No.	Mortality %	Related	Mortality No.	Mortality %	Cadaver	Mortality No.	Mortality %
1) Age >45	22	8	36	10	1	10	12	7	58
2) Age <15	20	3	15	15	1	7	5	2	40
3) Diabetes	9	1	11	8	1	12	1	0	0
4) Other problems	12	3	25	7	1	14	5	2	40
Total high risk	63	15	24	40	4	10	23	11	48
Total ideal	58	6	10	37	1	3	21	5	24
Summary	121	21	17	77	5	6	44	16	36

TABLE 2

Other High Risk Patients

Patient	Age	Problem	Donor	Outcome
GS	32	Gastroduodenal ulcer	Brother	Alive
AV	43	Gastroduodenal ulcer	Brother	Alive
JM	23	Gastroduodenal ulcer	Father	Died (5 months)
CS	17	Ileal bladder	Brother	Alive
PS	21	Previous ileal bladder	Cadaver	Alive
RB	19	Previous ureterostomies	Cadaver	Alive
PB	20	Polyarteritis nodosa	Husband	Died (5 months)
MB	26	LED	Father	Alive
AM	30	LED	Cadaver	Died (2 months)
DG	19	Goodpasture	Sister	Alive
DK	37	Angina pectoris	Brother	Alive (dialysis)
BB	34	Previous TBC	Cadaver	Alive

Summary: of 12 patients, 3 dead: 5 unrelated, 2 dead; 7 related, 1 dead.

TABLE 3

Multiple High Risk Factors (All Reported in Other Groups)

Patient	Age	Problem	Donor	Outcome
FS	47	Gastroduodenal ulcer	Cad-cad[a]	Alive (dialysis)
CP	46	Gastroduodenal ulcer	Cadaver	Died (10 months)
RRe	70	Gastroduodenal ulcer	Cadaver	Died (5 months)
CW	10	Outlet obstruction	Father	Alive
KL	13	Ileal bladder	Mother	Alive
VO	47	Myocardial infarction	Brother	Alive
AC	59	Myocardial infarction	Brother	Alive
SP	10	Cystinosis	Mother	Alive
LS	47	Bronchiectasis (prev. TBC)	Cad-cad	Died (3 months)
YH	47	Fibrotic lung (prev. TBC)	Cadaver	Died (4 months)
MMc	48	Diabetes	Son	Died (1 month)
RR	5	Wilms tumor	Cadaver	Died (5 months)
RK	55	Diverticulosis	Cadaver	Died (8 months)

Summary: of 13 patients (9 >45 years old) 7 dead (6 >45 years old): 6 related, 1 dead; 7 cadaver, 6 dead.

151

TABLE 4

All Other Problems

Problem	Total Mortality (%)		Related Mortality (%)		Cadaver Mortality (%)	
Gastroduodenal ulcer	6	50	3	33	3	66
Outlet problem	5	0	3	0	2	0
Coronary disease	3	0	3	0	–	–
Lung disease	2	100	–	–	2	100
"Hypersensitivity" disease	4	50	2	0	2	100
Other	5	60	2	50	3	66
Summary	25	40	13	15	12	67
All other high risk	38	13	27	7	11	27
Ideal candidates	58	10	37	3	21	24

TABLE 5

Causes of Deaths in Patients Receiving Renal Transplants at the
University of Minnesota 1968–1970 (Observation Time, June 30, 1971)

Patient	Age	Time after transplant (months)	No. transplant	Causes of death
MMc[a]	48	1	1st related	Rejection, encephalomalacia (diabetes)
AK	45	2	1st cadaver	Ureter leak, sepsis
AM[a]	24	2	1st cadaver	Pneumonia, LED
LS[a]	47	3	2nd cadaver	Pulm. absc. (bronchiect.)
WA[a]	6 wks	3	1st cadaver	Rejection, intest. fistula
MB	28	3	1st related	Cytomegalovirous inclusion disease
CJ[a]	61	3	1st cadaver	Staph pneumonia, empyema
YH[a]	47	4	1st cadaver	Influenza pneumonia (pulm. fibrosis, prev. TBC)
DC	40	4[b]	2nd cadaver	Dissecting aortic aneurysm
WR	23	5	1st cadaver	Pneumonia
PB[a]	20	5	1st unrelated	Cerebral bleeding (polyart. nodosa)

TABLE 5 (cont.)

Patient	Age	Time after transplant (months)	No. transplant	Causes of death
RRe[a]	70	5	1st unrelated	Pulmonary abscesses
JM[a]	25	5	1st related	Pulmonary abscesses
RR[a]	5	5	1st unrelated	Reop. (art. stenosis), peritonitis
RK[a]	55	8	1st cadaver	Perforated colonic diverticulum
CP[a]	46	10	1st cadaver	Repeat GI bleeding, peritonitis
SB[a]	8	11	1st related	Cerebral bleeding, hypertension
EB[a]	52	12	1st related	Rejection, septic shock
DR	37	13	1st cadaver	Herpes, GI bleeding
LK[a]	52	17	1st cadaver	Marasmus, infection (1 year dialysis)
LP	36	24	2nd cadaver	Sudden death (2 years dialysis)

[a] High risk patients (15 of 21).

[b] Six months after 1st transplant.

154

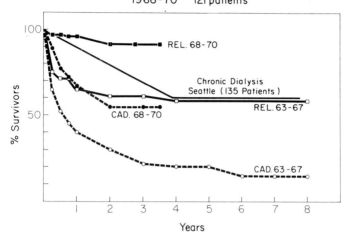

Survival Curves Dialysis-Transplantation
Transplants Univ. of Minn.
1963-67   83 patients
1968-70   121 patients

Fig. 1

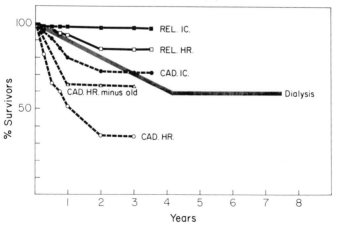

Survival Curves 1968-70 Transplantation Univ. of Minn.
Ideal Candidates (15-45 years, no systemic disease) 58 Patients
High Risk Patients (old, young, diabetes, systemic disease) 63 Patients

Fig. 2

155

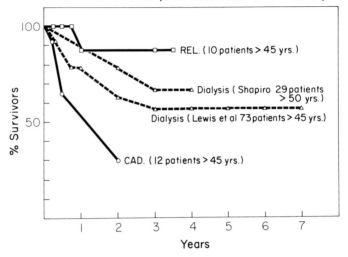

OLDER PATIENTS
Survival Curves Transplantation (Univ. of Minn.)-Dialysis
100
50
% Survivors
REL. (10 patients > 45 yrs.)
Dialysis (Shapiro 29 patients > 50 yrs.)
Dialysis (Lewis et al 73 patients > 45 yrs.)
CAD. (12 patients > 45 yrs.)
1
2
3
4
5
6
7
Years

Fig. 3

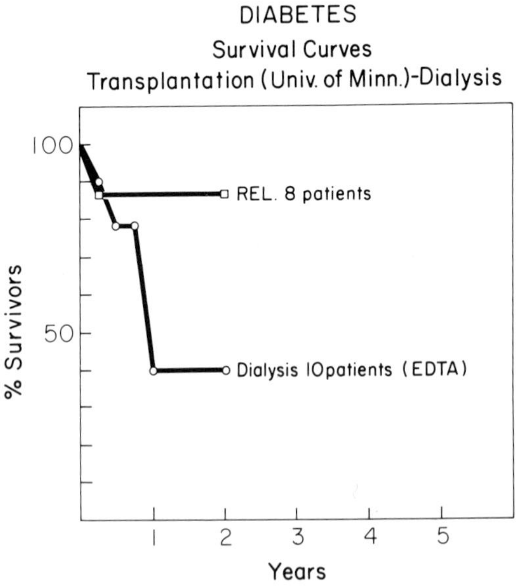

DIABETES
Survival Curves
Transplantation (Univ. of Minn.)-Dialysis
100
50
% Survivors
REL. 8 patients
Dialysis 10 patients (EDTA)
1
2
3
4
5
Years

Fig. 4

CHILDREN < 15 YEARS

Survival Curves Transplantation
(Univ. of Minn.1968-70) Dialysis

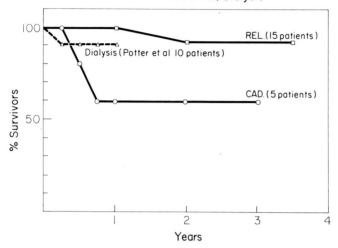

Fig. 5

OTHER PROBLEMS

Survival Curves Transplantation
(Univ. of Minn. 1968-70)

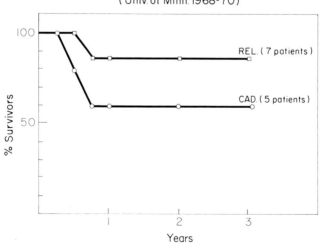

Fig. 6

157

THE SURGEONS' VIEW OF TISSUE
TYPING IN HUMAN TRANSPLANTATION

John E. Woods

Department of Surgery
Mayo Clinic
Rochester, Minnesota

This presentation presents the results of a recent telephone survey of a cross-section of the transplant centers in the United States. The questions asked related to the minimum grade of cross-match or of tissue-typing grade which was acceptable for transplantation. Query was also made as to any other unusual features that were pertinent in each particular institution. While the information presented was current at the time of the survey, rapid changes in the field of transplantation occur even on a monthly basis and thus stated policies or practices may now be different. The operating philosophy for the institutions contacted are presented below.

The first one is Boston City Hospital. Dr. Tony Monaco was the informant. Their practice is confined entirely to cadaver transplants. They do no living, related donors. All transplants done thus far have been "C" or "D" matches (1). They will accept two to four major antigenic mismatches. It was the opinion of Dr. Monaco that "D" matches were no worse than "C" matches. He mentioned that they have a fifty percent (50%) two year survival in their first ten patients on ALG and he felt that this had something to do with his results. One of twelve has died at six to twelve months in their most recent group.

At the Cleveland Clinic, in the case of both living related donor and cadavers they will do "D" matches. The informant, Dr. Bill Braun, stated that

159

four out of five of their longest cadaver survivors were "D" matches. He felt that failure was more often associated with a major mismatch at the first sublocus as opposed to the second. They do avoid doing transplants, however, where there are no matching antigens. They are using the routine cross-match. He mentioned that they have had no hyperacute rejection without detectable antibodies.

The third institution is the Medical College of Virginia. Dr. Jim Pierce indicated they will do "D" match in parents for living, related donors. They will do "D" match in siblings with one shared allele, but they will not transplant when there is a two-allele difference. In cadavers, they do "D" matches but they try not to do greater than two major mis-matches. They have a slightly different way of determining which matches are acceptable in their Southeastern Organ Exchange Group. A computer is used to check the chances of getting a better match and if there is a twenty percent (20%) or less chance of getting a better match than with the kidney in question, the transplant is performed. They are also putting emphasis on finding matching antigens and are doing cross-matching using kidney cells.

Looking at the Mayo Clinic, until very recently we were doing only "C" matches. A number of factors have altered our policy so that "D" matches are now accepted. In a number of instances patients ori-ginally thought to have received "C" match allografts were in actuality found to have received "D" or "E" match kidneys when newer typing sera became avail-able. The results were indistinguishable from cadaver kidney recipients with better matches. In addition, present data in the literature would seem to indicate that there is not a great deal to be distinguished between "C" and "D" matches. Further-more, with our present method of treating rejection with large doses of intravenous methylprednisolone, most rejections have been reversible. In fact, in recent experience the only rejection that we have not reversed using this method was a hyperacute rejection which will be mentioned with reference to cross-matching. Routine cross-matching is performed, but in addition, Milgrom's mixed agglutination technique has been used on occasion. In a recent patient, the routine cross-match was negative, but on a pre-transplant sample when Milgrom's technique was done retrospectively, it was positive. This patient underwent hyperacute rejection of the allo-graft.

At the New York University, Dr. Rapaport commented on the recently proposed concept of the Net Histocompatibility Ratio presented by him and Dr. Dausset. He said that in the article presenting the concept in Science, it might appear that only "C" matches were acceptable. In a recent review of some of Dr. Starzl's work, however, he felt that if the donor had two different HLA antigens that are cross-reacting, (i.e. that have overlap,) that donor and recipient are compatible. Speaking of Dr. Starzl's excellent survival data on cadaver transplants, with "C" and "D" matches included, Dr. Rapaport stated that these are broken down and the cross-reacting antigens are taken into consideration there is excellent correlation with tissue typing.*

At the Peter Bent Brigham Hospital, the informant was Dr. Bernie Carpenter. They will do a living donor, a "D" match; in fact, they feel that any living related donor, a "D" match or otherwise is preferable to a cadaver donor. This is the sentiment also expressed by Dr. Simmons this morning. With regard to cadaver donors, they will do "D" matches including two to four major mismatches. They found no correlation or no difference between the "C" and "D" matches. Mixed lymphocyte cultures are being performed as an educational project looking for mis-matched patients with lymphocyte stimulation.

Dr. Zoltan Lucas at Stanford reports that in living related donors, they will do "D" matches. If

---

* More recent analysis of Dr. Starzl's data has not confirmed this concept.

there are more than two siblings they will do a
genotype and attempt to look for the best donor. In
cadavers, they will do "D" matches. They're not concerned with mismatches. They do matching on all
patients, but they're guided by a very sensitive
method of cross-matching, the leukocyte binding
inhibition technique, the exact mechanics of which
have been reported elsewhere. They do place heavy
reliance on this method. If there are antibodies
present by this technique, the transplant is not
performed. In their experience there has been no
correlation between results and tissue match grade
except in identical siblings.

At the University of California in San Fran-
cisco, Dr. Kountz indicated that in both living
related donors and cadavers, only "C" matches or
better are acceptable. Their experience with "D"
match allografts has not been good. Kidney cells
are used in prospective cross-matching, which in
their opinion give more accurate results than those
obtained using lymphocytes.

According to Dr. Israel Penn at the University
of Colorado, in the living related donors, "D"
matches are acceptable in parent-to-child allografts.
A single haplotype difference is preferred in sibling to sibling transplants. They are hesitant to
transplant siblings with a two haplotype difference.
In cadaver donors, tissue type grade match is
disregarded aside from cross-matching and ABO compatibility. In their experience if anything, "C"
matches are slightly worse than "D" matches though
not statistically significantly different. They
continue to do prospective typing at this moment.

A member of the transplant team at the University of Michigan, who is attending this conference,
has indicated that "D" matches up to four antigen
differences are accepted for transplantation there.

At the University of Minnesota, Dr. Simmons has
already presented the philosophy in operation on this
subject. They have done "D" matches in cadavers,
including three to four major mismatches. The fact

is stressed that they would rather have a living related donor even with major mismatches than any cadaver donor.

The University of Utah is the other institution in this series which would do only "C" matches or better in both living related donors and cadavers. Dr. Larry Stevens stated that this was not based on bad experience with "D" matches, but was just on a theoretical basis. They are entirely guided by their tissue typer who has suggested this policy. They have also adapted the Net Histocompatibility Ratio of Rapaport and Dausset. For those not familiar with this ratio, it is a calculation which takes into account and weighs both compatibilities and incompatibilities as well as a factor for unknown compatibilities.

This data has not been presented in disparagement of tissue typing. We, in our own institution, have a great deal of confidence that tissue typing is going to present some very important answers. I think our decisions are based on a number of things, not the least of which is the desperate need for organs and the fact that we just can't afford the luxury of looking for donors who are better than "D". We currently have patients on dialysis who have been waiting over a year for a prospective donor of a good match. When a kidney becomes available, we will if possible use it for the recipient with the best match. If the best match is a "D", however, this will not deter us.

REFERENCES

1. M. R. Mickey, M. Kreisler, E. D. Albert, N. Tanaka and P. I. Terasaki. Tissue Antigens, 1, 57, (1971).

KIDNEY TRANSPLANTATION

Richard L. Simmons
Carl Magnus Kjellstrand
John S. Najarian

Departments of Surgery and Medicine
University of Minnesota Hospitals
Minneapolis, Minnesota

The technical knowledge necessary to perform
kidney transplants has been available since Carrel
and Guthrie developed the techniques of vascular
suture. It soon became apparent that more knowledge
than technique alone was needed before a transplant
would be successful because allografts were not
accepted as readily as autografts. Nonetheless, a
few attempts at renal allotransplantation and xeno-
transplantation in man were carried out in the first
half of the twentieth century.

In 1943 Medawar established the immunological
basis of allograft rejection (91) and Simonsen (153)
confirmed that the failure of renal allografts could
be attributed to immunologic differences. Between
the years 1951 and 1953 (59) Hume performed nine cadaver kidney transplants. In all of these transplants
function was adequate to maintain the patient for a
limited length of time, and one patient survived for
6 months. Some attempts were made to prolong the
life of these grafts with the use of steroids, but
insufficient doses were apparently utilized. In 1954
Murray et al. (100) successfully transplanted kidneys
between identical twins, thus confirming the technical feasibility of routine human renal transplantation. The discoveries by Schwartz and Dameshek that
6-mercaptopurine was immunosuppressive in rabbits
(138) and the subsequent demonstrations by Calne (19)

and Zukoski et al. (193) that immunosuppression would prolong renal allografts in dogs lead directly to the success of human renal allotransplantation. A number of comprehensive reviews have appeared that deal with the techniques, complications, and results of renal transplantation in man (59, 156, 164).

RECIPIENT SELECTION AND INDICATIONS
FOR TRANSPLANTATION

Criteria for Selection

The criteria for the selection of recipients of renal allotransplants have never been rigidly defined, but commonly accepted criteria include: (a) age, (b) failure to respond to good conservative management, (c) absence of reversible features, (d) normal lower urinary outflow tract, (e) absence of major extrarenal complications (e.g., malignancy, systemic disease, cerebral or coronary artery disease), (h) absence of active infection, (i) absence of severe malnutrition, and (j) absence of pancytopenia. Other groups use socioeconomic and psychiatric screening parameters to choose recipients for renal transplantation.

At the University of Minnesota there is only one primary indication for renal allotransplantation and dialysis - namely, renal failure that cannot be corrected by conservative measures. Most of the generally accepted contraindications to renal transplantation are unnecessarily exclusive. The only absolute contraindications are active infection or malignancy that cannot be brought under control, but many patients will have had mulitiple episodes of infection prior to transplantation and some patients will have had malignancies that are now cured.

Renal transplantation has been carried out for almost every imaginable renal disease. Results of transplantation in most cases justify the indications, although certain precautions should be understood.

Congenital or hereditary diseases of the urinary tract are obvious indications without contraindication. Of particular note is the high degree of success with congenital obstructive uropathy, including bladder neck obstruction and ureterovesical reflux and neurogenic bladders. A number of such patients were previously refused transplantation because of inadequate urinary outflow tracts. However, it is possible to correct many such abnormalities, especially those involving the bladder neck. After reconstruction of the bladder neck, such patients will be able to accept a kidney transplant with implantation of the donor ureter directly into the bladder despite the presence of diverticuli and trabeculation of the bladder.

Among the acquired diseases, most transplants are carried out for either chronic glomerulonephritis or chronic pyelonephritis. In fact, many patients do not present a classical history of either disease and the kidney disease is so far advanced by the time that biopsy is performed that the exact pathogenesis is indeterminant. Rather than assigning a definitive diagnosis suggesting an etiology, it is best that such patients be regarded as having end-stage renal disease of unknown etiology. Among the more specific glomerulonephritidies is Goodpasture's disease, in which antibodies to glomerular basement membrane can be detected by fluorescent techniques within the kidney. Such patients may or may not also have pulmonary hemorrhage and usually pursue a rather acute course of renal failure. It is generally agreed that serum titers of antiglomerular basement membranes should be performed and that the nephrectomy should precede transplantation in these patients. Transplantation should be delayed until the antiglomerular basement membrane has reached a very low level and the patient should be maintained on dialysis for several months (6 months to 1 year following nephrectomy.

The other glomerulonephritides may be less well defined. One that is becoming increasingly well understood is related to low complement levels within the blood stream and a proliferative membranoglomerulonephritis. Here, complement (beta 1C) can be detected in discrete fragments along the basement membrane without marked degrees of antibody deposition. Although the etiology of this disease is not well known, it seems not to be related to direct antikidney antibodies and delay in transplantation is not necessary. In the absence of well-defined disease, renal failure that follows an acute course complicated by a nonspecific glomerulonephritis should probably be treated by nephrectomy and a delay in transplantation, although prompt transplants have been made with success in such cases.

Most children with a nephrotic syndrome recover spontaneously or with steroid or immunosuppressive therapy. A number of patients, however, develop the nephrotic syndrome and progress toward terminal renal failure despite the use of steroids. Two such patients have received transplants at the University of Minnesota but both have undergone either rapid renal failure or gradual reappearance of the previous existent nephrotic syndrome. In the absence of further information some caution should be utilized in performing transplantation within this group.

Most patients with hypertensive nephrosclerosis present with gradual increases in hypertension and renal failure. A number of patients, however, presented with sudden onset of malignant hypertension and renal failure. Emergency nephrectomy can occasionally be carried out in such patients with resolution of the hypertension prior to transplantation.

Transplantation has been carried out in a number of patients with both benign and malignant tumors primarily arising within the kidney. Patients with benign tumors associated with tuberous sclerosis respond well to transplantation. It is best to maintain patients with malignant tumors of the kidneys on hemodialysis for several years prior to transplantation in order to avoid transplantation into patients with metastatic malignancies. Although individual

168

patients with diabetes and end-stage renal disease
have received renal transplants, no well-studied
series has yet been reported. At the University of
Minnesota, 21 patients with diabetes have received
kidney transplants from related living donors with
good renal function currently present in 16. No
increased problems in management of the diabetes or
infectious complications have been noted in these
patients and a gratifying cessation of the progression of gastroenteropathy and neuropathy previously
thought to be diabetic in etiology has been noted.
It is possible that such patients will not develop
recurrent diabetic glomerulosclerosis for many
years following transplantation and further trials
are certainly indicated.

Lupus erythematosus appears to involve the
kidney by means of a complex nephritis. Anti-DNA
antibodies combined with systemic DNA and are filtered out in the kidney leading to renal damage.
Extensive experience with transplantation for lupus
erythematosus and renal disease has not been obtained
but it is generally felt to be a satisfactory procedure. Other manifestations of lupus erythematosus
have been brought under control with the use of
immunosuppressive drugs. In contrast, polyarteritis
may not be amenable to transplantation, although
extensive trials have not been carried out.

Hemolytic uremic syndrome occurs in both children and adults. It is a disease of unknown etiology
in which renal failure follows massive hemolysis.
Although attempts have been made to treat the disease
with anticoagulation to counteract the disseminated
intravascular coagulation that occurs, few survivors
have been reported. Some patients may be amenable
to bilateral nephrectomy for this disease followed
by hemodialysis and ultimate transplantation.

A number of metabolic diseases, namely gout,
oxalosis, cystinosis, hyperoxaluria, nephrocalcino-
sis, and amyloidosis, have very little in common
except for the accumulation of abnormal deposits
within the kidney leading to or associated with

renal failure. Very little experience with transplantation in these diseases has been obtained. For
example, one patient with oxalosis had a poor result
following transplantation and several patients with
cystinosis underwent renal failure and transplant
failure of unknown etiology. However, a number of
other patients with cystinosis have been transplanted
with great success. Gout is not a contraindication
to transplantation. Patients with gout secondary to
uremia receive great benefit.

Two groups of patients require rather careful
individual scrutiny. These are patients with chronic
obstructive pulmonary disease in addition to their
renal disease. Such patients tolerate pulmonary
infections poorly and since pulmonary infections are
the primary cause of death in patients with renal
transplantation careful selection of these patients
is required. Heavy smokers should be allowed a long
period of time during which their smoking habit is
discontinued and prolonged physical therapy for
chronic pulmonary disease should be carried out in
order to evaluate the improvement that might be
obtained prior to transplantation. This is of
particular importance in chronic granulomatous
diseases, such as histoplasmosis, coccidiodomycosis,
and tuberculosis. Such diseases may remain latent
and inactive prior to the institution of immunosuppression and then be exacerbated in the presence
of the immunosuppressive drugs. Nevertheless, some
patients with tuberculosis have received successful
transplantations and tuberculosis development following transplantation has not uniformly resulted in
death or less of graft.

The social and psychological barriers to selection used by some groups seem most capricious. It
is extremely difficult to judge the psychological and
social stability of a patient who is dying of long-
term renal disease. Similarly, one cannot exclude,
out of hand, patients with coronary disease or
cerebral vascular accidents. Patients with peptic
ulceration frequently do quite well if surgical

170

correction of the peptic ulcer disease is carried
out prior to transplantation. Patients with severe
liver disease may be more susceptible to azathioprine
toxicity and liver disease thus remains a relative
contraindication.

In short, all transplantation centers are now
rapidly expanding their indications for transplantation and finding that the number of contraindications
has greatly diminished. Of the last 134 patients
evaluated with terminal renal failure for transplantation at the University of Minnesota, only three
patients have been refused either transplantation or
dialysis. One patient was diabetic with paraplegia
and had been bedridden for the previous 2 years; the
second patient was a 60 year old man with severe
emphysema, cirrhosis of the liver, and chronic
glomerulonephritis, and a third patient, a 56 year
old man, had active carcinoma of the bladder.

For the above reasons, patient selection is
relatively easy and special committees as utilized
in some centers may not be necessary. Recipient
selection at Minnesota is performed by the primary
dialysis physician with consultation with the
transplantation surgeons only if special problems
exist.

Workup of Potential Recipients and Timing of Dialysis

More important than the actual selection
technique of the potential recipient is the choice of
time for the institution of dialysis treatment. The
conservative management of renal failure will not
be discussed in detail here. In principle, homeo-
stasis can be maintained by manipulation of the
sodium, potassium, chloride, bicarbonate, and protein
intake. An occasional dialysis may be necessary for
exacerbations of renal failure secondary to infections in the urinary tract or elsewhere. Protein-
limited (high quality) diets described by Giodono
and Giovanetti are essential. It is even possible
to maintain patients in positive nitrogen balance

over several months and even years on this diet. The main problem, however, has been patient motivation, and near suicidal binges of eating are a constant problem over a long period.

It is generally agreed that dialysis should be instituted prior to the development of uremic complications. Once hypertension, pericarditis, cardiovascular failure, severe bone disease, bleeding, malnutrition, severe anemia, and neuropathy appear, management is markedly complicated and rehabilitation compromised. Ideally, the conservative management of patients treated for progressive renal functional deterioration should be in conjunction with nephrologists associated with dialysis and transplant centers. In this way, complication of severe uremia can be rapidly prevented by dialysis without the delays inherent in the referral process.

The main indication for the institution of dialysis has been a serum creatinine level greater than 15 mg% or a creatinine clearance less than 3 ml/min despite meticulous conservative care. It is obvious that there are exceptions to this rule. Some patients, particularly patients with polycystic kidney disease, with serum creatinine levels greater than 15 mg% can be maintained well for months on dietary management. Other patients will develop severe complications of uremia long before the serum creatinine level reaches that level, especially diabetic patients. The most pernicious of these complications is peripheral neuropathy. If there are signs of motor involvement, the patient should be dialyzed and transplanted without delay since very rapid progression of the disease can make it impossible ever to rehabilitate such a patient. Another indication for early dialysis-transplantation is uncontrollable hypertension, or hypertension that can be controlled only at the expense of severe orthostatic hypotension and other side effects. Severe anemia with anemic symptoms (dyspnea at the mildest exertion), severe bone disease (especially in children), and the failure to maintain his diet or

carry on his social and family obligations all should
lead to early dialysis and transplantation. There is
little to be gained by a delay of 3 to 6 months, and
lives may be lost in futile attempts at conservative
management.

Since some of the complications of uremia may
appear suddenly during conservative management, it is
extremely important that the patient be fully evaluated prior to the institution of dialysis, if possible. In addition to the medical evaluation, this
preparation should include interviews of the patient
and his family by the business office of the hospital, the rehabilitation clinic, and social service
in order to ameliorate the financial and social
difficulties that may accompany dialysis and transplantation. Rehabilitation of the patient can be
actively pursued even prior to the institution of
dialysis.

Preparation for Hemodialysis and Transplantation

Table 1 lists those studies that are performed
on all patients prior to transplantation. These are
similar to those performed by other groups. A check
list is very helpful in assuring the completeness of
the workup. Most of these studies are utilized as
baseline studies to assist with the management of the
patient on dialysis. A few of these studies deserve
special elaboration.

The urinary tract should be evaluated for
patency of its outflow and absence of ureterovesical
reflux. In general, a single test suffices, i.e.,
a voiding cystogram. With that test it is possible
to determine that the urethra is unobstructed, that
the bladder empties, that there are no abnormalities
of the bladder wall, and that there is no ureteral
reflux. Some patients with uremia will fail to
empty their bladder perfectly. Failure to empty the
bladder in the absence of obstruction disease would
indicate a repeat of the test after several weeks of
dialysis, by which time the urologic abnormality due

173

to uremia should have disappeared. Cystoscopy or retrograde pyelography are not generally indicated in the absence of obstructive disease when the bladder empties well. In some situations where neurogenic bladders are suspected or diagnosed, however, cystography, cystoscopy, and cystometric studies, along with bladder stimulation and bladder biopsy, may be indicated. Prostatic obstruction, urinary stricture, and bladder neck obstruction should be repaired prior to transplantation but after the patient has been dialyzed for several weeks.

It is very difficult or impossible to evaluate bladder emptying in the presence of ureterovesical reflux. Contraction of the bladder wall leads to reflux of the urine into the ureters, which then empty back into the bladder when the bladder wall is relaxed. It is necessary to remove both ureters at their ureterovesical junction prior to evaluation of the bladder for competence. Conversely, whenever ureterovesical reflux is present, one should reevaluate the bladder following nephrectomy and ureterectomy. It is not necessary to perform ileal bladder diversion on bladders that do not empty well because of ureteral vesical reflux when originally tested.

The upper gastrointestinal tract should be evaluated for the presence of preexisting peptic ulceration. Significant pathologic changes should be treated by surgical means in order to obviate the need for correction in the posttransplant period. These operations can usually conveniently be carried out at the time of pretransplant nephrectomy. Such precautions have almost completely eliminated upper gastrointestinal bleeding as a problem in the last 120 primary renal transplants at Minnesota.

Electromyography is very useful for documenting the progress or improvement of peripheral neuropathy. So many patients with uremia have hearing deficits that periodic audiograms should be carried out as well.

The procedures useful for histocompatibility testing have been extensively described in this volume and will be further discussed below.

It is obvious that dialysis frequently must be instituted prior to the completion of these studies. Most of the studies listed are primarily preparatory to transplantation. Dialysis is both a definitive therapy and the most important part of the preparation for transplantation. It should not be delayed in order to complete other studies, the results of which no longer exclude the patient from treatment.

Interrelationships Between Dialysis
and Surgical Procedures

No end-stage uremic patient should be operated upon without preceding dialysis. Chronic uremic patients exhibit a number of pathophysiological abnormalities that can be at least partially corrected by dialysis. These include coagulation defects, anemia, hypoproteinemia, edema, hypertension, and acid-base and electrolyte abnormalities. All except anemia improve even with short-term hemodialysis.

In order to bring the patient into optimal condition prior to any operation, careful planning of the sequence of dialysis and operation is necessary. Patients with end-stage renal disease are placed on dialysis for several weeks prior to nephrectomy and splenectomy. The dialysis is maintained on patients with living related donors for several weeks prior to transplantation. The patient should be dialyzed 2 days in a row before the day of any operation, thus making it possible to omit dialysis for 48 hrs after the operation (nephrectomy-splenectomy or when the transplant has not been successful), or no transplant can be carried out.

During the first of the two preoperative dialyses, transfusions of leukocyte-poor packed red blood cells should be performed to produce a hematocrit of 30 or more (higher hematocrits are necessary for patients with previous myocardial infarction, angina pectoris, old age, etc.). Transfusions should be performed on the first of the two preoperative

dialyses in order to minimize operative and postoperative hyperkalemia. The hyperkalemia resulting
from the transfused blood can be dialyzed off during
the second dialysis immediately prior to operation.
If the patient is hypoproteinemic, albumin can be
unfused during dialysis.

Only white blood cell (WBC) poor packed cells
should be given to these patients in order to minimize
sensitization against HL-A antigens. During the
last dialysis before the operations, the patients
are treated with regional heparinization, in order
to find out the patient's individual heparin requirements. The dose during this dialysis will be a
guideline for the dialysis taking place after the
operations.

SELECTION AND EVALUATION OF LIVING DONORS

The number of patients who receive kidneys from
cadaver donors is increasing with time. From the
recipient's point of view, however, it is preferable
that the donor be a biological relative. At the
present time, histocompatibility typing cannot
discern cadaver donors who will be more suitable
than a relative. At the present, even mismatched
sibling and parent kidneys survive with better
function for more prolonged periods than do closely
matched cadaver kidneys. Before the advent of histocompatibility typing, it was shown that kidneys from
sibling donors functioned better than kidneys from
parental donors. Because the genes governing the
expression of histocompatibility antigens are
situated at one (complex) locus, there will always be
one major allelic difference between the parent and
the offspring, whereas ¼ of siblings will be identical, ½ will have one allelic difference, and ¼ will
have two allelic differences. The genetic relationship may be even more complex since recent results
from larger centers suggest that siblings, parents,
and even aunts, uncles, and cousins' kidneys survive
equally well - all better than matched cadaver

transplants (164). A living related donor offers
other advantages to the recipient: The delay between
renal failure and rehabilitation is shorter, posttransplant renal function is usually immediate, and
there are fewer rejection episodes, so smaller doses
of immunosuppressive drugs are required.

The major blood group antigens (ABO) are strong
transplantation antigens. Although a number of
successful allotransplants have been carried out
across isoantibody barriers, it is generally unwise
to perform transplants into patients with known
preformed isohemagglutanins against the donor blood
type. The same rules apply to clinical transplantation that apply to transfusion, i.e., AB is the
universal recipient and O the universal donor. When
such blood type barriers are crossed, the most
violent type of hyperacute rejection reaction may
occur. There is no convincing evidence to suggest
that minor blood group factors (Rh, Duffy, Kell)
act as histocompatibility antigens.

Medical Evaluation of the Living Donor

The living related donor should be in perfect
health to minimize any risks inherent in an operation
of this magnitude. No deaths following renal donation from a healthy person have been reported.
Nevertheless, such deaths may occur in the future and
the utmost caution should be exerted not to harm or
diminish the renal reserve of a healthy volunteer.

Table 2 lists the examinations routinely carried
out on volunteer related donors: All preoperative
studies must be normal before the arteriogram is
performed to determine the status of the renal
arterial tree, and to rule out renal lesions. Multiple renal arteries are known to appear in a large
proportion of the population. It is preferable to
use the kidney on the side with the single renal
artery but a kidney with double renal arteries and
even triple arteries can be utilized (151).

177

Ethical Problems in the Selection
of Living Related Donors

Selection of a related donor is made on the
basis of histocompatibility testing when possible;
often, however, there is only one volunteer. The
ethical and social problems of donor selection have
been extensively discussed elsewhere but brief consideration is pertinent here.

In practice, the recipient is informed of the
risks and benefits of receiving a kidney from a
related donor. The recipient knows best which
relatives he can approach and which he cannot. When
a volunteer appears, he is blood typed and tissue
typed. If acceptable on these grounds, the risk of
donor nephrectomy is explained to him. The risk of
life in an otherwise perfectly healthy patient has
been estimated to be 0.5% (49). The long-term risk
has been estimated by actuarial statistics as equal
to risk incurred by driving a car 16 miles every
working day. Penn et al. (115) have demonstrated
that no long-term harm is done in the donation
process. Although the risks are small the pain,
anxiety, and loss of work time are real.

It is difficult to conceive of a living related
donor who is not subject to some family pressure to
donate (141). The fact that such pressures exist,
however, is only to admit that one has family and
role obligations within the society. When a person
freely volunteers to donate, both the benefits to the
recipient and the risks to the donor are explained.
No pressure is exerted to persuade or dissuade the
potential donor. He is not subjected to extensive
psychological interviews or testing. The early
studies of actual donors indicated a remarkable
favorable psychological response (30). Other
studies indicate much ambivalence and conflict within
the family (141). Further studies are needed to
clarify the attitudes and feelings of people who
donate or refuse to do so. On occasion, it is
necessary to fabricate a medical excuse to be used by

an otherwise medically immunologically compatible donor, when the potential donor expresses anxiety concerning his donation.

Sometimes it is necessary or advisable to utilize donors under the age of 21. This has frequently been necessary for identical twin transplants. The use of such donors, however, should be restricted to those circumstances in which other donors are not available. A court of law will also find it difficult to decide whether an adolescent should donate to his parents or siblings when family pressures may exist. Teenaged donors have been utilized when they insisted on donation and the court has agreed to the donation. No adverse psychological reactions have followed donation by these young people. The kidney registry reports that 38 kidneys have been transplanted from living donors aged 11 to 20 (105).

Unrelated persons are not generally encouraged to donate since the results are no better than that achieved with cadaver donors. It is possible that a pool of living unrelated donors may exist that could be typed and matched against a similar recipient pool in order to obtain ideal donors within unrelated populations. Such a system was tried at the University of California but with results no better than if cadaver donors were used (76). Prisoners, mental defectives, and psychiatric patients are not generally used as donors for the obvious reason that undue pressure might be exerted on these persons against their own best interests.

The purchase of organs, and its inevitable consequences, the selling of either living unrelated organs, or even the selling of a cadaver organs, must be discouraged. In addition to its obvious disadvantage (the rich will be the only ones capable of affording a transplant), it is likely that the related donor will be less willing to give if organs are available in the market place.

SELECTION OF A CADAVER DONOR

The ideal donor of a cadaveric kidney is one who (a) is young, (b) has remained normotensive until a short time before death, (c) is free of transmissible infection and malignancy, and (d) has died in the hospital after observation for a number of hours, during which time blood group and tissue type has been determined and urinary function assessed. Under these ideal conditions the donor kidneys can be removed within minutes to minimize the warm ischemia time. It is necessary, however, to compromise with a number of these ideal principles: The age of the donor is not important, and the kidney will even recover from long periods of shock and anuria. Even kidneys with hepatorenal failure have been used (74). A period of 2 hrs warm ischemia should not, however, be exceeded (20).

Criteria of Brain Death

The procurement of cadaver organs for transplantation has raised some serious moral, ethical, legal, and psychological problems. The first problem is to establish when death occurs. Since the decision is a clinical one, made by the physician in the interest of the patient (potential donor) it should be based primarily on clinical criteria of irreversible brain damage – fixed dilated pupils, absent reflexes, unresponsiveness to external stimuli, and the inability to maintain vital functions such as respiration, heart beat, and blood pressure without artificial means. The decision should be made by physicians who are not associated with the potential recipient in any way, either as referring doctor or as a member of the transplant team. The exact criteria vary between institutions and have been fully discussed by Schwab et al. (137), the Harvard Committee (52), and Juul-Jensen (65).

Juul-Jensen established four criteria of brain death: (a) The type of cerebral lesions must be established; the donors must therefore be selected among neurosurgical patients with severe trauma, vascular lesions, or tumors. Neuroradiological studies, arteriography revealing the absence of cerebral blood flow, and surgical exploration assist in the diagnosis of irreversible brain damage. (b) The level of consciousness must be that of deep coma, in which the patient does not respond to any form of external stimulus. Neurological examination must reveal dilated and reactionless pupils, absence of corneal and pharyngeal reflexes, no reaction to tracheal suction, absence of deep and plantar reflexes, and hypotonia. The patient must be without spontaneous respiration and must require controlled respiration. In this state, atropine will evidence no change in cardiac rhythm.

The above two criteria have generally been sufficient for most neurosurgeons to pronounce cerebral brain death after a period of observation and knowledge of the cerebral disease. A recent autopsy study confirmed that the brain damage in 24 consecutive cadaver donors was incompatible with recovery when these clinical criteria also were satisfied (95). Even so, Juul-Jensen (65) considers two more criteria, (c) a negative caloric test and (d) an isoelectric electroencephalogram (EEG), to be essential. Juul-Jensen feels that the isoelectric EEG is essential but points out that isoelectric EEG's have been described in anesthetized patients in hypothermia. He furthermore requires that the tests be repeated with a 24 hr interval where the EEG is recorded with normal amplification and double amplification with both a normal time constant and with an increased time constant (65).

These stringent electroencephalographic criteria are felt to be excessive by most parties (7, 140); vital signs will frequently fail before an isoelectric EEG will appear. A number of donors have been unnecessarily lost because of delay in the face of a destroyed brain.

A falling blood pressure has been used as a

criterion of brain death, but it is frequently the
result of dehydration of diuresis due to diabetes
insipidis. During the time that active therapy for
the cerebral lesions is completed, dehydration of the
patient may be extreme. This is aggravated by loss
of vasomotor tone, which produces hypotension. It is
possible to maintain almost all patients with total
brain death for prolonged periods with normal vital
signs using plasma and vasopressors; cardiac stimu-
lants are rarely required. Urinary output can likewise be maintained with hydration and diuretics.
Even the head injury patient who has been anuric and
in shock for may hours can be restored to hemodynamic
stability by repairing the relative hypovolemia.
Occasionally the electroencephalogram that was previously isoelectric will return; several patients
have recovered from coma merely by correcting the
hypovolemia. Therefore, cerebral death should not be
determined until such corrective measures have been
carried out. Then, with normal vital signs, a period
of observation for return of cerebral function can be
instituted. All decisions regarding the death of the
potential donor must be made by physicians who understand the criteria of brain death and who have had
no contact with the potential recipients. Various
administrative techniques have been utilized, the
best requiring determination of death by a team of
neurologists and neurosurgeons.

Preparations for Cadaver Donation

While awaiting final determination of brain
death, histocompatibility typing and cross matching
with potential recipients can be performed. The
absence of antibodies in the recipient that are cytotoxic to the peripheral blood or lymph node lymphocytes of the recipient is essential. This cross-
matching test should be performed using fresh recipient serum prior to any transplantation (166, 172).
Typing for HL-A antigens on the surfaces of leukocytes and/or kidney cells can also be carried out

within a few hours. There is poor correlation
between typing and the results of cadaver transplantation (174). In addition, unless the pool of recipients is extremely large, perfect matches will
almost never occur and close matches will be rare.
Therefore, if only well-matched donor kidneys are
utilized, kidneys will be wasted. In addition,
dialysis will be prolonged and the recipient will be
subjected to a greater risk of sensitization against
antigens in the population, thereby lessening his
chance of ever obtaining a good graft (22, 83). At
present it is probably best to use all kidneys
regardless of match, if the ABO blood type is compatible and if no preformed antibodies are present in
the recipient against the donor. These suggestions,
based on current typing specificities, will probably
undergo revision within the next few years. It
should be emphasized that the acknowledged value of
typing for sibling allografts is not in question
here.

The advances in organ perfusion and preservation
by surface cooling have alleviated the urgency of
cadaver transplantation considerably. It is possible
to harvest cadaver organs at the moment of death,
whatever criteria are utilized. Organs without
warm ischemic time can then be preserved with surface
cooling for several hours until the transplant recipients are prepared and the transplants carried out.
Even if a brief period of warm ischemia has occured,
the kidneys can be preserved by hypothermic perfusion
for more than 24 hours (9). If the kidneys perfuse
well under these circumstances, it is likely that
ultimate good renal function will be attained,
although a period of posttransplant dialysis may be
necessary. The use of preservation machines has
increased the availability of cadaver kidneys because
the kidneys can be transported for long distances.
In addition, cadaver kidneys that previously would
have been considered unusable because of prolonged
warm ischemia or anuria in the donor can be tested in
vitro with hypothermic perfusion to determine whether

adequate in vitro perfusion characteristics can be attained, and thereby adequate function predicted. The development of preservation also allows for more careful typing, matching, shipping, and sharing of organs between various centers (31, 62, 177). If histocompatibility typing is ever of practical importance in cadaver transplantation, preservation techniques will be essential to move the harvested organs to the recipient. Belzer reports the return of renal function in 120 consecutive cadaver kidneys perfused for 15 to 50 hrs (average 27 hrs) after warm ischemic intervals of 20 to 60 min (average 27 min) (personal communication, August 1971).

ORGAN HARVEST

Related Living Donors

The actual technique of the donor operation is not as crucial as those factors that maintain urinary output in the donated kidney and in the remaining donor kidney. Najarian et al. (102) first demonstrated that an active diuresis in the donor at the moment of renal artery occlusion foretold a prompt function in the recipient. Conversely, a soft cyanotic kidney in spasm after a difficult dissection frequently was slow to put out urine even if the period of ischemia had been short.

For these reasons, the urine output is monitored throughout the donor operation. The urine output should not fall below 1 ml/min/kidney. The patient is hydrated during the night prior to operation, and both colloid (5 ml/kg/hr) and crystalloid solutions (5 ml/kg/hr) are administered during the operation, with constant attention to the central venous pressure and the urine output. Mannitol and furosimide are given shortly before the kidney is removed. In addition, systemic heparinization is carried out 5 min before the renal artery is occluded. The heparin is then counteracted with protamine.

The donor operations has been well described in

Starzl's monograph (156). It is carried out through
a flank incision and the tip of the twelvth rib is
resected. The pleura must not be entered. The
peritoneum is retracted, the ureter identified, and
a length of ureter down to or below the pelvic brim
is dissected free. The ureter is then transected
(preserving its blood supply from the renal pelvis)
so that the urinary output of the donor kidney can
be observed throughout the operation. The remainder
of the ureter is dissected free up to the renal vein.
A large lumbar vein, the ovarian or testicular vein,
and the adrenal branch of the renal vein are doubly
ligated on the left side. There are no major
branches of the renal vein on the right side. Dissection on the renal vein is carried down to the vena
cava. The artery is not dissected free until the
dissection of the renal vein is complete.

The renal artery is dissected down to the aorta.
Arteriospasm and cessation of renal function is
frequently encountered if the periarterial dissection
is not gentle. Great care is taken not to divide
any arterial branches and careful study of the donor
renal arteriogram may be necessary during the operation to avoid dividing the polar arteries. When
a living donor with a double artery is utilized, both
arteries are dissected free with equal care and
small polar branches are preserved until it is
decided if they can be anastomosed. In living
related donors, a plaque of aorta encompassing the
origins of both renal arteries should not be taken
because the complete occlusion of the aorta may be
required, which may endanger the opposite kidney.
Instead, each artery is dissected free singly to its
origin on the aorta and double anastomoses are then
performed in the recipient (151).

When the renal arterial dissection is complete,
the kidney is replaced in the wound so that arterial
spasm will be relieved. The kidney is not removed
until urinary output from the donor kidney itself is
excellent. At that time the renal artery and vein
are sequentially clamped and divided. Care is taken

under these circumstances to leave an adequate cuff
of renal vein beyond the vascular clamp to keep the
vein from slipping out. Both vessels are oversewn.
If two veins are present, one is ligated on the
kidney because intrarenal venous anastomoses are
present.

Fluids are restricted postoperatively until the
possibility of pulmonary congestion caused by vigorous hydration is eliminated. An immediate postdona-
tion chest roentgenogram must be taken to detect
pulmonary congestion and small pneumothoraces.

Penn et al.(115) found complications in 47% of
238 consecutive renal donors (Table 3). Almost all
of the complications were mild and easily remediable,
and no deaths followed donor nephrectomy.

Donor postoperative renal function was also
studied by Penn et al. (115). In the immediate
postoperative period, transient elevations of blood
pressure were observed in ten patients (4%). Microscopic hematuria was occasionally observed in the
first few days after operation, and gross hematuria
was seen on three occasions. One donor had a fall
in creatinine clearance to 30 mg/min, and a rise in
blood urea nitrogen (BUN) to 55 mg% within one week
after nephrectomy. All of the abnormalities receded.
In 29 of the first 75 donors, there was a mean
increase in BUN and creatinine of 26% and 33% respectively. Clearance levels of creatinine were 70.5% of
the preoperative mean indicating a rapid 40% increase
in the function of the remaining kidney. No further
improvement in renal function occurred thereafter and
patients studied at 3 years had only 70% of their
preoperative renal function. The compensatory response is thus rapidly completed. These studies and
prolonged followups indicate that the health and
life expectancy of the donor population is not
adversely affected by donation. Kohler's study of
the survival of patients after unilateral nephrectomy for renal disease reached the same conclusion
(73).

Harvest from the Cadaver Donor

The technique of kidney harvest from a cadaver donor depends to a large degree on the status of the donor's circulation. If the cadaver is brain dead but with intact circulation and urine output, nephrectomy can be performed as in living donors, but by the transperitoneal route. The circulatory function of the cadaver can also be maintained by closed heart massage or artificial circulatory devices during the harvest procedure (154).

If the donor dies suddenly, the kidneys must be removed more rapidly to minimize ischemia time. The donor is heparinized, and both kidneys are removed together by clamping the aorta and vena cava above the origin of the renal arteries and veins and pulling the kidneys up together, prior to transection of the aorta and vena cava below the origin of the renal vessels and the ureters in the pelvis. The operation need not be done hastily for it only requires 10 min. Prompt cooling of the organs is required and both kidneys can be perfused with iced saline, Ringer's, or Collin's (24) solutions prior to storing them in the cold or perfusing them on preservation machines.

PREPARATION OF THE RECIPIENT FOR TRANSPLANTATION

Nephrectomy

Removal of the patient's diseased kidneys is desirable to (a) control hypertension, (b) eliminate a potential or real source of infection, (c) remove ureters from patients with ureterovesical reflux, and (d) eliminate the patient's diseased kidneys as potential pathogenetic agents in the recurrence of the primary disease. The latter reason is of theoretical importance only, since the recurrence of the glomerulonephritis in the transplanted kidney is not known to be aggravated by the presence of the diseased kidneys.

Many transplantation centers perform bilateral
nephrectomy at the time of the transplantation.
Others feel that is is better to stage the operations
and perform the nephrectomy sometime prior to transplantation in order to (a) minimize the surgical
stress at transplantation; (b) minimize the surgical
shock incurred, which might interfere with the function of the transplanted kidney; (c) apply the minimal surgical stress when immunosuppressant drugs are
utilized; (d) completely eliminate urinary tract
infection before immunosuppression is begun; and (e)
control hypertension prior to transplantation. Even
when hypertension is not evident prior to grafting,
hypertension occurs frequently enough during the
posttransplant course to necessitate the removal of
a potential source.

Splenectomy and/or thymectomy have also been
performed in kidney recipients prior to transplantation (117, 156). Thymectomy has fallen into disuse
since its performance was associated with the high
morbidity rate without improvement of renal functional survival (156, 163). Most groups still debate
whether splenectomy contributes to the well-being of
the recipient. There is no evidence that splenectomy
increases the functional survival of the graft (116),
although excision of a large portion of the bodies of
lymphoid mass was the original indication for
splenectomy. Splenectomy, however, seems to minimize
the leukopenia and thrombocytopenic effect of immunosuppressant drugs and allows larger doses of immunosuppressants to be utilized without incurring leukopenia and thrombocytopenia. There is even more
evidence that splenectomy may be a useful adjuvant
to immunosuppression in second transplants (117). At
the University of Minnesota Hospitals, bilateral
nephrectomy and splenectomy is performed routinely at
a separate stage 1 to 2 weeks prior to scheduled
transplantation from a related donor, or prior to
including a patient in the cadaver kidney waiting
list.

A number of techniques have been described for

the performance of the bilateral nephrectomy and/or
splenectomy in the transplant recipient. When this
is performed in the period immediately prior to the
transplantation, a midline incision can be made
through which the spleen and both kidneys can be
removed. Correction of ulcer diathese can be performed at the same time. Other operators use a
bilateral flank or posterior approach when the peritoneal cavity need not be opened to remove a spleen.
The only extra precaution to be taken at the time of
the recipient nephrectomy is to see if the ureter is
dilated. On rare occasions, reflux will be present
but not apparent on preoperative voiding cystography.
If ureters are dilated, total ureterectomy should be
performed.

When kidneys are removed at the time of transplantation, they are usually removed on the side of
the transplant through the transplant incision (156).
Contralateral nephrectomy is performed through a
flank incision. In small children, the nephrectomy
is usually postponed until the time of the transplantation, particularly when a transperitoneal
approach is required to fit an adult kidney into the
small child (104).

When two stage transplantation is carried out
(i.e., nephrectomy preceeding the transplantation by
a week or 10 days), the postnephrectomy management
is simple. Hyperkalemia is a recurrent postnephrectomy problem but it can usually be prevented if a
20% glucose solution is administered prophylactically
(with insulin if the patient has diabetes). Rectal
ion-exchange resins may be required to control
hyperkalemia. Dialysis can usually be postponed 2 or
3 days with these techniques. Delay in reinstituting
dialysis is preferred to avoid any anticoagulation
that might invite postoperative hemorrhage.

During preparation for transplantation, sepsis
from any source must be scrupulously removed.
Frequent sources of sepsis are (a) the hemodialysis
cannulas, if present, (b) the bladder in patients
with preexisting urinary tract infections, and

(c) the skin of patients with uremic dermatitis. The
bladder of the nephrectomized patient frequently
becomes infected and irrigations of the bladder with
neomycin should be performed several times weekly
prior to grafting (53).

Dialysis should be frequent and intense in the
immediate pretransplantation period. Recipients of
cadaver kidneys will have little preparation time
prior to transplantation. Many patients will be
maintained on systemic anticoagulants because of
clotting problems in hemodialysis shunts; the anticoagulants must be discontinued and vitamin K must
be administered. Patients on the cadaver list should
be maintained with fairly high hematocrits when compared with patients on chronic hemodialysis. On
admission, cadaver recipients should be checked for
pulmonary congestion, because several days may have
passed since the last dialysis. At this time, a
repeat cytotoxic cross match should be performed
against the donor leukocytes, using freshly drawn
serum.

TECHNIQUE OF RENAL TRANSPLANTATION

The technique utilized at the University of
Minnesota is similar to that described by Starzl
(156). The renal graft can be placed into either the
right or the left iliac fossa. Generally, the right
side is the best recipient site for either right or
left kidneys. The right common iliac and external
iliac vein appear to lie more superficially than do
the left, thus facilitating their dissection. Therefore, unless the right side has previously been
utilized in some way, it serves as the recipient site
for almost all kidney transplants.

An incision is made in the pubis to the twelvth
rib in a gentle curve, the muscles are divided; the
round ligament or the spermatic cord is divided; the
epigastric vessels are divided; and the peritoneal
contents are reflected. The host ureter is carefully
reflected onto the peritoneum, because it might prove

useful for pyeloureteral anastomosis in rare circumstances if the donor ureter is damaged. The dissection is carried along the entire length of the external and common iliac arteries to the bifurcation of the aorta and down the hypogastric artery to its smaller branches. The arterial system is then reflected medially and the dissection is carried along the iliac vein. The hypogastric venous branches are ligated and divided in order to provide considerable mobility of the venous system. Some surgeons do not free up the entire iliac venous system but leave it in situ.

The iliac vein is occluded superiorly and inferiorly and an incision of approximately 2 cm in diameter is placed in the iliac vein at approximately the level where the hypogastric veins enter. Fine vascular sutures are placed along the periphery of the orifice to prepare for the venous anastomosis. Usually, the hypogastric artery is utilized for the arterial anastomosis. The artery is divided distally and left clamped until the venous anastomosis is complete. The surgeon then brings the kidney from the donor and perfuses it with a solution of Ringer's lactate containing procaine and heparin to cool the kidney and flush it free of blood. The venous and arterial anastomoses can then be carried out.

On occasion, the hypogastric artery is totally or partially occluded by artheromatous plaques. In these patients, the side of the common or external iliac artery can be used for renal arterial anastomosis. If the side of the iliac artery is utilized, the hypogastric artery should be divided to release the medial attachment of the iliac artery. If this is not divided, tension at the renal arterial anastomosis will develop when the kidney falls laterally into the iliac fossa.

At the time the vascular anastomoses are completed, it is important that there be no deficit in blood volume. Hypovolemia interferes with the rapid resumption of renal function. Urine usually appears within a few minutes of completion of the vascular

anastomoses in related living donor kidneys; mannitol
and furosimide may be helpful in hastening the
appearance of urine.

Three methods are generally available for establishing urinary tract continuity. The preferred
method involves ureteroneocystostomy. Pyeloureterostomy (78) and ureteroureterostomy have also been
recommended but the incidence of urinary extravasation is far more common with that technique (181).
To perform ureteroneocystostomy the bladder is
opened, the trigone exposed, and two short transverse
incisions are placed just above the ureteral orifice
approximately 1.5 cm apart (156). Saline is injected
into the submucosal space to facilitate dissection of
the submucosal tunnel, and a catheter is passed
through the tunnel and then through the lateral-
posterior bladder wall. While the catheter lies in
the potential ureteral tract, the prosimal mucosal
incision is closed. The ureter is then pulled
through the tunnel and sutured to the mucosa. Care
is taken not to crush or manipulate the ureter during
any part of the operation. The Foley catheter is
irrigated free of clot and the bladder closed in
layers.

It is not necessary to either mark the kidney
poles with silver slips or to split the renal
capsule, because swelling of the kidney is not a
problem with current modes of immunosuppression;
changes in size of the kidney are not effective
early indicators of rejection. It is rarely necessary to suture the kidney in place except when blood
flow appears to be obstructed because of kinking.
Renal biopsy at this time can be useful where hyperacute rejection is suspected (71) but it is rarely
necessary in a primary transplant from a living
related donor.

Technique of Renal Transplantation in Children

The technique of renal transplantation in
children is identical to that in the adult if the

child is of adequate size, i.e., wieghs more than
20 kg. If the child weighs less than 20 kg and the
adult kidney is of normal size, the transperitoneal
approach is required. During this procedure the
nephrectomy and/or splenectomy can also be performed.
The kidney is placed in the retroperitoneal position
behind the cecum and anastomosed to the side of the
aorta and vena cava or common iliac vessels. After
the anastomosis is complete, the ureter is tunneled
in the retroperitoneal position and the bladder
anastomosis is performed in the usual manner. The
cecum is then replaced overlying the kidney. The
appendix is removed to obviate diagnostic difficulties that may occur if there is pain in the right
lower quadrant (104).

Anesthesia in the Anephric Patient

Certain precautions are necessary during any
operation on an anephric patient: In particular,
certain anesthetics are eliminated almost exclusively
by the kidney and should not be used (1). These
include the muscle relaxant gallamine triethiodide.
Both curare and succinylocholine are metabolized by
the liver but both may also be accompanied by prolonged paralysis in the postoperative period. In
the case of succinylcholine, a number of investigators have found that serum cholesterase is broken
down during hemodialysis. In such patients, succinylcholine would be expected to have prolonged
action (1). Aldrete et al. (1) have also found that
conduction anesthesia is not adequate for the transplant operation. They uniformly use inhalation
anesthesia combined with muscle relaxants. The
choice of inhalation anesthetic is not critical.
Halothane is most commonly used at both Denver and
Minneapolis.
In the administration of anesthetics and fluids,
it should always be assumed that the kidney will not
function immediately after transplantation, even if
the incidence of dialysis posttransplant is only less

than 10%. Similar thinking should be employed with regard to hyperkalemia in the uremic patient. Other concerns of the anesthesiologist are the loss of the hypertensive state after induction of anesthesia to normal levels and the low hematocrit in patients with chronic uremia. The hematocrit should be raised to 30 prior to transplantation; the normal decrease in blood pressure following induction of anesthesia is probably due to relaxation of the cardiovascular system in the face of uremic hypertension (1).

Technical Problems during Transplantation

Some attention should be paid to the technical problems that are occasionally encountered during renal transplantation.

Venous anastomosis:
The venous anastomosis is a simple prodecure. The right renal vein of the donor may be extremely short and the posterior wall quite friable. The short, relatively thin-walled right renal vein constitutes the major reason why the donor's left kidney is preferred. Great care must be taken to avoid excessive traction by the assistants in holding the kidney in position for the venous anastomosis to avoid tearing holes in the friable renal vein.

Arterial anastomosis:
The single renal artery seldom represents a technical problem. The end of the renal artery can be anastomosed to the side of the common or external iliac artery if the hypogastric artery is occluded or if there is a major discrepancy in size between the sizes of the vessels. Even young diabetic patients will have extensive disease of the iliac arteries and it is seldom possible to utilize the hypogastric artery in these patients.

Only four cases of bilateral multiple renal arteries were found in 34 cadavers by Ross and his colleagues (132). These multiple arteries appear to be even more frequent in volunteer or cadaver donors. In these circumstances, transplantation of the multiple arteries is necessary. When bilateral multiple arteries are present in living related donors, the choice of kidney is based on the following considerations (151): (a) Preference is given to the kidney of which both vessels are greater than 1 mm in diameter so that anastomosis is technically feasible. For example, if a small polar vessel is present on one side that cannot be anastomosed, the opposite kidney with two more equal sized vessels should be utilized instead of the vessel with the polar infarct. (b) Whenever possible, the left donor kidney is utilized because of its longer renal vein. (c) The kidney with the greater distances between the two arteries should be chosen as the graft to minimize the chances of inadvertently injuring one artery during dissection. Attempts to remove an aortic cuff encompassing both arterial origins should not be made for fear of occluding the contralateral renal arteries and in order to avoid slipping of the clamp from the aorta after removal of the kidney. Double anastomoses are sometimes technically impossible because bilateral small polar vessels are present; in such a case, a a kidney with a small polar infarct should be accepted.

The major renal artery is usually anastomosed to the end of the hypogastric artery. After anastomosis, this artery is immediately allowed to perfuse the major portion of the kidney. The smaller renal artery is then anastomosed to the side of the external iliac artery. Alternatively the primary anastomosis can be performed to the side of the aorta and the lesser anastomosis can be made to the side of the common iliac artery. Two major branches of the hypogastric artery can also be anastomosed to the renal arteries. During this anastomosis of the second vessel, blood frequently flows from the kidney through the lesser artery. When the bleeding is excessive, this artery can be temporarily occluded during the anastomosis (151).

ROUTINE POSTTRANSPLANT CARE

The management of kidney allograft patients in the early posttransplant period does not differ radically from the management of other postoperative patients. Vital signs are monitored frequently in the early postoperative period and the central venous pressure is utilized as a guide to blood volume. A Foley catheter is left in the bladder and it is not irrigated unless clots are thought to be occluding the catheter. The urine output is measured at least every hour. The volume of urine should be replaced with intravenous fluids. A convenient replacement solution consists of ½ normal saline with 5% dextrose and water and 10 meq of sodium bicarbonate per liter. Potassium need not be added to the intravenous fluids except in small children, whose urinary electrolytes should be replaced milliequivalent for milliequivalent. The urinary output in the early postoperative period may be enormous due in part to tubular dysfunction (54) but due primarily to the overhydrated state of even the best dialyzed patient. A creatinine clearance obtained on the evening of transplantation will confirm or contradict the presence or absence of obligatory diuresis associated with a high output renal failure. High creatinine clearances are almost never associated with obligatory diureses. When high output ischemic damage has been ruled out, fluid restriction can be practiced to keep from "chasing" the urinary output with intravenous fluids. The use of 1% dextrose and water with half-normal saline (as a intravenous infusion when urinary outputs are greater than 500 ml/hr) will diminish the osmotic diuresis due to glycosuria.

The Foley catheter can be removed almost any time after the first day. The tip of the catheter should be cultured at that time. Antibiotics may be necessary at this time to sterilize the urinary tract. Moderate hypertension is frequently seen in the early posttransplant period and a low sodium

diet and low doses of antihypertensive medication
(α- methyldopa, hydrachlorothiazide, or hydralazine)
are useful to counteract this tendency. Antacids
appear to be useful in preventing the appearance of
gastrointestinal ulceration of patients on immunosuppressive drugs.

The patient is allowed out of bed and begun on
oral fluids on the first postoperative day. Vitamin
supplements are usually continued for the first few
weeks.

Routine Posttransplant Laboratory Determinations

A 2 hour creatinine clearance is determined on
the second to fourth postoperative hours and once
more on the sixth to eighth postoperative hours.
These determinations are extremely useful in inter-
preting early oliguria. The hematocrit should be
followed at hourly intervals since rebleeding is a
rare but severe complication frequently associated
with oliguria and the onset of acute tubular necrosis
(ATN) can occur.

An I^{131} hippuran renogran (28, 51, 82) is
usually performed soon after transplantation along
with an intravenous pyelogram (IVP) (60) to establish a baseline picture of the transplanted kidney
and ureter. Determination of urea nitrogen (BUN),
serum creatinine, and creatinine clearance suffice to
estimate daily renal function. Serum electrolyte
determinations can usually be discontinued after
good renal function is established. Although urinary
electrolytes are helpful in the confirmation of
rejection episodes, they are expensive and not
necessary. Daily urinary lysozyme determinations
(106) are useful in the detection of early rejection
as are quantitative urinary protein determinations.
Blood glucose levels should be obtained weekly to
detect a possible rare case of steroid diabetes and
serum calcium levels. Daily leukocyte and platelet
counts are necessary to assay the state of the bone
marrow but direct bone marrow studies are rarely

necessary.

Routine Antibiotics

A number of centers utilize prophylactic antibiotics. The use of methicillin at the University
of Minnesota Hospitals has coincided with a decrease
in the incidence of wound infections to less than 1%.
Nystatin mouth washes can prevent oral moniliasis,
which was formerly a problem in the immunosuppressed
patient. The use of urinary antiseptics or sulfona-
mides is more controversial. They appear to be useful, at least until the bladder wounds have healed.

Prophylactic Immunosuppression

Standard immunosuppressive management at most
clinical transplant centers consists of azathioprine
with or without prednisone or antilymphocyte globulin. A number of centers also utilize prophylactic
local irradiation (58). So many factors are involved
in the success or failure of the transplant that the
differences in immunosuppression utilized at different centers cannot be evaluated. The present
regiment utilized at the University of Minnesota is
summarized in Table 4.

Antilymphocyte globulin (ALG)
Antilymphocyte sera are excellent immunosuppressive agents in animals. The widespread clinical
use of immunosuppressive drugs requires that the
following criteria be satisfied: (a) A high degree of
immunosuppressive activity should be present; (b) an
antigen should be found that is easily available and
does not elicit antibodies to red blood cells,
platelets, or glomerular basement membranes; (c) the
antibody preparation should be purified to evoke
minimal sensitization reactions over long periods;
(d) the route of administration should minimize both
toxicity and sensitization; and (e) a valid assay
should be available to predict the efficacy of the

product. These goals have not yet been attained
(104) but since Starzl introduced ALG to clinical
practice in 1967 (159) its efficacy has been widely
appreciated (86, 101, 176).

A cultured lymphoblast antigen that is used at
the University of Minnesota (103, 145) elicits a high
degree of immunity in horses against human lymphocytes. Hemagglutinins and thromboagglutinins are
present only in low titer, and prolonged intravenous
administration of this ALG does not result in anemia,
thrombocytopenia, or deposition of horse protein on
the glomerular basement membrane (183). In about
60% of the patients studied, no antibodies to the
horse gammaglobulin could be found. These patients
were rendered immunologically unresponsive to the ALG
when the intravenous route of administration was
used (36, 38). The ALG has been assayed in human
volunteers for its ability to prolong skin grafts
across strong histocompatibility barriers (146).
With doses that can double skin-graft survival in
man, a greatly decreased percentage of early rejection of transplanted cadaver kidneys has been noted
(145, 147).

Only a short course of high-dose ALG therapy is
required to achieve excellent clinical results.
There is probably a synergistic effect of ALG
priming with subsequent standard doses of azathioprine and prednisone (148, 180). Therefore, 2 days
prior to transplantation from a living related donor
the recipient is started on a 16 day course of 20
mg/kg of intravenous ALG. Recipients of cadaver
kidneys are given 30 mg/kg daily, beginning at the
time of transplantation.

ALG administration is stopped after 2 weeks to
avoid sensitization to horse globulin, which can
occur if therapy is prolonged (37). Prior induction
of tolerance to ALG by injections of small doses of
disaggregated gammaglobulin can be effective in
prolonging the action of the ALG in animals; in
humans they result in occasional sensitization and
inability to utilize the ALG at all (94). If prior

sensitivity to horse globulin has been present, a
goat ALG is utilized instead. Different preparative
techniques and different protocols have been utilized
with success in other centers (86, 101, 159, 176).

Azathioprine
        Azathioprine is the imidazole derivative of
6-mercaptopurine. Its efficacy in modifying or
preventing allograft rejection in experimental animals was demonstrated independently by Calne (19) and
Zukoski (193). Since 1963, it has formed the basic
agent in immunosuppressive therapy to which other
drugs have been added. Almost all transplant centers
continue to use azathioprine, although some substi-
tutes (e.g., cyclophosphamide) have also been tried
(160). The basic dosage utilized at the University
of Minnesota Hospitals are listed in Table 4. The
dose schedule should be modified if there is a progressive or sudden decrease in peripheral leukocyte
count or platelet count, or if there is a sudden or
progressive decrease in renal function. Azathioprine
toxicity is primarily directed at the bone marrow and
a fall of the peripheral leukocyte count may occur
rather precipitously in response to azathioprine
overdosage. Conversely, since excellent renal
function appears to be necessary for azathioprine
detoxification, any decrease in renal function
capacity will result in azathioprine toxicity and
leukopenia if the dose of azathioprine is not radically reduced. Therefore, it is important not to
raise azathioprine dosage during rejection or suspected rejection episodes because leukopenia will
frequently occur. This effect was first described
by Starzl et al.(156) and is not easily explained on
the basis of renal excretion of azathioprine.
        Azathioprine is administered for the life of the
graft. Its dose should not generally be reduced
unless there is evidence of toxicity. Intravenous
administration using one-half the oral dose is
occasionally indicated.

Prednisone

Prophylactic prednisone and methylprednisolone are now utilized at most centers, although several centers withhold prednisone until the first rejection episode. It is frequently possible to eliminate prednisone until the first rejection episode. It is frequently possible to eliminate prednisone from the regimen of patients with HL-A identical donors (A match) and it certainly can be eliminated in identical twins who will be given azathioprine in order to reduce the tendency for glomerulonephritis to recur in the isologous transplanted kidney. Prednisone dosage can be rapidly reduced during the first few weeks but then should be reduced slowly to avoid rejection episodes. Rapid reductions in the prednisone dose appear either to precipitate clinical rejection reactions or to make them clinically evident.

As the prednisone dose is reduced, reactive leukocytosis decreases. This may be interpreted at first as azathioprine toxicity but, unless the leukocyte count falls below normal levels, it may be related only to the decrease in prednisone dosage. Similarly, during a rejection reaction the increase in prednisone levels may induce a temporary leukocytosis that might mask potential azathioprine toxicity.

Methylprednisolone can be given intravenously in large doses with somewhat less adverse effect than oral prednisone because of its rapid excretion. Its immunosuppressive properties, however, appear to be prolonged, and high dose-short term intravenous methylprednisolone therapy is achieving some popularity both prophylactically and at the time of rejection (8).

A number of transplant groups (122) have successfully utilized alternate day prednisone therapy to reduce the side effects of daily prednisone. A few patients undergo rejection or hypoadrenalism and can not tolerate conversion to alternate day steroid treatment. It also seems ineffec-

tive in reversing rejection crises and should not be
instituted until renal function has stabilized.

Prophylactic local graft irradiation

There is no question that local irradiation to
the grafted organ is useful in counteracting rejection episodes (58, 66). There is less evidence that
prophylactic irradiation to the kidneys is of
clinical importance, although some centers utilize
150 R to the kidney on alternate days for a total of
three or four doses soon after transplantation (59).

Other immunosuppressants

Actinomycin C has not been found to be a useful
prophylactic immunosuppressant. Isoniozid, histadyl
(97), heparin (70), dipyridamole (70), cyclophosphamide (160), and methotrexate have also been utilized
at some centers for prophylactic immunosuppression.
Thoracic duct drainage (34, 174) to deplete the body
of small lymphocytes, extracorporeal irradiation of
the blood to kill lymphocytes (179), and intrarenal
infusions of immunosuppressant drugs (75, 84) have
been tried but have not been generally accepted.

COMPLICATIONS OF RENAL TRANSPLANTATION

Renal Failure

The most serious complication of renal transplantation is the failure of the graft to initiate
or maintain function. Although the causes of failure
can easily be defined, the differential diagnosis
may, at the time, be impossible. The functional
failure of the kidney is best examined in relation to
the time after transplantation: The kidney may (a)
never function, (b) have delayed onset of function,
(c) fail to function after a brief or prolonged time,
or (d) gradually lose its function over a period of
months or years. In each phase, four general diagnoses should be considered: (a) ischemic damage to the
kidney; (b) rejection of the kidney by reactions

directed against histocompatibility antigens on the
kidney; (c) technical complications; and (d) the
development of renal disease, either a new disease or
recurrence of the original.

The simplest and best assay for decreased renal
function is the frequent determination of blood urea
nitrogen and serum creatinine determinations, and the
determination of creatinine clearance. Occasional
renograms or intravenous pyelograms are also useful.
The differential diagnosis of renal malfunction,
however, may require retrograde pyelography, arteriography, and renal biopsy. On occasion, particularly
in patients with slow deterioration or renal function, the differential diagnosis may be impossible no
matter what method of study is utilized.

Early Anuria and Oliguria

Early anuria or oliguria is a major diagnostic
problem. The differential diagnoses must include
(a) hypovolemia, (b) thrombosis of the renal artery
or renal vein, (c) hyperacute rejection of the kidney
ney, (d) ischemic renal damage (acute tubular necrosis), (e) compression of the kidney (by hematoma,
seroma, or lymph), and (f) obstruction of the urinary
flow.

Differential diagnosis of early oliguria

The investigation of early posttransplant anuria
should be rapidly performed in a strict sequence.
The Foley catheter should first be irrigated and/or
changed to remove any question of catheter obstruction. Unfortunately, whatever the cause of anuria, a
clot can be obtained by bladder irrigation in the
first posttransplant day. The clot may not be the
primary cause of anuria, however, because blood will
clot within the bladder if the urine is not copious
enough to wash it out prior to coagulation. Therefore, even if a clot is present within the urinary
catheter, the urine output should be monitored for
the first 10 to 15 min after emptying of the bladder

to determine urine output adequacy.

If the obstructed catheter has not caused the clot, one must rule out hemorrhage into the wound, with resultant hypovolemia combined with compression of the kidney or displacement of the kidney by the hematoma. Repeated hematocrit determinations in the posttransplant period will usually make such a diagnosis obvious. Concomitantly, there will be an increase in abdominal girth and inability to palpate the kidney in the pelvic fossa. Hypotension and tachycardia may also be present and the central venous pressure will be low. A roentogenogram of the abdomen will reveal displacement of the intraperitoneal contents by a massive hematoma. The normal degree of ischemic damage to the transplanted kidney plus hypovolemia and compression of the kidney by a hematoma (and perhaps displacement and distortion of the renal vessels by the hematoma) all conspire to impair renal function. If anuria or severe oliguria is present, restoration of the blood volume will seldom suffice to restore renal function, even if furosimide or other diuretics are utilized. Many patients will require reexploration to control the bleeding point. After exploration, if the period of hypovolemia and renal compression has been relatively brief and diuretics have been utilized during ischemia, prompt restoration of renal function usually occurs. If heparin is not utilized during the transplant procedure, episodes of bleeding into the transplant wound are rare.

The diagnosis of bleeding is frequently apparent and obviates the need for the next step in the investigations sequence; the performance of an I^{131} hippuran renogram (28, 55, 82). The renogram will assess the blood flow to the kidney and the ability of the kidney to concentrate and excrete the hippuran. The results are never diagnostic. If the vascular phase and concentration is near normal, however, one can be relatively sure that the renal arterial and venous anastomoses are patent. Severe depressions of hippuran uptake by the kidney should

be promptly followed by a renal arteriogram. Arteriography should confirm patency of the renal arterial
anastomosis and clarify the diagnosis of hyperacute
rejection, in which case intravascular thrombosis of
the kidney will be seen.

Technical Complications

Thrombosis of the renal arterial anastomosis is
rare, appearing only in patients with extensive
atherosclerotic disease of the iliac vessels.
Partial obstruction due to torsion or kinking of the
vessels is more common and should be promptly
repaired. When the renogram demonstrates poor concentration of the hipurran, an arteriogram should be
performed to detect correctable technical complications.
Thrombosis of the renal vein occurs even more
rarely than thrombosis of the renal artery. When it
does occur, thrombosis of the artery ensues because
the collateral venous circulation of the kidney has
been interrupted by the transplant procedure. Partial thrombosis of the renal and iliac vein has
occurred. Usually, this is accompanied by swelling
of the ipsilateral lower extremity, fever, and evidence of pulmonary embolism. Patients with steroid-
resistant nephrotic syndrome who are prone to renal
vein thrombosis have developed recurrent steroid-
resistant nephrotic syndrome in the transplanted kidney with iliac vein thrombosis, but this syndrome
seldom occurs in the early posttransplant period.
One of the most common, and most frequently
fatal, complications following renal transplantation
was formerly urinary extravasation due to distal
ureteral necrosis. Rejection was seldom at fault,
and the problem can generally be avoided by (a)
shortening the ureter as much as possible; (b)
avoiding tension at the ureteroneocystostomy site;
(c) avoiding hematomas within the wound, which put
tension on the ureter and also interfere with collateral blood supply developing to the distal ureter;

(d) avoiding transperitoneal "clothes lining" of the ureter by always placing the ureter in the retroperitoneal position where tension will be minimal and the collateral blood supply can develop. Ureteral problems appear to be more common in diabetics.

Urinary extravasation from ureteroureterostomies and from pyeloureterostomies occurs much more commonly than that from ureteroneocystomies (181). Urinary extravasation from any site including from the bladder, usually becomes obvious within the first week after grafting although it has been ovserved more than 1 month following transplantation (88, 158). Whenever gross urinary extravasation appears, it is seldom confused with rejection.

Urinary extravasation is a serious complication leading to infection and frequently to death (181). It demands urgent reexploration with reimplantation of the ureter into the bladder, nephrostomy (107), or performance of a pyeloureterostomy to the host ureter. On occasion, the pelvis of the transplanted kidney may be involved and nephrectomy may be required. Delay in definitive repair will frequently lead to infection, the development of mycotic aneurysms, loss of the kidney and death. Obstruction to the ureteral urinary flow by granulomas at the ureteroneocystostomy may be confused with rejection. In these cases, the renogram will demonstrate prompt concentration of the hippuran but no excretion. Although this pattern is not specific, it tends to rule out hyperacute rejection. If the arteriogram is normal, cystoscopy and retrograde pyelography can be performed to determine if obstruction to the ureteral orifice is present. The ureteral obstruction may be incomplete, making the diagnosis very difficult. An infusion intravenous pyelogram with tomography may delineate a dilated ureter or one of normal caliber.

Technical errors can become manifest long after the immediate posttransplant period. Arterial stenosis, venous thrombosis, and late ureteral leaks and strictures are frequently confused with rejection.

Prior to any antirejection treatment, technical problems should be ruled out by arteriography, renography (35, 155), or intravenous or retrograde pyelography.

Hyperacute Rejection

Hyperacute rejection of the kidney (72, 157, 161, 184, 185) is almost surely mediated primarily by humoral antibody, with the subsequent participation of the complement, coagulation, and kinin cascade systems. Platelets, polymorphonuclear leukocytes, and vasospasm may also contribute. Hyperacute rejection occurs most frequently in patients who have demonstrable cytotoxic antibody directed against donor histocompatibility antigens. A lesser number of patients will reject renal allografts in the absence of demonstrable cytotoxic antibody (185) but a degree of subliminal sensitization that cannot be detected with current techniques may be present (83). Indeed, detectable cytotoxic antibody will appear and disappear at intervals in patients awaiting transplantation (21). The classic hyperacute rejection appears in patients who have received multiple transfusions or who have rejected a previous transplant. In these patients, the kidney will fail to regain its normal tugor and healthy pink color after the anastomoses are established despite patent anastomoses. Biopsy and histologic study at this time may reveal leukocytes in the glomerular capillaries, and intravascular renal thrombosis follows. On rare occasions, the intravascular coagulation will be so severe that a consumptive coagulopathy with a bleeding diathesis is produced (157). Definite evidence of a hyperacute rejection should be treated by immediate nephrectomy. A less acute rejection may occur, however, and renal function may not fail until a day or two following transplantation. In these patients an I^{125} hippuran renogram will show poor uptake of the isotope and arteriography will confirm the intrarenal vascular thrombosis. On occasion, such rejections may be confused with technical complications and arterial thrombosis. The detailed histologic changes and immunopathological changes have been discussed elsewhere (72, 161, 184, 185).

Since the advent and improvement of in vitro cytotoxic cross-match tests, antibodies against donor leukocytes can be detected prior to operation. Although transplantation has been successful in recipients who have preformed antibodies against donor tissue (53), the likelihood of this success is decreased and transplantation in the presence of a positive cross match should not be performed. Patients awaiting cadaver renal transplantation may develop detectable cytotoxic antibodies against certain potential donors, but not against others. Terasaki et al. (173) have shown that the incidence of success of transplants from any donor is reduced when such antibodies are found even if there are no detectable antibodies against the actual donor. Nevertheless, a large number of successful transplants have been carried out into patients with antibodies against antigens not possessed by the donor (166). Careful cross matching is therefore essential to any transplant program.

Acute Tubular Necrosis

The diagnosis of ischemic renal injury is one of exclusion. If all other causes of renal functional failure in the early posttransplant period have been ruled out, one must assume that the diagnosis is acute tubular necrosis (ATN) and that the kidney should recover. ATN is a misnomer, because biopsy of nonfunctioning viable kidneys frequently does not reveal necrosis of the tubules but merely hydropic changes within them. The term, in clinical parlance, refers to kidneys whose function is impaired secondary to ischemic or other nonspecific or unknown causes. ATN, then, occurs most commonly in cadaver transplant recipients when the donor has undergone long periods of stress resulting in hypotension and

oliguria. In addition, kidneys that sustain a period
of warm ischemia preceeding transplantation will fail
to function immediately. The term ATN implies the
expectation that function will return and that necrosis of the tubules is not too extensive. Kidneys
with warm ischemic intervals greater than 1 to 2 hrs
should not be utilized for transplantation because
function will seldom return to normal. Cold ischemia
is much better tolerated and preservation using
hypothermic pulsatile perfusion is now routine.
    ATN may present several clinical patterns.
Urine flow may be deficient from the moment of transplantation or the urine volumes may be initially good
but may be followed by oliguria and anuria. The
factors that contribute to the varying patterns are
not understood. In addition to warm ischemic time,
the amount of trauma engendered during donor nephrectomy that results in renal cortical spasm appears
to be important (102). ATN is far more frequent in
transplants from living related donors with double
renal arteries than with single renal arteries (151).
    ATN appears more often when kidneys from elderly
donors are utilized, and it is increased when hypovolemia and renal compression by hematoma ensues.
The I^{131} hippuran renogram may show an excellent
vascular phase and poor excretion or may be totally
flat depending on the severity of the damage. Once
the diagnosis of ATN has been made, however, the
function of the kidney can be followed by repeated
renogram.
    Almost all transplanted kidneys have undergone
some degree of damage secondary to trauma and
ischemia. A second trauma (i.e., hypovolemia,
hypoxemia, renal compression, bacteremia, allergic
reactions to ALG) that normally might not result in
ATN in normal kidneys may cause oliguria in transplanted kidneys. One must not diagnose rejection and
institute massive steroid therapy in the early posttransplant period without ruling out the possibility
that an additional insult to an already damaged kidney has occurred and that the diagnosis is not acute

rejection but ATN.

The severe oliguria accompanying many cases of ATN can be reduced by the immediate use of diuretics. Furosimide should be given in increasing doses as the diagnostic procedure progresses and as therapy (i.e., blood transfusions, bladder irrigations) is carried out. Even when the cause of ATN is finally discovered and corrected, the use of furosimide during the period of oliguria appears to improve the subsequent recovery of the kidney. If a diuretic response is achieved at any furosimide dose up to 15 mg/kg, a constant infusion of a mixture of 20% mannitol and 0.2% furosimide slowly over the following 24 hrs, may help to maintain the diuresis. One should be cautious about giving greater than 15 mg/kg furosimide to an anuric patient since deafness and/or gastrointestinal ulceration may result.

The long term management of the patient with ATN is simple. Urinary flow will resume in almost all cases within 2 or 3 weeks, but anuria for as long as 6 weeks with total recovery has been observed. I^{131} hippuran renograms are useful in following improvement prior to resumption of urinary flow. A number of studies have shown that the long-term function of renal transplants is independent of the presence or absence of oliguria in the early post-transplant period. One should reemphasize that the dose of azathioprine should be reduced (1.5 mg/kg) during renal functional failure to prevent leukopenia.

Dialysis is maintained intermittently during the period of oliguria. It is possible that rejection will occur during this period and, therefore, empirical antirejection therapy may be undertaken if improvement is not seen in the first 2 or 3 weeks.

Rejection

Technical errors may not become evident for several weeks postgrafting and any trauma can aggravate the degree of ATN in a previously damaged kidney. Most renal failures appearing after the first posttransplant week, however, can be attributed to rejection.

As histocompatibility matching has improved and new immunosuppressants have been developed, the acute rejection episodes that formerly appeared in the first month following transplantation are seen less and less frequently. Nevertheless, the majority of patients will sustain at least one acute rejection episode during the first 3 to 4 months following transplantation. Clinical rejection is rarely an all-or-nothing reaction and the first episode seldom progresses to complete renal destruction. In fact, evidence from renal biopsy data would suggest that rejection is progressing at all times in almost all allograft recipients, regardless of their renal function. The functional changes induced by rejection appear to be in large part reversible; therefore, the recognition and treatment of the rejection episode prior to the development of severe renal damage is of extreme importance. Even with prompt treatment the creatinine clearance may be permanently impaired, however slightly, following each clinical rejection episode.

Differential diagnosis of renal allograft rejection

Classic renal rejection is characterized by oliguria, enlargement and tenderness of the graft, malaise, fever, leukocytosis, hypertension, weight gain, and peripheral edema (59). Laboratory studies have shown lymphocyturia (108), red cell casts, proteinuria, immunoglobulin fragments (55), fibrin fragments in the urine, complementuria (81), lyso-zymuria (6, 139), decreased urine sodium excretion, renal tubular acidosis (12, 40, 45), and increased lactic dehydrogenase in the urine. The level of the blood urea nitrogen increases, as does serum creatinine and lactic dehydrogenase, the serum com-plement level is unstable (139). Special tests have revealed an increased spontaneous lymphocyte trans-formation in the peripheral blood (110). Creatinine clearance is obviously decreased; renograms will show slow uptake of the hippuran and slow urinary excretion. An intravenous pyelogram may be normal or it may also show some increased blunting of the calices. The renal cortical blood flow (80, 130) is also decreased during rejection and an arteriogram may show narrowing of the cortical vasculature with irregularity of the distal vessels. The classical renal rejection responds to increased prednisone doses (and occasionally to ALG infusion) and local irradiation.

Unfortunately, almost all of the above findings are also present in patients with several different maladies; obstruction or a leak at the ureter, hemorrhage with consequent ATN, infection, or partial obstruction of either the artery or the vein to the kidney. Biopsies of the kidney can be useful in attaining a true differential diagnosis (69, 112), but frequently there are signs of rejection within the kidney that are simultaneous with urinary obstruction or infection. Merrill recently reviewed problems of diagnosis and management of rejection in allografted kidneys (93), and classified the relative value of these symptoms and signs (Table 5). There seem to be no findings in typical acute allograft rejection that are specific and the differential diagnosis depends on the experience and clinical acumen of the physician.

The most important parameter to follow is the serum creatinine level. Unlike the blood urea nitrogen (BUN), which is sensitive to a number of changes (steroid administration, fever and high protein diet), serum creatinine levels are relatively stable for each patient. The creatinine clearance is more sensitive but it depends on a carefully timed collection of urine. The most reliable confirmatory test of renal functional deterioration (whatever the cause) is the radio renogram (28, 57, 82). When compared with previous renograms, the early signs of rejection are a decreased excretory rate and a slight delay in the vascular phase. These changes

are probably related to decreased cortical blood
flow and may appear prior to changes in serum
creatinine. More sophisticated modes of evaluating
the disturbances in renal blood flow that always
occur in transplant rejection have been described,
but they have not yet achieved widespread clinical
acceptance (77, 80, 130, 134, 135).

The most reliable clinical signs of renal functional deterioration are a slight decrease in
urinary output, slow weight gain, small increases in
diastolic blood pressure, and edema of the lower
extremity on the side of the graft. A peripheral
leukocyte count and a serum creatinine level should
be determined to confirm renal functional deterioration. A renogram and intravenous pyelogram should
be promptly performed and compared with those
obtained at the peak of renal function (usually
prior to discharge from the hospital). In the face
of poor renal function, tomograms during intravenous pyelography may outline a normal ureter. If
ureteral obstruction cannot be ruled out, a retrograde pyelography can be carried out, although it
may be difficult to cannulate the ureteral orifice.
Finally, arteriography may reveal (a) characteristic
changes of decreased concentration of dye flowing
into the kidney, (b) decreased nephrogram effect, or
(c) an irregularity of the cortical vasculature and
intralobar vasculature characteristic of rejection.

Many of the signs and the differential diagnoses
of renal functional failure depend on the length of
time that has passed since grafting and on the clinical condition of the patient: Increases in serum
creatinine during the first 2 weeks following transplantation are less often due to kidney rejection
than they are due to infection or technical errors.
Episodes appearing in the period from 2 weeks to
3 months posttransplant are more often due to
rejection, although ureteral stenosis, urinary leak-
age, arterial stenosis, venous thrombosis, and infection may also occur in this period. A high degree of
correlation exists between the appearance of an

213

infection and renal functional deterioration. It would seem, in fact, that mild infections may trigger renal allograft rejection (152).

A number of rejection signs are difficult to interpret: An unexplained fever may be related either to the rejection episode or to the infection that coincides with clinical rejection. Unexplained fever frequently appears in children following transplantation, but it must not be assumed that it represents rejection, which requires steroid therapy. Leukopenia may appear in a patient whose peripheral white blood cell count had been stable on moderate doses of azathioprine. Such leukopenic episodes frequently precede evidence of clinical rejection and may represent the sequence of rejection, decreased renal function, decreased azathioprine clearance, and bone marrow suppression even before the serum creatinine rises. For this reason it is dangerous to increase azathioprine dosage at the time of rejection, regardless of the peripheral white blood cell or platelet count. Proteinuria and development of the nephrotic syndrome have been described in patients with chronic rejection. Proteinuria also occurs in patients with a nephrotic syndrome who develop recurrence of their original disease.

One of the signs of rejection that was long thought to be the most reliable is the renal functional response to antirejection therapy, especially increased doses of steroids. A true rejection episode responds to steroids with a prompt diuresis, weight loss, resolution of edema, correction of hypertension, and return of the serum creatinine level and renogram to normal. Unfortunately, because steroids act to decrease inflammation and edema of whatever type, the renal functional deterioration associated with mild infections and ureteral obstruction all respond to high doses of steroids. We have reported several patients with renal arterial stenosis who responded several times to antirejection therapy before the renal arterial stenosis was finally discovered and repaired (150).

Renal biopsy should be a definitive diagnostic tool. Both open biopsy and needle biopsy techniques have been described and the histological changes of rejection are characteristic (79, 85, 119, 129, 131). A normal kidney biopsy is diagnostic, but a biopsy that reveals renal damage may merely reflect acute rejection, a chronic on-going process, exacerbation of the preexisting renal disease, or damage due to infection or radiation. Therefore, the interpretations of even classic rejection in such kidneys is difficult.

Infection and rejection

Simmons et al. (152) have recently described a number of apparent allograft rejection episodes that are preceded or accompanied by episodes of rather mild local or systemic infection. In only one case was the infection severe enough to be life threatening. A number of other patients have illustrated the concurrence of systemic and local infections associated with deterioration of renal allograft function (152). In each case, the infection, however mild, preceded the deterioration of renal function. Several possibilities could explain the coincidence: (a) It is most likely that the infectious agent acts as a nonspecific adjuvant upsetting the immunologic balance that exists between donor organ and host. Endotoxins, tubercle bacilli, and other microbial agents and products have long been known to act as adjuvants to the immunologic responses (191). (b) It is also possible that antigens are produced by the infecting agent that cross react with histocompatibility antigens, thus altering the specific unresponsive state (120, 121). (c) A third possibility is that immune complex nephritis may result from the combination of the infecting agent and the antibodies elicited by the infection. Whatever the case, appearance of mild infection in a renal transplant recipient suggests that renal functional deterioration may follow. Conversely, the appearance of a rejection episode should prompt a search for underlying infection. An increasing number of studies have revealed cytomegalic inclusion virus in the patients during rejection episodes (26, 126). Whether the virus led to a clinical infection that in turn acted as an adjuvant for renal allograft rejection is unknown. A systemic search for viruses in immunosuppressed transplant recipients is required to confirm the hypothesis.

When infection and rejection coincide in a transplant patient, it is difficult to know whether the rejection should be treated or whether it will spontaneously remit when infection is controlled. Frequently it is necessary to treat both the infection and the rejection, thus possibly rendering the patient increasingly susceptible to the infecting agent. The dilemma is not easy to solve, but when a clear-cut infection precedes or coincides with the rejection episode, it is best to withhold anti-rejection therapy for several days until the infection is brought under control.

Treatment of rejection

Most institutions have developed a standard rejection regimen for allografted kidneys (Table 6). In addition, actinomycin C or D (200 µg/day) have been suggested for repeated rejection episodes, even though there is no real evidence that it is effective in man. ALG is an excellent immunosuppressant in man and it will also reverse on-going allograft rejection in dogs, but it is of less use in patients already on large doses of other immunosuppressive drugs. In some circumstances, however, ALG appears to improve the function of acutely or chronically rejecting allografts in patients who cannot tolerate more steroid therapy. This standard rejection regimen can be repeated as many as three times within a 2 month period in patients for whom rejection appears to be unremitting. It can be repeated more often than that if rejection episodes will ultimately result in death unless the kidneys are removed and immunosuppression stopped (149). This decision is frequently subtle and difficult, particularly in patients who have deterioration of renal function over a period of months or years.

Williams et al. (188) have classified prognosis into four groups, depending on the number of rejection episodes and the time that they occur. Group 1 includes those patients who had no rejection episodes and no proteinuria. Such patients had 100% long-term function. Group 2 includes those patients with one acute rejection episode; long-term function was 87%. Group 3 patients had two or more acute rejection episodes, and only 50% long-term function. Group 4 patients had rejection episodes lasting over 30 days, or rejection episodes within the first week or after the fourth month. The long-term function of related transplants in these patients was only 27%. Thus, the early onset of rejection episodes, their frequency in the early posttransplant period, or their appearance late following transplantation are relatively grave prognostic signs. In such patients it is relatively easy to make the decision to remove the grafted kidney in the face of recurrent rejection because the chance of saving the kidney over the long term is poor, and their lives may be saved by its removal at an early period of time.

Renal Failure Due to Recurrent Disease

Human renal isografts have been performed in man for 20 years (39). Even though such transplants do not encounter the severe immunologic barriers to success that allografts do, they have not been uniformly successful. Recipients of renal isografts whose original disease was glomerulonephritis frequently develop a lesion in the graft identifiable as glomerulonephritis. An original disease of rapidly progressive glomerularnephritis is associated with the earlier and more frequent appearance of glomerular lesions on the isografts, and subsequent progression to chronic renal failure. In contrast, a slowly progressive glomerulonephritis is correlated

217

with lower instances of glomerular lesions in isografts and a greater opportunity for survival.
Glomerulonephritis of the isograft rarely appears in
recipients whose primary disease was not categorized
as glomerulonephritis.

The recurrent disease in the isografts in some
respect resembles the late-onset glomerular lesion of
the allografted kidney; the nephrotic syndrome may
occur in either situation. The glomerulonephritis
of isografts is associated with basement membrane
and mesangial deposition of IgG, complement, and
fibrinogen. The presence of preformed antiglomerular
basement antibodies as well as immune complexes has
been implicated in the pathogenesis of the recurrent
disease. The high recurrence rate of glomerulonephritis in isografts and the apparent low rate in allografts is thought to be due to the relative universal
use of immunosuppressive therapy in the latter group.
Genetic predisposition to glomerulnephritis may
exist among the donor-recipient pairs in the isograft
series.

Although experience is limited, prophylactic
immunosuppression appears to have merit in the
prevention and treatment of recurrent glomerulonephritis in isografts. There seems to be no relation to
the time in which the recipient's diseased kidneys
are removed and the time of transplantation. It is
also not known whether the bilateral nephrectomy
hastens the disappearance of antiglomerular antibodies or actually prolongs their circulatory life.

The general strategy is not to delay allotransplantation or isotransplantation after the nephrectomy of patients with proven glomerulonephritis
unless the disease is of acute onset or there are
high circulating titers of antiglomerular basement
membrane (anti-GBM) antibody present. If the disease
is of recent onset with rapid progression to failure,
nephrectomy is performed and the titer of anti-GBM
antibody followed until it falls to neglible quantities. At that time, transplantation should be
carried out with immunosuppressive coverage in both

isogenic and allogenic recipients. Patients with
Goodpasture's disease respond well to this treatment
(47).

Because of the nonspecific changes that can
occur as consequences of chronic rejection and antirejection treatment, there is still active debate
about the incidence of recurrent nephritis in renal
allotransplants. In patients with complex nephritis,
either of unknown etiology or secondary to lupus
erythematosis, it is possible that precipitation of
complexes on the transplanted kidney glomerular basement membrane will reactivate the disease. It is
also possible that complexes of antibody will be
filtered with streptococci, other bacteria, viruses,
or ALG. Alternatively, direct binding of antibody
with the GBM may take place not only as a consequence
of preexisting anti-GBM antibodies, but also secondary to GBM binding by ALG or by the development of
Masugi nephritis. In general, however, most of the
glomerular changes in allotransplants can be considered to be part of the rejection process.

COMPLICATIONS OF IMMUNOSUPPRESSIVE THERAPY

The complications of immunosuppressive therapy
in recipients of renal allotransplants are almost
impossible to distinguish from the complications of
recurrent rejection. Patients who do not develop
rejection episodes do not generally suffer major
complications of immunosuppressive therapy. The
dose of steroids can be reduced in such patients to
easily tolerated levels (0.1 to 0.25 mg/kg prednisone per day), the ALG is stopped after a short
period of time, and azathioprine toxicity can be
avoided as long as renal function is normal. Conversely, the patient who requires repeated large
doses of prednisone to avoid further rejection
episodes or who suffers diminished renal function in
the presence of high doses of azathioprine will
develop potentially lethal complications. The major
complications all relate to a relative inability to

respond effectively to a large variety of pathogenic,
and even normal, saprophytic organisms. There may
be, moreover, a decrease in the normal capacity to
destroy mutant, potentially neoplastic cells.

Infections

Infection is the most serious complication of
immunosuppression and is the most common cause of
death in renal transplant recipients. Table 7
summarizes the causes of death reported to the
National Kidney Registry for 1940 renal allotrans-
plant recipients who died since 1963. The causes
of death were frequently complex but sepsis was mentioned in 47% of the cases, whereas rejection in
the absence of sepsis accounted for less than 10%.
These data, however crude, confirm the findings of
most investigators who have reported smaller series
of more carefully documented patients. Table 8
illustrates that the incidence of early posttransplant death is decreasing at a faster rate than is
the rate of transplant rejection. These data suggest
that kidneys are being removed and the patients are
being placed on dialysis rather than continuing in
vain attempts at immunosuppression.

Simmons et al. (144) have reported that 46 of
52 deaths following transplantation in the years
1963 to 1969 were related to septic complications.
Most of the deaths prior to 1967 occurred in the
first 3 months after transplantation. The most
common organisms responsible were Staphyloccus
aureus and Klebsiella pneumoniae. Since the advent
of penicillinase-resistant penicillins, however,
staphylococci have ceased to be a major problem;
Klebsiella and Pseudomonas are now more often the
lethal agent. With the control of staphylococci,
deaths in the first month following transplantation
became quite rare. All investigators have confirmed
the relative frequency of lethal infection due to
organisms that are normally only weakly pathogenic.
As antibiotics eradicate the pathogens, opportunistic

organisms colonize the susceptible host (5, 56, 98, 125, 127). Hill et al. (56) have pointed out that it takes these organisms longer to kill than usual, and deaths due to these opportunistic organisms are seldom seen before the second posttransplant month. In Hill's series of 67 deaths reported in 1967, the protozoan pneumocystis carinii was found in the lungs of ten patients. Cytomegalovirus was found in almost half of the patients who died following transplantation. However, pulmonary insufficiency caused by Pneumocystis carinii was considered to be present in only two of the ten patients (56) with the organism, and Cytomegalovirus apparently was not the cause of death in the 30 patients who showed evidence of this virus. Cytomegalovirus appeared to represent a common subclinical infection in patients treated with immunosuppressants, but its significance in relation to other more lethal infections is unknown. Pneumocystis carinii, of course, in itself can cause severe pulmonary insufficiency and has been responsible for a number of deaths, but both cytomegalovirus and Pneumocystis infections are usually accompanied by other bacterial and fungal invaders if the infections are to prove fatal (56).

Fungal infections are common in all series (21, 127, 128, 144). The pathogens most frequently found are Candida and Aspergillosis, but fatal infections due to tuberculosis, Cryptococcosis, Nocardiosis, Histoplasmosis, and Murcomycosis, as well as other organisms, have all been reported. These infections are frequently mixed. For example, in our series (144) all the patients with Aspergillosis were also infected with Candida and one patient with Nocardiosis also had Pneumocystis carinii, Candida, and Cytomegalovirus. Thus, mixed infections with fungal agents and superimposed bacterial infections are frequently the cause of death in patients with immunosuppressants.

Prevention of Infection

Eliminating septic sites
 The incidence of severe, near fatal infections
can be reduced through a number of precautions, which
have been previously discussed. The most important
precaution is to eliminate all sources of infection
prior to transplantation, especially those in the
urinary tract and shunt site. Other sources of
infection should be sought by routine preoperative
cultures of nasopharynx, throat, sputum, urine,
stool, and hemodialysis cannula sites. If any source
is found, it should be eliminated by the appropriate
use of surgical drainage or antibiotic therapy.

Technical problems
 Technical problems clearly predispose to sepsis.
Urinary extravasation frequently leads to wound
infections. Abscesses deep to the transplant are
difficult to drain and mycotic aneurysms may develop
at sites of anastomosis or in the iliac vessels
(112). In addition, the inadequately drained infections become the source of repeated septicemias. The
initially susceptible organisms are replaced by
opportunistic organisms as repeated courses of antibiotic therapy are administered. It is frequently
necessary to remove the kidney to obtain control of
the infection.

Role of the relationship between donor and
recipient in the development of infection
 Recipients of cadaver renal transplants do less
well than the recipients of living related donors,
despite the use of histocompatibility typing in the
selection of cadaver donors. Organs from unrelated
donors elicit more frequent and more vigorous rejection reactions. They require such large doses of
immunosuppressive drugs that the patient's resistance
even to saprophytic organisms is eliminated. Consequently, if repeated rejection can be avoided, there
is little danger that life will be lost because of

infection. Rejection can be best avoided by using
organs donated by living related donors whenever
possible.

The role of leukopenia in the development
of lethal infections
    Almost all patients who die of infection develop
leukopenia (especially neutropenia) at some time
(144, 149). Therefore, the advent of leukopenia is
a poor prognostic sign. The patient who develops
more than one or two episodes of leukopenia during
his course of treatment will almost uniformly
develop a severe infection. Leukopenia can be prevented by careful reduction in azathioprine dosage
when the leukocyte count or platelet count falls and
when renal function is lost for whatever reason. The
use of other bone marrow depressants (e.g., chloram-
phenicol) should be scrupulously avoided in patients
already on azathioprine therapy.

Prophylactic antibiotics
    It is difficult to prove that the use of prophy-
lactic antibiotics is of any value. Most transplant
centers maintain patients on urinary antiseptics or
sulfasoxaxole until the urinary tract has healed.
Other centers utilize antistaphyloccal antibiotics
because staphylococci were frequently lethal in the
early days of transplantation. The use of bladder
irrigations with antibiotic solutions prior to transplantation do minimize the incidence of urinary tract
infections following transplantation (53). Similarly,
the early removal of the catheter when renal function
has been established (1 to 3 days posttransplant)
appears to be useful in reducing the incidence or
urinary tract infections. Urine cultures should be
performed biweekly in the posttransplant period.
Whenever colony counts greater than $10,000/m^3$ are
found, specific antibiotic treatment should be
instituted.

Isolation precautions

Gowns, masks, and gloves were formerly used to
minimize infections in the initial postoperative
care. Most transplant units have discontinued their
use because they restrict access to the patient,
impose psychological stresses, and are probably
ineffective against viral, fungal, or endogenous
bacteria.

Diagnostic Problems Associated with
Infections in Immunosuppressed Patients

A high index of suspicion is essential for the
early diagnosis of a potentially fatal infection in
patients treated with immunosuppressants. Any
illness, particularly febrile illnesses, should be
suspect and the patient should be admitted for diagnostic study on the basis of minimal symptoms. No
symptoms lasting more than a day or so should be
attributed to insignificant upper respiratory infections. Most significant infections, however, will
be characterized by fever and systemic toxicity.
The peripheral white blood count is of little
assistance. Routine cultures of the nose, throat,
sputum, blood, and urine should be performed whenever
fever is present. Particular attention should be
paid to the urinary tract and wounds: Wounds in
these patients may reveal hidden infections months
and even years after the incisions apparently heal
(98).

The concurrence of mild infections with apparent
rejection episodes has been mentioned previously:
Sudden deterioration of renal function should therefore also suggest an occult infection (152).

Pulmonary infections

Although it is clear that the factors previously
listed tend to predispose to the development of
lethal infection, there appears to be no factor that
predisposes specifically to any one type of infection. Urinary tract infections, although common, are

usually minor and can be brought under control without great difficulty (10, 79, 87). Septicemia seldom appears after the first few weeks and is usually associated with wound infection. The most lethal infections involve the lung. Most lung infections will appear as regional infiltrates on chest roenogenograms and will be accompanied by symptoms exactly like those of pneumonia.

The prompt choice of proper therapeutic modality in these desperately ill patients depends on precise determination of the etiologic agent responsible for the infection; this may be extremely difficult. Mixed infections are the rule and bacterial infection is present in almost every case of fungal disease. The organism that is usually treated is the one that is most easily cultured from the sputum but it may or may not be the organism that is causing the infection, particularly in the patient who is already on antimicrobial therapy. The infecting fungi and protozoa, in particular, are seldom present in sputum or tracheal aspirates. In addition, Rifkind has pointed out that Sabouraud's medium is utilized for isolation of fungi not because of its particular suitability for these organisms, but because of its inhibitory effect upon the bacterial flora (127). More suitable media are available for each of the common infecting fungi. Thus, it is possible that fungi may not be found by routine techniques. In Rifkind's series, the infecting fungal agent was isolated from the sputum in only six of the 14 patients who died with fungal pneumonias (127). In the University of Minnesota Hospital series, none of the patients who died with fungal diseases was diagnosed by routine techniques (144).

The pattern of skin tests is of little use in the diagnosis of opportunistic infections. Their development takes too long and delays the institution of therapy. In addition, all delayed hypersensitivity responses may be obliterated in these patients. Patients with known tuberculosis have had negative tests while being treated with immunosuppressants;

the skin tests for blastomycosis, coccidiodomycosis, and histoplasmosis are frequently negative during the acute disease. One should not be deceived by the use of four skin tests that do not even include the most common fungal agents, which may infect these patients (Candida, Aspergillus, Cryptococcus).

When pulmonary infiltrates are present, cultures of sputum and tracheal aspirates should be performed and appropriate antibiotic therapy instituted. If there is no response to therapy, needle biopsy or open pulmonary biopsy should be performed immediately. However, needle biopsy carries the risk of pneumothorax, bronchopleural fistula formation, and contamination of the needle tract. In addition, its yield of positive information is small in these patients because the biopsy is limited to small areas of the lung, whereas multiple organisms may be infecting multiple areas. It is frequently necessary to perform open pulmonary biopsy.

When open pulmonary biopsy is necessary, a significant piece of involved pulmonary tissue should be taken. If multiple areas are involved, multiple wedges should be taken. Fresh imprints on slides should be made of the lung tissue and these should be stained with Gram stain, acid-fast stain, silver methenamine, and Giemsa stain (for fungi and Pneumocystis carinii). Frozen sections should also be made, since some fungi can be identified on pathologic sections and the typical proteinaceous alveolar infiltrates associated with Pneumocystis carinii can be identified. Sections of lung should be cultured both aerobically and anaerobically for bacteria. Multiple media should be utilized for fungal cultures, which should be incubated aerobically and anaerobically for prolonged periods. Viral isolation techniques, if available, should also be utilized.

A few opportunistic infections have rather typical clinical patterns that should raise suspicion. Aspergillus frequently appears in a classic form. The upper lobes are almost uniformly involved and the lesion usually appears as a rounded or oval shadow that is not particularly dense, a portion of which is circumscribed by a thin crescentic line (23, 109). Cavitation is frequently present. Even in the patient treated with immunosuppressants, the progress of this aspergillosis may be slow. Its early appearance in the upper lobes is classic, even though it may later spread to other areas of the lung with multiple abscesses and cavitation. It should be emphasized that most lower lobe abscesses are of bacterial origin even in immunosuppressed patients.

The other fungi may be present as relatively soft, bulky, nodular infiltrates that are not diagnostic one from the other, although the patterns do suggest a nonbacterial origin. The early nodules may be indistinct and require tomography for definition. Rarely, patients will die of milliary tuberculosis, histoplasmosis, or cryptococcosis. In these cases, the lungs will reveal multiple miliary nodules on roengenograph examination.

One classic pattern that is readily recognized and can usually be diagnosied on the basis of the patient's history, physical examination, and chest roenogenogram is Pneumocytis carinii pneumonia (29, 125). This organism may accompany other infections but may itself cause respiratory insufficiency and death. The patients will usually have severe shortness of breath, low-grade fever, and a dry nonproductive cough. The degree of dyspnea far exceeds the other signs of toxicity and there may be cyanosis in the absence of any sputum or fever. On examination, there may be bronchial breathing but no rales or areas of consolidation. The chest examination is almost diagnostic. There is a uniform bilateral alveolar infiltrate extending from the hilum to the periphery of the lung. As the infiltrate progresses, an air bronchogram appears, caused by the opacity of the remainder of the lung. This pneumonia consists of a thick proteinaceous intraalveolar exudate composed primarily of the organisms themselves. There is minimal inflammatory

change. Severe physiologic arteriovenous shunting
results in profound hypoxemis and cyanosis. If
recognized early, this pneumonia can be treated and
cured, because it may run an indolent course. The
diagnosis is confirmed by either open or closed lung
biopsy. The rather time-consuming silver methenamine
stain has been replaced by the Giemsa stain on imprints of the fresh lung.

Viral pneumonia, especially that associated
with Cytomegalovirus isolation, also appears in a
rather reproducible clinical pattern. The patient
presents with fever without respiratory symptoms
some deterioration of renal function or hepatic
function may also be evident. The chest roengeno-
gram reveals an interstitial pneumonia that is most
pronounced in the lower lobes and perihilar areas.
Lung biopsy may be necessary for confirmation but
Cytomegalovirus can be cultured from the sputum and
urine of some patients.

Neurologic Complications of Sepsis

Not only are multiple organisms frequently
involved in life-threatening infections in patients
treated with immunosuppressants, but multiple sites
may be involved as well. Rifkind has pointed out
that the neurologic manifestations of systemic
fungal infections may be due not only to the generalized toxicity involved in any systemic infection but
are also frequently due to fungal abscesses within
the central nervous system (CNS). Because the CNS
manifestations were primarily behavioral and seizure
disturbances, specific diagnostic measures were not
brought into play to localize the infections prior
to death. It is important to bear in mind that
pneumonias coincident with neurologic problems are
frequently due to fungal diseases, particularly
Aspergillus (128). The use of arteriograms, brain
scans, echograms, and electroencephalograms may be
essential in localizing a CNS abscess requiring
drainage.

Problems in Differential Diagnosis of Infection

Pulmonary embolisms

Although pulmonary infiltrates usually represent infection, pulmonary embolisms secondary to thrombosis of the common iliac vein have resulted in death. Despite the multiple pulmonary infiltrates, no pathogenic organisms can be cultured. If pulmonary biopsy can be performed in these circumstances the diagnosis can be made early enough to save the patient.

Transplant lung

A syndrome of arterial hypoxemia of obscure etiology has been referred to as "transplant lung." Minimal physical signs are present and chest roenogenograms show a variety of patterns ranging from a normal appearance to patchy bilateral pulmonic infiltrate (57). The classic picture is accompanied by an episode of transplant rejection and responds to the administration of prednisone. A number of etiologies have been suggested (such as a diffuse vasculitis and autoimmune reaction against pulmonary tissue). Weight gain is often excessive and the correlation of pulmonary changes with rejection (both of which respond to prednisone) suggests that the rejection episode is most likely accompanied by interstitial pulmonary edema. Fluid retention, weight gain, and oliguria are frequent consequences of rejection and may result in pulmonary edema as well as the more obvious peripheral edema. It is important to rule out infection in these patients because similar syndromes can be produced by Pneumocystis carinii or Cytomegalovirus pneumonia.

Transplant fever

Obscure fevers are common following transplantation. Classic rejection episodes are accompanied by fever but with more efficacious use of immunosuppressive agents and histocompatibility testing, fever is now less often present. Fevers frequently go

undiagnosed and are explained away by low-grade
urinary tract infection, allergic reactions to ALG,
or drug sensitivities. They may well be symtomatic
of virus infections (5, 126) and may precede apparent
rejection episodes. Withdrawal of large doses of
steroids (59) does not seem to be a common cause of
transplant fever any more. Despite these exceptions,
fever still strongly suggests sepsis, and a vigorous
campaign of diagnostic procedures to determine the
site and etiology of sepsis is uniformly carried out.

Other Infections

A number of other infections are common in
recipients of renal transplants. These infections
include herpes zoster, which is usually localized and
painful but does not progress to systemic involvement (124). Localized herpes simplex infection has,
however, progressed to death (96).

Hepatitis has been a problem at some centers,
presumably as a consequence of multiple blood transfusions received during dialysis, but it is probably
more a direct result of transplantation from a
cadaver kidney. Fatalities occasionally occur. Reed
et al. (123) described a high incidence of Australia
antigenemia in transplant patients, but clinical
hepatitis among the staff far exceeds that in transplant recipients. Immunosuppressive drugs may well
interfere with the expression of the viral disease
without interferring with viremia. Patients with
deficiencies in immunologic responsiveness tend to
have mild anicteric hepatitis and persistant antigenemia. The evidence that clinical hepatitis may
be a manifestation of an antigen-antibody reaction
supports these observations (123).

Jaundice does not necessarily indicate hepatitis.
Azathioprine toxicity may present itself as icterus.
Reduction of azathioprine dosage usually leads to
recovery and increasing azathioprine doses lead to
recurrence. Rejection has occasionally followed the
permanent reduction of azathioprine dosage to low

levels in these patients.

Treatment of Infections in Immunosuppressed Patients

The principal aim of the treatment of sepsis in the immunosuppressed patient is to save his life. The discontinuation of immunosuppression may kill the grafted kidney and one is hesitant to surrender the kidney unnecessarily. The decision to discontinue the therapy is made even more difficult because even this drastic measure does not guarantee a reversal of the infection. Such patients may have accumulated an irreversible degree of immunosuppression that is unresponsive to sacrifice of the kidney, reinstitution of hemodialysis, and appropriate antibiotic therapy. The degree of immunosuppression may be so great that rejection of the kidney may not occur even when the regimen is stopped.

The decision is less difficult when the infections develop while the patient is chronically rejecting his transplants. In such cases, the continual use of repeated courses of antirejection therapy in the face of recurrent infection will lead to the patient's death (144, 149). This is also true in the patient whose renal function is deteriorating over a period of months and years.

Although it is clear that azathioprine must be discontinued when rejection and significant infection are present, it is less clear how rapidly one should diminish steroid dosage in such patients. Generally, steroids should be decreased stepwise over a period of 3 to 4 days to maintenance levels of approximately 0.2 to 0.3 mg/kg until the infection is under control.

If immunosuppressive therapy is stopped, renal functions usually deteriorate slowly, but if accelerated rejection takes place, the kidney should be removed. The rapid death of the kidney apparently produces a toxic state characterized by stupor and coma. Diffuse electroencephalographic changes become apparent and the symptoms can be relieved only by prompt transplant nephrectomy.

Actual resistance to antibiotic therapy is not the major problem in the infected patients: Most bacteria are sensitive to available antimicrobials. The inability to diagnose the precise etiologic agent and the failure to deliver the antibiotic into the sequestered abscesses are two of the greatest problems. Lung abscesses due either to fungal or bacterial infection are common, and surgical drainage may be necessary even in these acutely ill patients (68, 111).

Fungi have recently proven to be highly sensitive to nonnephrototoxic doses of amphotericin B. Amphotericin is not dialyzable by hemodialysis, but it is cleared by the kidney; consequently, loading doses followed by small incremental doses are utilized in patients with renal failure. It is increasingly apparent that the sensitivity of fungi to amphoteracin is such that low doses will be effective; renal toxicity need not therefore be a threat. A newer fungal agent, 5-fluorocytosine, has been developed. This drug is known to be effective against Candida and Cryptococcus and may well be effective against other fungi as well. The drug is presently restricted to treating recurrent fungal diseases that have not responded to amphotericin (172). Nocardia, which is actually a bacteria rather than a fungus, responds readily to sulfadiazine.

Pneumocystis carinii is highly susceptible to pentamadine isethionate. Despite its ability to eradicate the organism, pentamadine is seldom curative in transplantation patients because such patients cannot eradicate the proteinaceous alveolar infiltrate following the death of the organism. Even when effective, the clinical response is slow. Pentamadine is hepatotoxic and nephrotoxic and may cause hypoglycemia and hypocalcemia.

Noninfectious Complications of Immunosuppression

Malignancy

Malignancy is a frequent concomitant of renal

immunosuppression (171). The deeper malignancies could not be effectively treated by this approach, and led to death in eight of nine epithelial and ten of 17 mesenchymal tumors (118).

It is generally agreed that agressive conventional malignancy therapy should be employed and that as much immunosuppression as can be safely eliminated should be discontinued. Complete cessation of immunosuppression would not be expected to result in the cure of these neoplasms as they would if the neoplasms had been inadvertantly transplanted from allogeneic donors. Arbitrary discontinuance of immunosuppressive drugs is therefore not advised, although cautious reduction in dosage may assist conventional therapy.

An unanswered question is why a high incidence of malignancy is seen in some transplant centers and not in others. It is possible that some apparently insignificant differences in the immunosuppressive regimen plays a role here. It is generally agreed that immunosuppression of all types predisposes to the development of malignancy not only in these patients, but also in children with congenital immunological deficiencies and other patients on immunosuppressive therapy.

Cushing's disease

Most transplant patients on steroid therapy undergo a series of changes that are referred to as iatrogenic Cushing's syndrome. The rate of its development is a result of the dose of steroid and number of rejection episodes. The appearance of the face is altered by rounding, puffiness, and plethora: Fat tends to be redistributed from the extremities to the trunk and face. There is also an increased growth of fine hair over the thighs and trunk, and sometimes the face. Acne may increase or appear and insomnia and increased appetite are noted; however, the underlying metabolic changes that accompany the obvious changes can be serious by the time the latter actually appear. The continuing breakdown of protein

and diversion of amino acids to glucose increases the
need for insulin and results in weight gain, fat
deposition, muscle wasting, thinning of the skin with
striae and bruising, hyperglycemia, growth suppression (in children), and sometimes the development
of steroid diabetes, cataracts, and osteoporosis.
Some patients develop a myopathy, the nature of which
is unknown.

The Cushingoid changes may on rare occasions
represent such a psychological problem that transplant nephrectomy will be necessary on that basis
alone. Women are more severely affected and the
psychological problems are greater. These problems
can be enormous in children who grow less well and
most particularly in small girls on chronic steroid
therapy who seem to grow very little after age 13.
The male psyche tolerates steroids better; the
plethora and broad faces give most men a healthy
look.

Steroid diabetes

Steroid diabetes is an occasional complication
of chronic steroid administration, even when the
steroid doses are not high. This may represent
exacerbation of the prediabetic state. The diabetes
is frequently mild and may be controlled by oral
hypoglycemic agents alone. The onset of diabetes,
however, is frequently insidious, and the patient may
have diabetic acidosis before the diabetic state is
discovered and controlled.

Gastrointestinal bleeding

Gastrointestinal bleeding due to reactivation of
a preexisting ulcer or diffuse ulceration of the
gastrointestinal tract is an almost uniformly fatal
complication of renal allografts and frequently
causes death (98). The relative contribution of
progressive uremia and repeated massive steroid
administration in the pathogenesis of gastrointestinal hemorrhage is unknown, but when bleeding
appears it is severe and difficult to control by

nonoperative means. Occasionally the intramesenteric arterial infusion of vasopressin and gastric cooling provide effective treatment (168).

During moderate doses of steroid therapy, episodes of GI bleeding can be almost totally prevented by the use of antacids between meals. Magdalate (Riopan) is a useful antacid since it is required in only small doses. In patients with recurrent rejection who require many episodes of high steroid dosage, antacid therapy must be intensified with each increase in steroid administration. Magnesium-containing antacids, however, are contraindicated in patients with poor renal function since hypermagnesemia will result.

Other intestinal complications

Penn et al. (115) reported a number of colonic complications, including diverticulitis, bleeding, and ulceration associated with immunosuppressive treatment. A syndrome of acute cecal ulceration with GI bleeding has also been reported in transplant patients (168).

Cataracts

Cataracts are common in patients who have sustained several rejection episodes and high steroid doses. The cataracts, which develop slowly, appear to be independent of the absolute prednisone dosage.

Azathioprine toxicity

The complications attributable to azathioprine primarily relate to depression of bone marrow function. Signs of hepatic dysfunction occasionally will require the reduction of azathioprine dosage (azathioprine has also been associated with temporary hair loss).

Thrombosis and thromboembolic phenomena

Thrombophlebitis may occur in the transplant recipient, particularly on the side of the graft where the venous anastomosis may become partially

or completely thrombosed. This has occurred in
patients who previously had steroid-resistant nephrotic syndrome and may be related to recurrence of
the disease.

When attention is focused on the immunological
and infectious phenomena, thrombophlebitis and pulmonary embolism may be difficult to diagnose.
Swelling of the leg on the side of the transplant
site is a frequent sign of rejection associated with
increases in weight, pulmonary infiltrates, and
slight increases in serum creatinine. When the
differential diagnosis is difficult, a femoral veno-
gram is indicated (23, 25, 32). The diagnosis of
pulmonary embolisms may also be difficult and
multiple pulmonary infiltrates should not be
treated as fungal pneumonia based on sputum cultures
alone.

Hypertension

Many of the patients who come to renal transplantation are already hypertensive. Hypertension
can usually be controlled with dialysis and, if more
refractory, with nephrectomy. Most patients will
develop hypertension soon after transplantation but
the posttransplant hypertension is mild and easily
controlled with dietary salt restriction and drugs.
The hypertension seems to be due not only to prednisone but also to failure to regulate the normal salt
and water balance in the early posttransplant
period (11, 14, 42). The transplanted kidney can
secrete renin (13, 182). The antihypertensive drugs
can usually be stopped as maintenance levels of
prednisone are reached. Hypertension returns with
rejection but significant hypertension may be due to
renal arterial stenosis and arteriography may be
necessary for the differentiation.

Disorders of calcium metabolism

Patients frequently come to transplantation with
renal osteodystrophy. Alterations in vitamin D
metabolism and secondary hyperparathyroidism are

prominent factors in the pathogenesis of skeletal disease (57). Long-standing acidosis may likewise be contributory (18). The resulting osteoporesis, osteomalacia, and ostitis fibrosa cystica in the child can lead to growth restriction, epiphysiolysis, skeletal deformities, and pathological fracture (48). The bone disease in some cases can be arrested with pharmacological doses of vitamin D, aluminum hydroxide, or by total or subtotal parathyroidectomy.

Hemodialysis can correct the uremic state, but the bone disease may actually progress if the stimulus to parathormone secretion is not effectively eliminated. Great attention should be directed toward keeping the dialyzate calcium concentration at a level (6 to 7 mg%) that does not promote calcium loss from the blood. Again, parathyroidectomy may be indicated if osteitis fibrosa cystica is progressive and cannot be reversed by maintaining the calcium concentration in the serum at normal or slightly elevated levels (18).

Parathyroidectomy performed in the patient with renal failure or on hemodialysis may help to arrest progressive bone disease. Frequently, however, the calcium levels will remain high and will only fall after renal transplantation. Conversely, if prompt transplantation from a related donor is planned, or if the cadaver list is short, transplantation by itself will usually lead to the reversal of the hyperparathyroid state. The hypercalcemia of the immediate posttransplant period can be managed with a high phosphate diet, low calcium intake, and furosimide diuretics. Even patients with flagrant osteoitis fibrosis cystica with metastatic calcification will respond to transplantation alone without parathyroidectomy. Parathyroidectomy seems primarily indicated for patients on chronic hemodialysis in whom transplantation is not planned.

Careful studies of calcium and phosphorus metabolism after renal allotransplantation have been carried out by Alfry et al. (2). They found that hypercalcemia, hypophosphatemia, and increased renal phosphate clearance was present in over 50% of their patients, suggesting the diagnosis of hyperparathyroidism. Alfry et al. (2), however, suggest that hypophosphatemia is an effect of steroid therapy and that the hypercalcemia is an effect of depletion of body phosphate stores secondary not only to the effect of steroids on phosphate stores but to the intense antacid therapy with aluminum hydroxide. Posttransplant tertiary hyperparathyroidism may then be an artifact that can be reversed by the administration of phosphate-containing antacids. In fact, posttransplant hypercalcemia is not associated with elevated parathormone levels (63), and parathyroidectomy will rarely be indicated after successful transplantation.

Musculoskeletal complications

The most disturbing complication of successful renal transplantation is avascular necrosis of the femoral heads and other bones. Its occurrence is most closely correlated with the dosage of steroid used (46). Transient rheumatoid symptoms may precede changes visible by radiography by several months. The bone changes apparently occur secondary to steroid osteopenia or osteonecrosis with resulting microfractures. Alterations in lipid metabolism caused by fluctuating high levels of steroids likewise appear to be important in explaining the pathogenesis (17). The treatment is for the most part symptomatic. It is doubtful that bone lesions can revascularize sufficiently to restore normal architecture in the presence of maintenance steroids. Should symptoms increase in the hip and bone destruction progress, replacement arthroplasty may be indicated.

Migratory arthralgia, myalgia, and tendonitis are common in our experience. It has been suggested that antiallotype (61) antibodies may be a factor in joint and soft tissue changes. Again, the treatment is symptomatic.

Occasionally the development of synovitis may

occur secondary to the presence of fungal infections
in the joint. Associated skin lesions resembling
erythema nodosum should alert one to this possibility
(61). Bacterial infection may occur in joints as
well as in the bursae; they must be promptly recognized and surgically drained.

Serum sickness with arthralgias and arthritis
can be seen after ALG therapy and are usually controlled with antihistamines and steroids.

Pancreatitis

Pancreatitis may appear suddenly and unexpec-
tedly in renal allograft recipients; it may occasionally be fatal. Its cause is obscure and it has
been attributed variously to corticosteroid therapy,
Cytomegalovirus or hepatitis virus (59). The
clinical course is sometimes accompanied by increases
in serum creatinine, which may or may not be related
to rejection. Most cases subside with conventional
therapy and do not recur.

Erythremia and anemia

The transplanted kidney is apparently fully
capable of manufacturing and secreting erythropoietin
(99). During rejection, the serum level may be
increased. Erythremia also (169) may appear but
apparently it is not related to elevated erythropoietin levels.

Anemia usually is not present except in association with uremia or immunodepression secondary
to azathioprine toxicity. A microangiopathic hemolytic anemia has also been thought to be induced by
the vascular changes within the chronically rejecting
organ.

RESULTS OF RENAL TRANSPLANTATION

Transplant Registry Results

The results presented here are those of the
Ninth Report of the NIH/ACS Human Renal Transplant

Registry (Tables 7-13) (105). All the data reported
to the registry are analyzed collectively. Although
large numbers allow precise analysis, the reported
results are neither as good as those of the most
experienced centers, nor as poor as those centers
with the worst records. The report, therefore,
should be thought of as an average of performance
achieved by groups reporting to the registry.

The data for calculations in this report were
derived from 5794 transplantations reported to the
registry. These include 3661 transplants performed
in the United States from 96 institutions, and 2133
reported from 96 centers elsewhere.

The distribution of the ages of recipients is
shown in Table 11; Table 9 illustrates the sources of
donor kidneys since 1953. Cadaver donors are utilized more frequently, whereas parent and siblings
are used as donors at approximately the same rate as
previously. Volunteer unrelated donors are no
longer being utilized.

The mortality data from the registry has previously been described (Table 7). Tables 8, 9, and
11 illustrate survival of first renal transplants
followed for more than 2 years. It is clear from
this data, pooled from first transplants performed
around the world, that the kidneys from living
related donors survive much better than do those
from cadaver donors. This has been a fairly consistent finding throughout all the years of renal
transplantation. It is also clear that the improvements in results seen in the early days following
transplantation has now leveled off and that the
results of transplantation are not much better than
they were in 1968. The results of cadaver transplantation have improved slightly.

Table 9 also compares the results of transplantation from cadaver transplants performed since
1968 with those performed from less closely related
donors, including aunts, uncles, and cousins. The
results from other related donors are certainly
better than the results from unrelated donors but are

less satisfactory than kidneys from siblings or
parents. Some large centers have found, however,
that aunts, uncles, cousins, and children are as
satisfactory as siblings and parents (164).

Table 10 reports the results of renal transplantation according to the primary renal disease of the
recipient. The registry data suffers from an overwhelming preponderance of patients with a diagnosis
of glomerulonephritis. This diagnosis is frequently
based on the absence of evidence of infection in an
end-stage kidney, the pathogenesis of which is unde-
finable. The diagnosis of glomerulonephritis does
not, therefore, necessarily imply a specific disease.
The table reveals, however, that there are no great
differences in survival or function among the different primary renal diseases. There are several
exceptions to this rule however, i.e., patients with
familial nephritis, who are usually children or
adolescents, appear to have better survival. Far
less good survival is seen in patients with malignant
hypertension and cancer of the kidney.

Table 11 reports results of all renal transplantations since 1955 grouped by recipient ages. The
2 year functional survival appears to depend largely
on the age of the recipient. Although the transplantation of children less than 5 years old does not
appear to be highly successful, in the age range from
6 to 40 years there is only a slight decline with
increasing age. After age 40, there is a sharp drop
in survival in recipients of sibling transplantation,
and after age 50 there is a sharp drop in the survival of recipients of cadaver transplants. The
question may be raised whether older recipients
receive the kidneys of older donors. Registry data,
however, can show no difference in functional renal
survival in kidneys transplanted from cadavers of
age 11 to 20 or cadavers of age 40 to 60.

The Transplant Registry has the advantage of
pooling the data from both large and small transplant
centers. The main disadvantage is not being able to
discriminate some of the factors that determine

success or failure in transplantation. Three of
these factors seem to be the most pertinent: (a) The
importance of histocompatibility typing and cross
matching; (b) the importance of ALG as an immunosuppressant; and (c) the importance of recipient
selection.

The Importance of Histocompatibility
Typing and Cross Matching

The technique and results of histocompatibility
typing are discussed elsewhere in this volume. Once
HL-A was established as the major human transplantation system (exclusive of the A and B antigens), it
seemed only a matter of time before information about
individual HL-A specificities could be translated
into steadily improved donor selection. This has not
proved to be the case. The assignment of HL-A
alleles within families is a relatively simple procedure. The demonstration that certain alleles are
more immunogenic than others is also possible within
families, but the demonstration that certain individual specificities are of greater significance in
graft rejection than others has not yet been accomplished. In fact, there is more confusion of
thought at the present time regarding the importance
of histocompatibility matching than would have seemed
possible a few years ago when the clear association
between HL-A compatibility in families and transplant
success was first established. The area of HL-A
typing remains a controversial one but certain facts
do appear to be clear: (a) Cross matching, in which
cytotoxic antibodies against donor antigens are
detected, is a valuable clinical technique. When
cytotoxic antibodies are present, the donor should
not be utilized. More controversy exists about
whether any patient who displays antibodies against
other individuals in the population will have a
worse prognosis upon receiving a kidney from an
individual against whom he has no demonstrable cytotoxic antibodies. Success in such circumstances is

less likely than if the recipient has no cytotoxic antibodies against any other member of the population (172). Successful transplantation has been carried out in many cases in which a recipient with multiple cytotoxic antibodies has received a kidney from a donor to whom he is not sensitized (16). The sensitivity of the cytotoxicity test for the detection of anti-HL-A antibodies has been questioned and other techniques have been suggested as being more sensitive indicators of antibody activity (83). In practice, however, most centers utilize the cytotoxic techniques against donor peripheral blood leukocyte.

(b) Genotyping in families in the search for sibling donors of identical HL-A configuration should be practiced when possible. HL-A identical siblings, while not as successful as monozygotic twins, have a significantly higher rate of long-term transplant success than other siblings. A number of rejection episodes are fewer, and immunosuppressive drugs can be reduced to low, relatively nontoxic levels (50, 64, 133, 167, 190).

(c) Histocompatibility typing from parent to child has not demonstrated any significant difference between the well-matched parent and the poorly matched parent (174). All such parents will differ from their children by at least one haplotype, i.e., by two histocompatibility antigens, unless the parents share antigens.

(d) Histocompatibility typing to select the best aunt, uncle, cousin, or grandparent donor has not been practiced widely enough to suggest that it is useful.

(e) Histocompatibility typing in the selection of cadaver donors is a controversial area. The largest cooperative series, collected by Terasaki, has revealed no significant difference between well-matched and poorly matched donors except when all four HL-A antigens of donor and recipient are perfectly matched, confirming the impression of most of the larger transplant centers in the United States (174). This failure to correlate HL-A tissue typing

with results of transplantation from unrelated donors
suggests several possible explanations. The first
explanation is that the HL-A locus is even more complex than thought. Thus, there may be more antigens
determined by the two subloci that are as yet undetected by current serological techniques. Second,
the fact that many grafts survive for a long time in
spite of obvious serological incompatibilities may be
explained by numerous cross reactions existing
between the different products of the same HL-A
locus, i.e., certain antigenic specificities that
appear to be serologically different are effectively
the same (27). Third, the generally accepted two-
sublocus hypothesis for the HL-A histocompatibility
system is incorrect (3) and there may actually be
a transplantation locus closely linked to the HL-A
locus. Thus, the fact that HL-A correlates well with
transplantation success between siblings would only
mean that the transplantation locus and the HL-A
locus are closely linked and that recombination in
one generation is rare. Lastly, a third transplantation sublocus has been suggested.

In practice, delay in cadaver transplantation
subjects potential recipients to multiple blood
transfusions and sensitizes them to antigens within
the population. This practice may be more inhibitory
to transplantation success from a cadaver donor than
would be ignoring the typing results (excluding the
ABO system) and utilizing every kidney that became
available, regardless of the histocompatibility
match of the recipient. As the problem becomes
better defined, revision of this working plan will
certainly be necessary.

Transplantation Results in Ideal-Risk
and High-Risk Patients

As kidney transplantation has evolved, most
transplant groups have selected recipients from
among candidates with end-stage renal disease. Those
patients who do not become recipients are either

244

referred for dialysis or are offered no treatment at all. This selection process has been justified by the facts that facilities and trained personnel are in limited supply, that transplantation is expensive, and that only those patients who are ideal risks should be chosen so that the maximum number of patients will benefit from the limited capacity for transplantation available. Medical and social criteria have, therefore, excluded thousands of patients from dialysis and transplantation because of undocumented fears that psychological, surgical, and immunosuppressive stress would not be tolerated.

Some centers have studied the results of transplantation in those patients who might be considered as high risk from the stresses of the transplantation process. We have previously compared the survival of kidneys transplanted from living related donors or cadavers in ideal-risk recipients and high-risk recipients at the University of Minnesota during the period 1968 to 1970. The ideal-risk recipients were defined as patients ranging in age from 17 to 44 years, with primary renal disease without complicating intercurrent disease or systemic disorder of any type. They had normal lower urinary tracts, had never bled from the gastrointestinal tract, and were free of infection and malignancy. The remaining high-risk patients included (a) children aged 3 to 16 years, (b) adults older than 45, (c) patients with diabetes (d) patients with abnormal lower urinary tracts, (e) patients who had bled from gastrointestinal ulcers, (f) those who had severe psychological disorders leading to their rejection by other dialysis and transplantation centers, and those with (g) severe myocardial disease, (h) lupus erythematosus, (i) polyarteritis nodosa, (j) cystinosis, (k) inactive tuberculosis, or (1) hypertensive encephalopathy. Many patients occupied positions in more than one high-risk category. Recipients of related kidneys had an 88% chance of long-term (greater than 2 years) renal function based on life table computations. Recipients of unrelated transplants in the ideal-risk group had a 70% chance of such long-term function. Recipients of related kidneys in the high-risk group were no more likely to reject their kidney in the 2 years following transplantation than were the ideal-risk patients. However, high-risk recipients of cadaver transplants had only a 33% chance of maintaining normal renal function for 2 years. This is less than one-half the number achieved in ideal-risk recipients.

Elderly patients who receive transplants from cadavers are the highest risk group of transplant patients (143). The Transplant Registry reported similar results (Table 10). Many patients over 45 will die of sepsis even if renal function remains normal. The problem does not appear to be as great in the older patient with a related kidney who is not subject to increased doses of steroids with multiple rejection episodes. However, the older patient with an unrelated kidney who usually requires several periods of elevated steroid doses is truly a high-risk patient.

Transplantation in Patients with
Abnormal Lower Urinary Tracts

It has been axiomatic that a normal bladder and lower urinary tract is required for transplantation. Kelly et al. (67), however, have transplanted kidneys to the ileal bladders of patients with uncorrectable lower urinary tracts. This practice has been continued at the University of Minnesota. More than one half of these patients are living and well with normal renal function, several more than 5 years posttransplant. There is no question, however, that such patients are subjected to a greater risk because the problems of the ileal loops, ureterointestinal anastomoses, and atonic dry bladders (43, 44) frequently compound the problems of transplantation.

Such transplants are normally carried out in several stages. At the first stage, the kidneys,

246

ureters, and spleen of the patient with a neurogenic
bladder are removed. At the second, an ileal loop
is constructed, the most proximal end being placed in
the retrocecal or retrosigmoid position. At the next
stage, the kidney transplant is carried out and the
ureteral ileal loop anastomosis is performed. Following transplantation, a loopogram should reveal
that the anastomosis is widely patent with free
reflux into the pelvis of the kidney. Such studies
should be carried out periodically in order to rule
out the development of stenosis and infections in the
dry bladder.

Patients without neurogenic bladder, regardless
of reflux, should have bladder neck obstructions of
either congenital origin or due to stenosis repaired
prior to transplantation. After repair of the
obstruction, the bladder can be utilized as in
normal patients.

Diabetes

Diabetics are not generally accepted for transplantation. Twenty-one diabetics have received
renal transplants at the University of Minnesota
since January 1968, 14 from related donors. Eleven
of the 14 are alive with good renal function, and
four out of seven who received cadaver transplants
are also alive and well with good renal function.
Such patients, however, are subject to slightly more
increased risk than are nondiabetic recipients of
comparable kidneys. The hypogastric vessels are
frequently obstructed with atherosclerosis in
diabetic recipients; consequently, end-to-side
anastomoses to diseased vessels are required. Technical failure may be more common in this group. Such
patients seem to have increased incidence of ureteral
complications, perhaps due to defects in wound heal-
ing. Although traditionally prone to the ravages of
infectious complications, only two patients died of
infectious complications after primary renal transplantations.

247

One of the most remarkable results following transplantation in diabetics is to see the improvement in diabetic neuropathy. The intestinal symptoms disappear and motor and sensory function of the lower extremities returns. Diabetic neuropathy may be aggravated by the presence of uremia. The retinopathy associated with diabetes also appears to be relieved and vision returns to the occasional patient with severe retinal changes. This may merely represent loss of the hypertensive component of the diabetic retinopathy.

Transplantation in Children

Renal failure in children is a common cause of death; however, young children have not been traditionally considered ideal candidates for renal transplantation, although excellent results have been reported by a number of investigators. The small caliber of vessels and active social behavior of children make their management on hemodialysis extremely difficult. Long-term immunosuppressive therapy is also thought to interfere with normal growth with resultant social problems. Long-term hemodialysis is seldom satisfactory, and a parent is almost always willing to donate a kidney. The Renal Registry statistics (Table 11) reveal that patients above the age of 5 do extremely well posttransplant, confirming the impression of several large pediatric transplant groups (33, 41, 104, 187). Several infants have been transplanted, and at least one has survived for more than 1 year. The growth of children following transplantation has been the subject of several studies (104). Most allografted children grow slightly slower than normal. The adolescent growth spurt is absent in the transplanted children and adolescent growth is particularly depressed in girls.

This early cessation of growth causes the typical appearance of transplanted girls, who are short and more Cushingoid than the boys. Attempts to

correlate the amount of first-year posttransplant
growth with the kidney donor, renal function, or
prednisone dosage have been unsuccessful (104). No
such correlations can be made, even though it is
generally felt that prednisone interferes with
growth.

Sexual maturation in boys appears to be normal,
although the period of observation has been short.
Similarly, some girls have failed to menstruate at
the usual age despite relatively normal renal function and only moderate doses of prednisone. Most
girls have resumed menstruating if previously mature,
or they undergo a normal menarch upon reaching age
13 or 14.

Results of Multiple Transplants

A number of studies have shown that second and
third transplants are less successful than the first
(Table 12). The rejection of one transplant will
apparently sensitize the patient to a number of
histocompatibility antigens that are shared by other
potential donors within the population. The development of cross-matching techniques has increased the
chances of finding a second donor to whom the recipient is not sensitized.

Table 13 summarizes the results of second transplants in patients who rejected the first transplant.
Here it is clear that recipients of related kidneys
after having lost the first related kidney have a
much better chance of maintaining function for 2
years in the second kidney than do patients who
receive a cadaver kidney after rejecting a related
kidney. Similarly, patients who receive a related
transplant after rejecting a cadaver transplant have
a much better chance of success than those who
receive a cadaver transplant after rejecting a first
cadaver transplant. There is no difference, however,
between recipients of cadaver transplants, whether or
not a related or cadaver transplant was rejected the
first time. Patients who lost the first kidney for

technical reasons also seem to tolerate a second
graft better than patients who rejected their first
kidney graft.

Rehabilitation

The results of a survey performed at the University of Minnesota in December of 1970 are shown in
Table 14. This survey included only patients surviving transplantation. Almost all the children had
returned to their previous activities and were in
school. By 1 year posttransplant, 90% of the adults
were performing most of their customary activities.
These figures support the generally held opinion that
transplantation restores most patients with renal
failure to good health.

Some problems do remain in the posttransplant
patients, but uremic neuropathy (4, 15), pericarditis,
anemia, and malaise are relieved; however, cataracts,
weakness, and musculoskeletal disorders are common.
The sexual and reproductive functions of both males
and females (92, 117) return to normal as soon as
the steroid doses are reduced to maintenance levels.
Congenital defects in the offspring of patients on
potentially teratogenic drugs has not proven to be a
problem (117, 170).

REFERENCES

1. J.A. Aldrete, W. Daniel, J.W. O'Higgins, J.
   Homatas, and T.E. Starzl, Anesth. Analg. (Cleveland) 50, 34 (1971).
2. A.C. Alfrey, D. Jenkins, C.G. Groth, W.S. Schorr,
   L. Gecelter, and D.A. Ogden, N. Engl. J. Med. 279,
   1349 (1968).
3. B. Amos, Transplant. Proc. 3, 71 (1971).
4. A.K. Asbury, N. Engl. J. Med. 284, 1211 (1971).
5. S.L. Balakrishman, D. Armstrong, A.L. Rubin, and
   E.H. Stenzel, J. Amer. Med. Ass. 207, 1712 (1969).
6. B. Ballantyne, W.G. Wood, and P.M. Meffan, Brit.
   Med. J. 2, 667 (1968).

7. H.K. Beecher, N. Engl. J. Med. 281, 1070 (1969).
8. P.R.F. Bell, K.C. Calman, R.F.M. Wood, J.D. Briggs, A.M. Paton, S.G. MacPherson, and K. Kyle, Lancet 1, 876 (1971).
9. F.O. Belzer, R.W. Reed, J.P. Pryor, S.L. Kountz, and J.E. Dunphy, Surg., Gynecol. Obstet. 130, 467 (1970).
10. W.M. Bennett, C.H. Beck, H.H. Young, and P.S. Russell, Arch. Surg. 101, 453 (1970).
11. S.E. Bergentz, R. Olander, F. Kissmeyer-Nielsen, T.S. Olsen, and B. Hood, Scand. J. Urol. Nephrol. 4, 143 (1970).
12. O.S. Better, G.G. Alroy, C. Chaimowitz, and I. Sisman, Lancet 1, 110 (1970).
13. M.D. Blaufox, A.E. Birbari, T.B. Hickler, and J.P. Merrill, N. Engl. J. Med. 275, 1165 (1966).
14. M.D. Blaufox, E.J. Lewis, P. Jagger, D. Lauler, R. Hickler, and J.P. Merrill N. Engl. J. Med. 280, 62 (1969).
15. C.F. Bolton, M.A. Baltzan, and R.B. Batlzan, N. Engl. J. Med. 284, 1170 (1971).
16. W.E. Braun, N. Engl. J. Med. 280, 1303 (1969).
17. J.F. Bravo, J.J. Herman, and C.J. Smyth, Ann. Intern. Med. 66, 87 (1967).
18. N.S. Brickner, E. Statopolsky, E. Reiss, and L. V. Avioli, Arch. Intern. Med. 123, 543 (1969).
19. R.Y. Calne, Lancet 1, 417 (1960).
20. R.Y. Calne, Brit. Med. J. 2, 565 (1969).
21. P.P. Carbone, S.M. Sabesin, H. Sidrausky, and E. Frei, III, Ann. Intern. Med. 60, 556 (1964).
22. J. Caseley, V.K. Moses, E.A. Lichter and O. Jonasson, Transplant. Proc. 3, 365 (1971).
22a. B.O. Cerilli, Personal communication (1971).
23. S.E. Clarke, J.A. Kennedy, J.C. Hewitt, J. McEvoy, M.B. McGeown, and S.D. Nelson, Brit. Med. J. 1, 154 (1970).
24. G.M. Collins, M. Bravo-Shugarman, and P.I. Terasaki, Lancet 2, 1219 (1969).
25. L.G. Coolste, H. Bostrome, G. Magnusson, G. Skogsberg, and B. Werner, Scand. J. Urol. Nephrol. 5, 80 (1971).

26. J.E. Craighead, J.B. Hanshaw, and C.B. Carpenter, J. Amer. Med. Ass. 201, 99 (1957).
27. J. Dausset, and J. Hors, Transplant. Proc. 3, 1004 (1971).
28. J.B. Dossetor, S.M. Sweig, S. Treves, and W.M. Ross, Can. Med. Ass. J. 102, 1373 (1970).
29. S.B. Feinberg, R.C. Lester, and B.A. Burke, J. Radiol. 76, 594 (1961).
30. C.H. Fellner, and S.H. Schwartz, N. Eng. J. Med. 284, 583 (1971)
31. H. Festenstein, R.T.D. Oliver, A. Hyams, J.R. Moorhead, A.J. Pirrie, G.C. Pegrum, and I.C. Balfour, Lancet 2, 389 (1969).
32. J.E. Figueroa, L.M. Cortez, P.T. DeCamp, and J. L. Ochsner, Brit. Med. J. 1, 288 (1971).
33. R.N. Fine, R.M. Korsch, Q. Stiles, H. Riddell, H.H. Edelbrock, L.P. Brennan, C.M. Grushkin, and E. Lieberman, J. Pediat. 76, 347 (1970).
34. J.C. Fish, H.E. Sarles, A.R. Reemers, K.R.T. Tyson, C.O. Canales, G.A. Beathard, M. Fukushima, S.E. Ritzmann, and W.C. Levin, Surg., Gynecol. Obstet. 129, 777 (1969).
35. E.W.L. Fletcher, J.W. Lecky, and H.C. Gonick, Clin. Radiol. 21, 144 (1970).
36. H. Gewurz, A.W. Moberg, D. Johnson, R.L. Simmons, and J.S. Najarian, Transplant Proc. 3, 747 (1971).
37. H. Gewurz, A.W. Moberg, R.L. Simmons, R.A. Good, R.J. Pickering, and J.S. Najarian, Int. Arch. Allergy Appl. Immunol. 39, 210 (1970).
38. H. Gewurz, A.W. Moberg, R.L. Simmons, R. Soll, B. Pollara, and J.S. Najarian, Int. Arch. Allergy Appl. Immunol. 39, 113 (1970)
39. R.J. Glossock, D. Feldman, E.S. Reynolds, G.J. Dammin, and J.P. Merrill, Medicine (Baltimore) 47, 411 (1968).
40. B. Goldberg, S.R. Lynch, H.I. Goldman, A.J. Meyers, J.A. Myburgh, I. Cohen, and K.I. Furman, S. Amer. Med. J. 44, 699 (1970).
41. L.L. Gonzalez, L. Martin, C.D. West, R. Spitzer, and P. McEnery, Arch. Surg. 101, 232 (1970).

42. J.A. Greene, Jr., A.J. Vander, and R.S. Kowal-
    czyk, J. Lab. Clin. Med. 71, 586 (1968).
43. M. Gross, and C.A. Moore, J. Urol. 103, 612
    (1970).
44. K. Guerrier, D.J., Albert, and L. Persky, Arch.
    Surg. 103, 63 (1971).
45. A.Z. Gyory, J.H. Stewart, C.R.P. George, D.J.
    Tiller, and K.D G. Edwards, Quart. J. Med. 38,
    231, (1969).
46. C.G. Halgrimson, F.T. Rapaport, P.I. Terasaki,
    K.A. Porter, G. Andres, I. Penn, C.W. Putnam,
    and T.E. Starzl, Transplant Proc. 3, 140 (1971).
47. C.G. Halgrimson, C.B. Wilson, F.J. Dixon,
    I. Penn, J.T. Anderson, D.A. Ogden, and T.E.
    Starzl, Arch. Surg. 103, 283 (1971).
48. M.C. Hall, S.M. Elmore, R.W. Bright, J.C.
    Pierce, and D.M. Hume, J. Amer. Med. Ass. 208,
    1825 (1969).
49. J. Hamburger and J. Crosnier, In "Human Trans-
    plantation"(F.T. Rapaport and J. Dausset, eds.)
    p. 37. Grune & Stratton, New York, 1968.
50. J. Hamburger, J. Crosnier, B. Descamps, and D.
    Rowinska, Transplant. Proc. 3, 260 (1971).
51. H.E. Hansen and A. Sell, Acta Med. Scand. 188,
    205 (1970).
52. Harvard Medical School Committee, J. Amer. Med.
    Ass. 205, 337 (1968).
53. W.F. Heale, P.J. Morris, R.C. Bennett, P.J. Mor-
    tensen, and A. Ting, Med. J. Aust. 2, 382 (1969).
54. L.W. Henderson, K.D. Nolph, J.B. Puschett, and
    M. Goldberg, N. Engl. J. Med. 278, 467 (1968).
55. G. Hermann, V. Zuhlke, and P. Faul, Eur. Surg.
    Res. 2, 55 (1970).
56. R.B. Hill, B.E. Dahrling, T.E. Starzl, and D.
    Rifkind, Amer. J. Med. 42, 327 (1967).
57. C.A. Hubay, D. Gonzalez-Barcena, L. Klein, V.
    Frankel, R.E. Eckel, and O.H. Pearson, Arch.
    Surg. 101, 181 (1970).
58. D.M. Hume, H.M. Lee, G.M. Williams, H.J.O. White,
    J. Ferre, J.S. Wolf, G.R. Provt, Jr., M. Slapak,
    J. O'Brien, G.J. Kilpatrick, H.M. Rauffman, Jr.

and R.J. Cleveland, Ann. Surg. 164, 352 (1966).

59. D.M. Hume, J.P. Merrill, B.F. Miller, and G.W. Thorn, J. Clin. Invest. 34, 327 (1955).

60. T.J. Imray, and E. Gedgaudas, Radiology 95, 653 (1970).

61. R. Irby, and D.M. Hume, Clin. Orthop. Related Res. 57, 101 (1968).

62. M. Jeannet, A. DeWeck, P.C. Frei, P. Grob, and G. Thiel, Helv. Med. Acta 35, 239 (1969-1970).

63. J.W. Johnson, R.S. Hattner, C.L. Hampers, D.S. Bernstein, J.P. Merrill, and L.M. Sherwood, J. Amer. Med. Ass. 215, 478 (1971).

64. O. Jonasson, E.A. Lichter, W.M. Hamby, R.D. Smith, C.L. Gantt, and Nyhus, L.M. Arch. Surg. 101, 219 (1970).

65. P. Juul-Jensen, "Criteria of Brain Death: Selection Donors for Transplantation." Munksgaard, Copenhagen, 1970.

66. H.M. Kauffman, Jr., R.J. Cleveland, J.J. Dwyer, H.M. Lee, and D.M. Hume, Surg., Gynecol. Obstet. 120, 49 (1965).

67. W.D. Kelly, F.K. Merkel, and C. Markland, Lancet 1, 222 (1966).

68. J.W. Kilman, C. Ahn, N.C. Andrews, and K. Klassen, J. Thorac. Cardiov. Surg. 57, 642 (1969).

69. P. Kincaid-Smith, Lancet 2, 849 (1967).

70. P. Kincaid-Smith, Lancet 2, 920 (1969).

71. P. Kincaid-Smith, P.J. Morris, B.M. Saker, A. Ting, and V.C. Marshall, Lancet 2, 748 (1968).

72. F. Kissmeyer-Nielsen, S. Olsen, V.P. Petersen, O. Fjelborg, Lancet 2, 662 (1966).

73. B. Kohler, Acta Chir. Scand. 91, Suppl. 94, 1 (1944).

74. M.H. Koppel, J.W. Coburn, M.M. Mims, H. Goldstein, J.D. Boyle, and M.E. Rubine, N. Engl. J. Med. 280, 1367 (1969).

75. S.L. Kountz, and R. Cohn, Lancet 1, 338 (1969).

76. S.L. Kountz, H.A. Perkins, R. Payne, and F.O. Belzer, Transplant. Proc. 2, 427, (1970).

77. S.L. Kountz, L.E. Truex-Earley, and F.O. Belzer,

Circulation 41, 217 (1970).
78. G.W. Leadbetter, A.P. Monaco, and P.S. Russell, Surg., Gynecol. Obstet. 123, 839 (1966).
79. D.A. Leigh, Brit. J. Urol. 41, 406 (1969).
80. D.H. Lewis, S.-E.Bergentz, U. Brunius,H. Ekman, L.-E. Gelin, and B. Hood, Scand. J. Urol. Nephrol. 2, 36 (1968).
81. B.S. Linn, P. Portal, and G.B. Snyder, Life Sci. 6, 1945 (1967).
82. M.K. Loken, R.E. Linnemann, and G.S. Kush, Radiology 93, 85 (1969).
83. Z.J. Lucas, N. Coplon, R. Kempsom, and R. Cohn, Transplantation 10, 522 (1970).
84. Z.J. Lucas, J.M. Palmer, R. Payne, S.L. Kountz, and R.B. Cohn, Arch. Surg. 100, 113 (1970).
85. G.H. Malek, and W.A. Kisken, Amer. J. Surg. 119, 334, (1970).
86. J.A. Mannick, R.C. Davis, S.R. Cooperband, A.H. Glasgow, L.F. Williams, J.T. Harrington, T. Cavallo, G.W. Schmitt, B.A. Idelson, C.A. Olsson, and D.C. Nabseth, N. Engl. J. Med. 284, 1109 (1971).
87. D.C. Martin, Arch. Surg. 99, 474 (1969).
88. D.C. Martin, M.M. Mims, J.J. Kaufman, and W.E. Goodwin, J. Urol. 101, 680 (1969).
89. D.A. McIntosh, J.J. McPhaul, Jr., E.W. Peterson, J.S. Harvin, J.R. Smith, F.E. Cook, Jr., and J.W. Humphreys, Jr.,J. Amer. Med. Ass. 192, 1171 (1965).
90. C.F. McKhann, Transplantation 8, 209 (1969).
91. Medawar, P.B. J. Anat. 78, 176 (1944).
92. I.R. Merkatz, G.H. Schwartz, D.S. David, K.H. Stenzel, R.R. Riggio, and J.C. Whitsell, J. Amer. Med. Ass. 216, 1749 (1971).
93. J.P. Merrill, Transplant. Proc. 3, 287 (1971).
94. A.W. Moberg, H. Gewurz, R.L. Simmons, and J.S. Najarian, Lancet 2, 214 (1970).
95. A. Mohandas, and S.N. Chou, J. Neurosurg. 35, 211 (1971).
96. J.Z. Montgomerie, D.M.O. Becroft, M.C. Croxson, P.B. Doak, and J.D.K. North, Lancet 2, 867

(1969).

97. T.C. Moore, Surg., Gynecol. Obstet. 133, 75 (1971).

98. T.C. Moore, and D.M. Hume, Ann. Surg. 170, 1 (1969).

99. G.P. Murphy, E.A. Mirand, and J. Grace, Ann. Surg. 170, 581 (1969).

100. J.E. Murray, J.P. Merrill, and J.H. Harrison, Surg. Forum 6, 432 (1955).

101. J.A. Myburgh, B. Goldberg, A.M. Meyers, P.J.P. van Blerk, L. Gecelter, C.J. Mieny, S. Browde, M. Shapiro, A. Zoutendyk, and C.G. Anderson, Brit. Med. J. 3, 670 (1970).

102. J.S. Najarian, P.P. Gulyassy, R.J. Stoney, G. Duffy, and P. Braunstein, Ann. Surg. 164, 398 (1966).

103. J.S. Najarian, R.L. Simmons, H. Gewurz, A.W. Moberg, F.K. Merkel, and G.E. Moore, Fed. Proc., Fed. Amer. Soc. Exp. Biol. 29, 197 (1970).

104. J.S. Najarian, R.L. Simmons, C.M. Kjellstrand, R. Vernier, and A. Michaels, Ann. Surg. (1972) (in press).

105. Ninth Report of the Human Renal Transplantation Registry. Prepared by the Advisory Committee to the Human Renal Transplant Registry. J. Amer. Med. Ass. 220, 253 (1972).

106. R.E. Nobel, J.S. Najarian, and H.D. Brainerd, Proc. Soc. Exp. Biol. Med. 120, 737 (1965).

107. C.A. Olsson, J.A. Mannick, G.W. Schmitt, B.A. Idelson, L.F. Williams, J. Lemann, J.T. Harrington, and D.C. Nabseth, Amer. J. Surg. 121, 467 (1971).

108. B.S. Ooi, and P. Kincaid-Smith, Med. J. Aust. 2, 667 (1970).

109. N.G.M. Orie, G.A. DeVries, and A. Kikstra, Amer. Rev. Resp. Dis. 82, 649 (1960).

110. G. Pappas, G. Schroter, L. Brettschneider, I. Penn, and T. Starzl, J. Thorac. Cardiov. Surg. 59, 882 (1970).

111. J.R. Parker, F.G. Ellis, J.S. Cameron, and C.S. Ogg, Proc. Eur. Dialysis Transplant. Ass. 7,

331 (1970).
112. A. Pasternack, Lancet 2, 82 (1968).
113. J.E. Payne, B.G. Storey, J.H. Rogers, J. May, and A.G.R. Sheil, Med. J. Aust. 1, 274 (1971).
114. I. Penn, L. Brettschneider, K. Simpson, A. Martin, and T. Starzl, Arch. Surg. 100, 61 (1970).
115. I. Penn, C.G. Halgrimson, D. Ogden, and T. Starzl, Arch. Surg. 101, 226 (1970).
116. I. Penn, E. Makowski, W. Droegemueller, C.G. Halgrimson, and T. Starzl, J. Amer. Med. Ass. 216, 1755 (1971).
117. J.C. Pierce, and D.M. Hume, Surg., Gynecol. Obstet. 127, 1300 (1968).
118. J.C. Pierce, and D.M. Hume, Transplant, Proc. 3, 127 (1971).
119. K.A. Porter, J.B. Dosseter, T.L. Marchioro, W.S. Peart, J.M. Randall, T.E. Starzl, and P.I. Terasaki, Lab. Invest. 16, 153 (1967).
120. F.T. Rapaport, A.S. Markowitz, and R.T. McCluskey, J. Exp. Med. 129, 623 (1969).
121. F.T. Rapaport, R.T. McCluskey, T. Hanaoka, and T. Shimada, Transplant. Proc. 1, 981 (1969).
122. W.P. Reed, Z.J. Lucas, and R. Cohn, Lancet 1, 747 (1970).
123. W.P. Reed, Z.J. Lucas, R. Kempson, and R. Cohn, Transplant. Proc. 3, 343 (1971).
124. D. Rifkind, J. Lab. Clin. Med. 68, 463 (1966).
125. D. Rifkind, T.D. Faris, and R.B. Hill, Jr., Ann. Intern. Med. 65, 943 (1966).
126. D. Rifkind, N. Goodman, and R.B. Hill, Jr., Ann. Intern. Med. 66, 116 (1967).
127. D. Rifkind, T.L. Marchioro, S.A. Schneck, and R.B. Hill, Jr., Amer. J. Med. 43, 28 (1967).
128. D. Rifkind, T.E. Starzl, T.L. Marchioro, W.R. Waddell, D.T. Rowlands, and R.B. Hill, Jr., J. Amer. Med. Ass. 189, 808 (1964).
129. R. Rock, W. Rosenau, and J.S. Najarian, Surg., Gynecol. Obstet. 125, 289 (1967).
130. S.M. Rosen, N.K. Hollenberg, J.B. Dealy, and J.P. Merrill, Clin. Sci. 34, 287 (1968).

131. W. Rosenau, J.C. Lee, and J.S. Najarian, Surg., Gynecol. Obstet. 128, 62 (1969).
132. J.A. Ross, E. Samuel, and D.R. Millar, Brit. J. Urol. 33, 478 (1961).
133. D.T. Rowlands, P.M. Burkholder, E.H. Bossen, and H.H. Lin, Amer. J. Pathol. 61, 177 (1970).
134. J.R. Salaman, Brit. Med. J. 1, 232 (1971).
135. D. Sampson, Lancet 2, 976 (1969).
136. S.A. Schneck, and I. Penn, Arch. Neurol. 22, 225 (1970).
137. R.S. Schwab, F. Potts, and A. Bonazzi, Electro-encephalogr. Clin. Neurophysiol.15, 147 (1963).
138. R. Schwartz, and W. Dameshek, Nature (London) 183, 1682 (1959).
139. I.H. Shehadeh, C.B. Carpenter, C.H. Monterio et al., Arch. Intern. Med. 125, 850 (1970).
140. J. Shillito, Jr., N. Engl. J. Med. 281, 1071 (1969).
141. R.G. Simmons, K. Hickey, C.M. Kjellstrand, and R.L. Simmons, J. Amer. Med. Ass. 215, 909 (1971).
142. R.L. Simmons, W.D. Kelly, M.B. Tallent, and J. S. Najarian, N. Engl. J. Med. 283, 190 (1970).
143. R.L. Simmons, C.S. Kjellstrand, T.J. Busel-meier, and J.S. Najarian, Arch. Surg. 103, 290 (1971).
144. R.L. Simmons, C.M. Kjellstrand, and J.S. Najarian, In "Critical Surgical Illness" (J.E. Hardy, ed.), p. 559. Saunders, Phila-delphia, Pennsylvania, 1971.
145. R.L. Simmons, A.W. Moberg, H. Gewurz, R. Soll, and J.S. Najarian, Transplant. Proc. 3, 745 (1971).
146. R.L. Simmons, A.W. Moberg, H. Gewurz, R. Soll, M.B. Tallent, and J.S. Najarian, Surgery 68, 62 (1970).
147. R.L. Simmons, and J.S. Najarian, Kidney 4, 1 (1971).
148. R.L. Simmons, A.J. Ozerkis, and R.J. Hoehn, Science 160, 1127 (1968).
149. R.L. Simmons, M.B. Tallent, C.M. Kjellstrand,

and J.S. Najarian, Amer. J. Surg. 119, 553
(1970).

150. R.L. Simmons, M.B. Tallent, C.M. Kjellstrand,
and J.S. Najarian, Surgery 68, 800 (1970).

151. R.L. Simmons, M.B. Tallent, C.M. Kjellstrand,
and J.S. Najarian, Surgery 69, 201 (1971).

152. R.L. Simmons, R. Weil, III, M.B. Tallent, C.M.
Kjellstrand, and J.S. Najarian, Transplant.
Proc. 11, 419 (1970).

153. M. Simonsen, J. Buemann, A. Gammeltoft, F.
Jensen, and K. Jorgensen, Acta Pathol. Microbiol. Scand.32, 1 (1953).

154. D.B. Skinner, M.H. Newman, and R.A. Squire,
J. Surg. Res. 10, 287 (1970).

155. W.A.B. Smellie, M. Vinik, T.A. Freed, and D.M.
Hume, Surg., Gynecol. Obstet. 127, 777 (1968).

156. T.E. Starzl, ed. "Experience in Renal Transplantation." Saunders, Philadelphia, Pennsylvania, 1964.

157. T.E. Starzl, H.J. Boehmig, H. Amemiya, C.B.
Wilson. F.J. Dixon, G.R. Giles, K.M. Simpson,
and C.G. Halgrimson, N. Engl. J. Med. 283, 383
(1970).

158. T.E. Starzl, ·C.G. Groth, C.W. Putnam, I. Penn,
C.G. Halgrimson, A. Flatmark, L. Gecelter, L.
Brettschneider, and O.G. Stonington, Ann. Surg.
172, 1 (1970).

159. T.E. Starzl, C.G. Groth, P.I. Terasaki, C.W.
Putnam, L. Brettschneider, and T.L. Marchioro,
Surg., Gynecol. Obstet. 127, 1023 (1968).

160. T.E. Starzl, C.G. Halgrimson, I. Penn, G. Mar-
tineau, G. Schrofer, H. Amemiya, C.W. Putman,
and C.G. Groth, Lancet 2, 70 (1971).

161. T.E. Starzl, R.A. Lerner, F.J. Dixon, C.G.
Groth, L. Brettschneider, and P.I. Terasaki,
N. Engl. J. Med. 278, 642 (1968).

162. T.E. Starzl, T.L. Marchioro, V. Zuhlke, and L.
Brettschneider, Med. Times (Port Wash., N.Y.)
95, 196 (1967).

163. T.E. Starzl, K.A. Porter, G. Andres, C.G. Groth,
C.W. Putnam, I. Penn, C.G. Halgrimson, S.J.

Starkie, and L. Brettschneider, <u>Clin. Exp.</u>
<u>Immunol</u>. <u>6</u>, 803 (1970).

164. T.E. Starzl, K.A. Porter, G. Andres, C.G. Halgrimson, R. Hurwitz, G. Giles, P.I. Terasaki,
I. Penn, G.T. Schroter, J. Lilly, S.J. Starkie,
and C.W. Putnam, <u>Ann. Surg</u>. <u>172</u>, 437 (1970).

165. L.E. Stevens, A. Bloomer, G.D. Lower, R. Mad-
dock, and K. Reemtsma, <u>Ann. Surg</u>. <u>168</u>, 578
(1969).

166. J.H. Stewart, J.R. Johnson, A.M. Sharp, A.G.R.
Sheil, K.M. Wyatt, and J.M. Johnston, <u>Lancet 1</u>,
176 (1969).

167. D.L. Stickel, H.F. Seigler, D.B. Amos, F.E.
Ward, J.C. Gunnells, A.R. Price, and E.E.
Anderson, <u>Ann. Surg</u>. <u>172</u>, 160 (1970).

168. D. Sutherland, R.S. Frech, R. Weil, J.S. Najarian, and R.L. Simmons, <u>Surgery</u> (1972)(in press).

169. J.D. Swales, and D.B. Evans, <u>Brit. Med. J</u>. <u>2</u>,
80 (1969).

170. M.B. Tallent, R.L. Simmons, and J.S. Najarian,
<u>J. Amer. Med. Ass</u>. <u>211</u>, 1854 (1970).

171. M.B. Tallent, R.L. Simmons, and J.S. Najarian,
<u>Amer. J. Obstet. Gynecol</u>. <u>109</u>, 663 (1971).

172. D. Tassel, and M.N. Modoff, <u>J. Amer. Med. Ass</u>.
<u>206</u>, 830 (1968).

173. P.I. Terasaki, M. Kreisler, and R.M. Mickey,
<u>Postgrad Med. J</u>. <u>47</u>, 89 (1971).

174. P.I. Terasaki, and M.R. Mickey, <u>Transplant</u>.
<u>Proc</u>. <u>3</u>, 1057 (1971).

175. N.L. Tilney, and J.E. Murray, <u>Transplantation</u>
<u>5</u>, 1204 (1967).

176. J. Trager, J.L. Touraine, D. Dries, and F.
Berthoux, <u>Transplant. Proc</u>. <u>3</u>, 749 (1971).

177. W.S. Tunner, E.I. Goldsmith, and J.C. Whitesell,
<u>J. Urol</u>. <u>105</u>, 18 (1971).

178. J.J. van Rood, J. Freudenberg, A. van Leeuwen,
H.M.A. Schippers, R. Zweerus, and J.L. Terpstra,
<u>Transplant. Proc</u>. <u>3</u>, 933 (1971).

179. E. Weeke, and S.F. Sorensen, <u>Transplant. Proc</u>.
<u>3</u>, 387 (1971).

180. R. Weil, III, and R.L. Simmons, <u>Ann. Surg</u>. <u>167</u>,

239 (1968).
181. R. Weil, III, R.L. Simmons, M.B. Tallent, R.C. Lillehei, C.M. Kjellstrand, and J.S. Najarian, Ann. Surg. 174, 154 (1971).
182. T.H. West,J.G. Turcotte, and A. Vander, J. Lab. Clin. Med. 73, 564 (1969).
183. N.G. Westberg, R.L. Simmons, L. Raij, A.W. Moberg, C.M. Kjellstrand, and J.S. Najarian, Transplantation
184. R. Wilbrandt, K.S.K. Tung, S.D. Deodhar, S. Nakamoto, and W.J. Kolff, Amer. J. Clin. Pathol. 51, 15 (1969).
185. G.M. Williams, B. dePlanque, R. Lower, and D. Hume. Ann. Surg. 170, 603 (1969).
186. G.M. Williams, D.M. Hume, R.P. Hudson, P.J. Morris, K. Kano, and F. Milgrom, N. Engl. J. Med. 279, 611 (1968).
187. G.M. Williams, H.M. Lee, and D.M. Hume, Transplant. Proc. 1, 262 (1969).
188. G.M. Williams, H.J. White, and D.M. Hume, Transplantation 51, Suppl., 837 (1967).
189. R.E. Wilson, E.B. Hager, C.L. Hampers et al. N. Engl. J. Med. 278, 479 (1968).
190. V.A. Wonham, H.J. Winn, and P.S. Russell, N. Engl. J. Med. 284, 509 (1971).
191. D.J. Yashphe, Isr. J. Med. Sci. 7, 90 (1971).
192. C.F. Zukoski, D.A. Killen, E. Ginn, B. Matter, D.P. Lucas, and H.F. Seigler, Transplantation 9, 71 (1970).
193. C.F. Zukoski, H.M. Lee, and D.M. Hume, Surg. Forum 11, 470 (1960).

Table 1

Workup of Potential Recipients
of Renal Transplantation

General
    History and physical examination
    Chest x ray
    EKG
    Electrophoresis
    (FBS)

Hematological
    RBC
    WBC
    Indices
    Platelet count
    Bleeding-clotting time
    PT, PTT, TT

"Allergic" potentially complicating
    Electrophoresis
    LE test
    FANA
    Complement
    ASO
    Rheumatoid factor
    Antiglomerular basement antibodies

Renal
    Flat plate of abdomen (kidney size) (Tomography)
    Creatinine clearance
    24 hour protein excretion
    (Electrophoresis/urine, protein excretion
        selectivity)
    Electrolyte status in blood
    (Electrolyte status in urine)
    Urinalysis x 3
    Urine culture x 3
    Renal biopsy (nephrectomy specimen)

Table 1, continued

Signs of hyperparathyroidism
    Bone x ray (hands, skull, clavical, lamina dura)
    Ca, PO_4, Mg, alkaline phosphatase

Hypertensive workup
    Chest x ray (heart size)
    EKG
    Ophthalmic examination
    Serial blood pressure

Urologic evaluation
    Voiding cystogram
    (Retrograde pyelography)
    (Cystometrography)
    (Bladder biopsy)
    (Bladder stimulation)

Upper gastrointestinal x ray

(Colon x ray)

Typing
    ABO
    Blood pedigree
    Tissue typing including serial cytotoxic
        antibody determinations

(Pulmonary function studies)

Infectious workup
    Chest x ray
    (PPD-fungal skin tests)
    Urine culture
    Blood culture
    Skin-nose-throat culture
    Feces culture
    (Sinus-teeth x-ray-ENT consultation)

Financial-Social Rehabilitation
    (Psychological-psychiatric)

Table 2

Protocol for Living Related Donor Workup

---

1. History and physical examination

2. Hematology
    Hematocrit, leukocyte count, differential
    count, platelet count

3. Coagulation
    Prothrombin time, partial thromboplastin
    time, thrombin time

4. Chemistry
    Serum Na^+, K^+, Cl^-, CO^{2-}, SGOT, bilirubin,
    uric acid, Ca^{2+}, P, BUN, creatinine, fasting
    blood sugar, glucose tolerance test

5. Urine
    Urinalysis, 24 hour urine for creatinine
    clearance

6. Microbiology
    Clean catch urine culture x 2

7. Immunology
    Blood type (major and minor), tissue typing,
    leukocyte cross match for recipient anti-
    donor and leukocyte antibodies. VDRL;
    Australian antigen

8. x ray
    Chest x ray: PA and lateral, intravenous
    pyologram, renal arteriograms

9. Isotope
    Bilateral renogram

10. Electrocardiogram

Table 3

142 Complications in 112 (47%) of 238
Living Related Kidney Donors[1]

Complication	Number of cases
Atelectasis or pneumonitis or both	33
Small pleural effusion	12
Pneumothorax	26
Urinary retention	7
Urinary tract infection	24
Hepatic dysfunction	4
Gastric distention or intestinal ileus or both	4
Wound infection	4
Transient nerve palsies	4
Hematoma of deltoid muscle	2
Deep-vein thrombosis and possible sma small pulmonary embolus	3
Prolonged incisional pain	3
Transient hypertension	10
Transient hematuria	3
Nephrocalcinosis	1
Acute glomerulonephritis	1
Suspected acute tubular necrosis	1

[1]Data taken from Penn et al. (115).

Table 4

Prophylactic Immunosuppression for Renal
Transplantation at University of Minnesota

Antilymphoblast globulin (ALG)
1. 30 mg/kg intravenously daily for cadaver
    recipients for 2 weeks
2. 20 mg/kg intravenously daily for related
    recipients for 2 weeks

Azathioprine (Evening dose after checking leukocyte
    count)
1. Preoperative dosage is 5 mg/kg/day for 2 days
2. First and second postoperative days: 5 mg/kg
3. Third through sixth postoperative days:
    4 mg/kg
4. Seventh postoperative day: 3 mg/kg, maintain
    at 2 to 3 mg/kg
5. Adjust at all time with respect to WBC,
    platelet count, and renal function
6. Caution: Reduce dosage to 1.5 mg/kg for
    severe renal functional impairment

Prednisone
1. Related kidney
    a. 0.25 mg/kg every 6 hrs beginning 36 hrs
        prior to transplant
    b. first and second postoperative days:
        1 mg/kg/day
    c. third through sixth postoperative days:
        0.75 mg/kg/day
    d. seventh through ninth postoperative days:
        0.5 mg/kg/day
    e. reduce level slowly to achieve a main-
        tainance dose of 0.15 to 0.25 mg/kg/day

Table 4, continued

---

2. Cadaver kidney
   a. 0.5 mg/kg every 6 hrs on first 3 post-operative days (total dose 20 mg/kg)
   b. 1.5 mg/kg/day for the next 3 days
   c. 1.0 mg/kg/day for 3 days
   d. 0.75 mg/kg/day for 3 days
   e. 0.5 mg/kg/day until discharge
   f. reduce dose slowly to achieve a main-tainance dose of 0.3 to 0.4 mg/kg

Methylprednisone
   1. 20 mg/kg/day intravenously on evening of transplantation and on first 2 postoperative days

---

Table 5

Clinical and Laboratory Signs of Rejection[1]

Sign	Reliability[2]
Clinical manifestations	
Fever	3
Leukocytosis (imuran)	3
Malaise	4
Tenderness	4
Increase in size, induration	4
Hypertension	4
Oliguria	4
(NRF decreases Na increases OSMOL)	5
Swelling of leg, testicle	4

Table 5, continued

Urine	
Lymphocyturia	1
RBC cast	3
Proteinuria	3
(Selective)	4
Fibrin fragments	3
Lysozyme	3
Na wasting	4
Tubular acidosis	4
LDH increase	2
Blood	
Urea	3
Platelet count	?
Spontaneous lymphocyte trans- formation	?
Suppression PTH lymph, trans- formation	?
Creatinine	4
Platelet clumping	?
Complement decrease	2
LDH increase	3
Tests of Function	
Creatinine clearance	3
Arteriogram	4
Hg scan	3
Renal biopsy	3
Renogram	5
Intravenous pyelogram	3
{ 133Xe intrarenal distribution	
Blood flow	5
Radio hippuran disappearance	3

[1] Data taken from Merrill (93).

[2] Reliability in diagnosis rated on a scale 1 to 5; most reliable is 5.

Table 6

Standard Antirejection Therapy at the
University of Minnesota

Therapy

Solumedrol: 20 mg/kg/day intravenously x 3

Prednisone: 2 mg/kg x 3 days
then 1.5 mg/kg x 3 days
then 1.0 mg/kg x 3 days
thereafter reduce prednisone slowly
to a maintenance dosage

Azathioprine: regulate dose to prevent leukopenia, do not increase

Irradiate kidney transplant: 150 R every other
day for 3 doses

Adjuncts

Reinstitute antacid therapy

Reinstitute oral Nystatin (100,000 U bid) to
prevent mucosal candidasis

Reduce protein and fluid intake if renal function is significantly impaired

Table 7

Causes of Renal Recipient Death Reported
to NIH/ACS Transplant Registry
(All Transplants Through 1970)

Cause	Number of cases
Sepsis	582
Sepsis and rejection	188
Sepsis and technical	72
Sepsis and immunosuppression	28
Sepsis, rejection and technical	23
Sepsis, rejection, and immunosuppression	16
Sepsis, immunosuppression, and technical	8
Sepsis, rejection, immunosuppression, and technical	5
Immunosuppression	45
Immunosuppression and technical	8
Immunosuppression and rejection	4
Immunosuppression, rejection, and technical	2
Rejection	174
Rejection and technical	16
Technical	121
Unrelated to transplant	120
GI hemorrhage and ulceration	75
Myocardial infarction	71
Cerebro-vascular accidents	30
Tubular necrosis	21
Cardiac arrest	20
Pancreatitis	20
Pulmonary embolus	19
Diffuse vasculitis	14

Table 7, continued

Cancer	19
Unknown	239
Total deaths	1940
a. Deaths related to sepsis	922
b. Deaths related to immuno-suppression	116
c. Deaths related to rejection	428
d. Deaths related to technical factors	255

Table 8

Kidney Transplant Registry One and Two Year Survival
Related[1] and Cadaver Donors by Year of Transplant[2]

Donor type	Year of Transplant	Sample size	One year Living (%)	One year Function (%)	Two year Living (%)	Two year Function (%)
Related	1940–1966	687	64.9	60.5	59.4	54.0
	1967	306	80.0	74.7	74.8	67.8
	1968	368	83.5	76.2	80.5	71.8
	1969	362	80.0	72.0	76.1	66.2
	1970	160	88.9	76.9	88.9	76.9
Cadaver	1940–1966	721	41.1	34.7	33.7	27.3
	1967	393	56.1	43.7	48.5	36.3
	1968	623	56.1	43.9	48.6	36.1
	1969	747	65.7	52.3	59.2	44.7
	1970	462	69.1	51.1	69.1	51.1

[1]Monozygotic twins not included.

[2]Data taken from the Ninth Report of the Human Renal transplantation Registry (105).

Table 9

Calculated Patient Survival and Transplant Function
Considering Donor Source and Date of Transplant[1]

Donor type	Year of transplant	Sample size	One year		Two year	
			Living (%)	Function (%)	Living (%)	Function (%)
Cadaver	1953–1966	640	42.6	36.0	35.2	28.6
	1967	344	56.8	45.3	49.5	38.3
	1968	534	57.2	45.0	49.5	36.9
	1969	644	66.7	54.0	60.6	46.6
	1970	408	70.2	52.5		
Aunts, uncles, cousins, grand- parents	1953–1966	20	63.1	60.0	63.1	60.0
	1967	15	63.4	53.3	63.4	53.3
	1968	10	88.8	88.8	88.8	88.8
	1969	11	79.1	54.5	79.1	54.5
	1970	1	–	–		

[1]Data taken from the Ninth Report of the Human Renal Transplantation Registry (105).

273

Table 10

Effect of Primary Renal Disease on Results of
Renal Transplantation: Cadaver Donor Only[1]

Disease	Sample size	One year Living (%)	One year Function (%)	Two year Living (%)	Two year Function (%)
Glomerulonephritis	1,447	56.7	45.0	48.6	36.8
Pyelonephritis	404	57.6	45.4	52.2	39.0
Polycystic kidneys	166	63.2	52.6	54.2	44.1
Malignant hypertension	82	42.7	36.6	40.1	34.3
Familial nephritis	32	71.0	60.4	59.6	50.7
Congenital, non-obstructive	30	54.4	46.6	54.4	46.6
CA of kidney	9	50.4	44.4	37.8	33.3
Lupus nephritis	5	57.1	40.0	57.1	40.0
Diabetic glomerulo-sclerosis	3	66.6	66.6	22.2	–

[1]Data from the Ninth Report of the Human Renal Transplantation Registry (105).

Table 11

Results of Renal Transplantation Considering
Donor Sources and Recipient Ages[1]

Donor type	Recipient age group	Sample size	One year		Two year	
			Living (%)	Function (%)	Living (%)	Function (%)
Sibling	6-10	1	100.0	100.0	100.0	100.0
	11-20	68	87.4	84.6	83.3	76.7
	21-30	267	83.3	77.1	77.0	70.2
	31-40	285	82.1	75.5	78.6	70.9
	41-50	132	75.8	66.7	65.1	56.3
	51-60	16	65.0	65.0	53.1	53.1
Parent	0-5	6	30.0	30.0	30.0	30.0
	6-10	51	78.3	69.5	75.3	66.9
	11-20	415	73.6	67.1	67.8	58.9
	21-30	326	70.8	65.3	66.9	59.8
	31-40	105	59.9	54.8	58.5	53.6

Table 11, continued

41–50	10	75.0	58.2	75.0	58.2
51–60	1	—	—	—	—
Cadaver					
0–5	30	51.3	40.0	44.5	25.8
6–10	40	52.7	42.4	45.2	36.3
11–20	316	65.0	48.8	58.2	40.9
21–30	659	60.6	47.7	53.8	40.5
31–40	725	58.1	47.3	49.7	38.9
41–50	576	51.8	43.1	45.0	36.3
51–60	147	48.6	39.8	36.5	27.7
61–99	7	18.1	18.1	18.1	18.1

[1]Data from the Ninth Report of the Human Renal Transplantation Registry (105).

Table 12

Results of Renal Transplantation: Comparison of Results of Multiple Transplants

Transplant number	Year of transplant	Sample size	One year		Two year	
			Living (%)	Function (%)	Living (%)	Function (%)
1	1953-1966	1488	52.8	47.1	46.8	40.7
	1967	656	68.0	58.6	61.8	51.5
	1968	906	68.7	58.1	63.0	51.5
	1969	1010	71.6	60.3	66.4	53.6
	1970	567	75.9	59.3		
2	1953-1966	113	37.4	32.3	28.7	24.0
	1967	55	63.9	43.6	55.6	34.5
	1968	96	53.6	40.7	47.2	33.7
	1969	100	59.2	43.7	49.8	34.7
	1970	52	64.3	50.3		
3	1953-1966	6	33.3	33.3	33.3	33.3
	1967	7	24.7	14.2	24.7	14.2
	1968	9	39.2	22.2	39.2	22.2
	1969	12	50.1	28.3	50.1	28.3
	1970	5	80.0	20.0	—	

[1]Data from the Ninth Report of the Human Renal Transplantation Registry (105).

277

Table 13

Results of Renal Transplantation:
Results in Second Grafting Following Failure of a First Graft[1]

Donor relationship	Sample size	One year		Two year	
		Living(%)	Function(%)	Living(%)	Function(%)
Transplant 1: related Transplant 2: related	23	90.3	81.4	84.1	70.5
Transplant 1: related Transplant 2: cadaver	87	51.3	37.3	43.1	28.7
Transplant 1: cadaver Transplant 2 related	30	70.0	62.9	65.6	58.9
Transplant 1: cadaver Transplant 2: cadaver	234	46.7	35.1	37.2	25.9

[1]Data from the Ninth Report of the Human Renal Transplant Registry (105).

Table 14

Rehabilitation after Renal Transplantation at the University of Minnesota

Adults

Condition of patient	Time posttransplant (months)			
	0-3	3-6	6-12	12+
Well and doing most things I did before illness	4=50%	4=50%	19=76%	39=78%
Well but not performing many customary activities	4=50%	2=25%	5=20%	6=12%
Up most of the day but quite restricted in activity	0	2=25%	1= 4%	4= 8%
Confined to a wheelchair or to bed	0	0	0	1= 2%
	n=8	n=8	n=25	n=50

Children

Condition of patient	Time posttransplant (months)			
	0-3	3-6	6-12	12+
Well and doing most things I did before illness	0	3=100%	4=80%	17=94%
Well but not performing many customary activities	0	0	1=20%	1= 5%
Up most of the day but quite restricted in activity	0	0	0	0
Confined to a wheelchair or to bed	0	0	0	0
	n=0	n=3	n=5	n=18

IMMUNE SUPPRESSION AND THE INCIDENCE OF MALIGNANCY

Charles F. McKhann

Departments of Surgery and Microbiology
University of Minnesota
Minneapolis, Minnesota

Several techniques can be used to suppress the
general immune response, including whole body irradiation, thymectomy, the administration of steroids and
immunosuppressive drugs, and, more recently, the use
of antilymphocyte globulin. All of these have been
applied to tumor systems and all have indicated that
a normal intact immune response is of value in controlling the development and growth of malignancy.
In immunologically depleted animals, carcinogen-
induced tumors occur in larger numbers, after shorter
latent periods, and with an accelerated growth rate,
and virus-induced tumors occur earlier and grow more
rapidly.

"Experiments in nature" have provided valuable
information about many biological systems that normally function almost too perfectly to be analyzed.
The study of disease has often provided the key to
understanding normal function. In attempts to assign
to the immune system the role of a natural defense
mechanism against malignancy, immunologic deficiency
diseases of man have also provided supporting evidence. Among the other fates befalling a child with
diseases of immunologic deficiency is the markedly
increased likelihood of malignancy, particularly of
the reticuloendothelial system. The incidence of
leukemia, lymphoma, reticulum cell sarcoma, etc. in
children with the acquired type of hypogammaglobulinemia, ataxic telangiectasia, and the Wiscott-Aldrich
Syndrome is far higher than that in the normal child

of the same age (Table I)(1).

Deliberate suppression of the immune response in order to facilitate organ transplantation provides another group of patients for clinical evaluation of the incidence of malignancy. Here again, the number of tumors encountered is far above that of the same age adjusted population. The tumors so far encountered are frequently of the reticular endothelial system, particularly reticulum cell sarcoma (2,3). One interpretation is that this tumor ordinarily appears frequently in the normal population but is usually suppressed by the normal immune response. It must be noted, however, that the agents used to suppress the immune response, including Imuran, Prednisone, actinomycin D, and antilymphocyte globulin, all have the reticuloendothelial system as their primary target. Any toxicity of these materials that directly causes the production of malignant cells is expected to produce tumors of this system. At the present time, the incidence of malignancy is far too low to be of concern for the patient who needs organ transplantation and no single agent can be singled out as being more frequently associated with malignancy than any other.

References

1. Gatti, R.A., and Good, R.A. Cancer 28, 89 (1971).
2. McKhann, C.F. Transplantation 8, 209 (1969).
3. Penn, I. Personal communication.

Table I

Incidence of Primary Malignancy in Immunologic
Deficiency Diseases and Renal Transplant Patients

Disease	Incidence of Malignancy	Type of Malignancy
Wiscott-Aldrich Syndrome [a]	8/52 (15%)	lymphoreticular sarcoma
Ataxic relangiectasia [a]	15/150 (10%)	lymphoma, lymphoreticular sarcoma, reticulum cell sarcoma, Hodgkin's disease, cancer.
Brutons agammaglobulinemia [a]	5/50 (10%)	acute lymphatic leukemia
Renal transplant patients	37/37,000 (1.0%)	reticulum cell sarcoma, lymphoma, carcinoma
Normal children (2-10 years)	7/100,000	
Normal young adults	22/100,000	

[a] Estimates made by Robert Good, M.D. and Richard Gatti, M.D., Department of Pediatrics, University of Minnesota (Review in Reference 1)

THE BIOLOGY OF KIDNEY ALLOGRAFT TRANSPLANTATION

John E. Foker and John S. Najarian

Department of Surgery
University of Minnesota Medical School
Minneapolis, Minnesota

Kidney transplantation is becoming increasingly successful both as a treatment of severe renal disease and as a contributor to immunobiological knowledge. Transplanted kidneys have now provided over 3000 patient-years; along with this clinical benefit, however, the rejection reaction has become a relatively frequent immunological disease. Rejection, however, is not a purely one-way reaction and the transplanted kidney is capable of considerable response to it. Both the development of immunity and the biological capabilities of the kidney cells are important to the fate and performance of the grafted kidney.

KIDNEY ANTIGENICITY

An early, if not first, event in an immune reaction is the host's recognition that a tissue cell, or molecule is foreign (antigenic). Although a transplanted kidney presents many potential antigens to the recipient, cellular antigenicity is relatively confined. The main determinants are components of the cellular membranes, which in turn are thought to be composed of a mosaic of subunits (1). Whereas the as yet hypothetical subunit may range in size from a single lipoprotein molecule to a specific aggregation of several different molecules, the arrangement of antigens supports the existence of distinct groupings on the cell surface. Recent work

285

utilizing ferritin-tagged antibodies to locate antigen by electron microscopy has found them in discrete topographical areas (2). Kidney cells should prove to be structurally analogous to the leukocytes investigated in this study.

Studies in both man and the guinea pig indicate that antigens are predominantly, if not entirely, protein (3, 4). If classical antibody response is a valid analogy, then a single amino acid substitution or deletion between comparable membrane subunits in host and donor could be sufficient to produce incompatibility.

Presumably, antigens are associated with particular subunits but the structural and functional contributions made to them are unknown. The major determinant of transplantation antigenicity in man is the expression of the complex HL-A genetic locus (5). A large but uncertain number of codominant alleles compete for this site. In addition to the HL-A system, other loci control transplantation antigens, which have varying but lesser potential antigenicity (6). Both the large number of possible alterations and the complex behavior of the cistrons involved have hindered precise analysis.

Why one subunit controlled by one complex genetic locus expresses most of the antigenicity of a cell is unexplained. Less latitude for diversity may be available to other components of the membrane, and they may be relatively constant from person to person. Experimentally, determinants have been found that are antigenic to other species but not within the species of origin; they are therefore probably uniform from one individual to another (4).

Studies in the mouse have allowed the intriguing observation that, whereas both major and minor antigenic determinants are expressed on most cells, the amount can vary from cell type to cell type (7). This raises the provocative question of the functional role of these antigens. It seems unlikely that the complex antigenicity is fortuitous but it is not proven that the function is to make the individual nearly unique to aid recognition of foreign material.

Genetic diversity may not be the only factor, and the determinants of antigenicity may also be subject to phenotypic variation within a tissue population. Both the apparent incompatibility seen in exchanging skin grafts between monozygotically derived armadillo offspring and the antigenic modulation found in some tumor tissue indicates that foreignness may not always be genetic in origin (8, 9).

When applied to the kidney, antigenicity includes both transplantation and renal antigens. The extensive and incompletely fathomed transplantation antigens are of major importance in rejection. Kidney cells may not be the only source of transplantation antigens in a renal graft and a recent study indicates that the scattering of donor leukocytes present in a transplanted kidney are a potent source of antigenicity (10). In addition, components of unique kidney structures, such as the tubule cell brush border and the glomerular basement membrane, have been shown to be antigenic experimentally but their role in rejection is unknown (11-13).

ANTIGEN AVAILABILITY

Antigens in the transplanted kidney seem to be available to the host in at least two ways. Certainly an immediate consequence of kidney transplantation is the shedding of antigen. Within 10 min of transplantation, plasma from the renal vein will sensitize a third party and inhibit cytotoxic antibody (14-17). Both the antigenic quality and quantity may vary, and consequently the ability of consecutive plasma samples to immunize differs. Normal maintenance of cellular membranes may involve the inadvertent release of antigenic molecules. These membranes are increasingly being recognized as dynamic structures, and a continuous turnover of the subunits, including the antigenic determinants, is likely. The general nature of antigen release is supported by the presence of glomerular basement membrane antigen in the urine of normal individuals (18). In any case, Davies (19) has shown that antigenic molecules are not tightly bound to the cell surface and transplantation stresses may increase normal losses. The pattern observed following transplantation stresses may increase normal losses. The pattern observed following transplantation suggests both ischemia and rejection exacerbate the release, although greatly prolonged ischemia did not further increase antigen shedding, experimentally (14, 15).

The apparently inevitable release of antigen should sensitize the host whenever the recipient recognizes the foreign tissue. However, the physical state of the antigen is an unknown factor. In some experimental systems where the antigen is present in soluble form, the tendency to immunize is less than when the antigen is aggregated and easily engulfed by the phagocytic cells (20, 21). Even this distinction is not rigid, and multiple injections of whole spleen cells of the donor strain have prolonged kidney allografts in the rat (22). In both forms, antigen injections were more effective in selectively inhibiting immunity when combined with the suppressive effects of passively administered antidonor antibody. Considerable effort is now being expended on determining how blocking antibodies can be elicited by antigen injections and thus parry the rejection mechanism.

The host may not be dependent on released antigen and recognition may come from the passage of lymphocytes through the foreign kidney. Medawar (23) has postulated that the contact of circulating lymphocytes with endothelial antigen is sufficient to induce sensitization on their return to the lymph node. Experimentally, lymphocytes perfused through an allogeneic kidney tend to remain there (24). Strober and Gowans (25) found that as little as 1 hr of recycled perfusion sensitized lymphocytes and transferred greater immunity to unsensitized animals than plasma controls.

Our experiments on antigen release seemingly produced different results. The white cell effluent was far less able to transfer immunity than the plasma (14, 15). The apparent discrepancy between the two studies may be a function of experimental differences. By recycling the lymphocytes, Strober and Gowans (25) exposed them repeatedly to the antigen, and the immunogenic capacity of their plasma controls was assayed by the less efficient intravenous route. Alternatively, the possibility exists that they merely washed out the immunogenically potent donor leukocytes.

ANTIGEN PROCESSING

Upon reaching the lymph follicle, antigen is filtered out and adheres to the interdigitating surfaces of the dendritic reticular cells (26, 27). Such an exposed position presumably facilitates antigen processing and initiation of events leading to cell sensitization.

Nossal and associates (26, 27) have studied the travels of microgram quantities of ^{125}I labeled Salmonella adelaide flagellums after injection into rats. By combination electronmicrograph and radioautography, the ^{125}I was found to be taken up by both the medullary and cortical areas of lymph node follicles. In contrast to the immunogen taken up by the medullary macrophages, the immunogen in the follicular area was retained in an extracellular location for as long as 3 weeks. It was most frequently found at or near the surface of fine cellular processes, usually in the branches of dendritic reticular cells. An important finding would seem to be that the antigen-containing processes of the reticular cells often interdigitate with the equally fine processes of lymphocytes. The long residence of immunogens on these exposed positions could allow the development of immunity among the neighboring lymphocytes. Evidence of this development is the finding of transformed lymphocytes in the area.

These transformed cells are identical morphologically to lymphocytes responding to antigens in vitro. When the rats had been previously sensitized to the flagellum antigen the number of these responding cells in the cortical area was greatly increased.

Admittedly, these morphological events are the response of an experimental animal to a bacterial flagellar immunogen, but nonetheless, the events should be applicable to histocompatibility immunogens arriving at a lymph node. It is not clear, however, whether the lymph node represents a mere way station for the antigen, which happens to be structurally advantageous for the development of immunity, or whether it possesses unique conditions for essential cell-to-cell contact. The ensnarement of the immunogen on the surface of the dendritic reticular cell may only enhance the chance of contact with a receptive lymphocyte. Alternatively, the role of this cell may be more complex and may include either the physical preparation of the immunogen or a function as an inducer cell to the differentiation of the lymphocytes.

At the cellular level the production of immunity is proving to be complex. Although lymphocytes alone are the seat of immunological recognition, there is evidence that the development of immunity requires an interaction of macrophages and lymphocytes (28, 29). The role of the macrophage has not yet been precisely defined but it seems to consist of ingestion and perhaps processing of the antigens prior to contact with the lymphocytes. Schmidtke and Unanue (29) have shown uptake of antigens by the macrophage, which then retained them both within the cell and on the macrophage surface for long periods of time. The membrane-bound material was further shown to be responsible for the immunogenicity of the antigen.

Other workers have suggested that the macrophage does more than present the antigen on its surface. The macrophage may process the antigen to a molecule that is more stimulatory to the lymphocyte. Macrophages, after exposure to antigen, contain an RNA

fraction that, when incubated with lymphocytes, has
converted them into specific antibody producers (30).
The RNA is required for the activity of this preparation, but whether it is an early intermediate in the
development of immunity or a final mRNA molecule
coding for antibody is unknown. Evidence for an
mRNA component comes from Adler et al. (30), who were
able to induce antibody production with the same
allotype as the source of the RNA. This may prove to
be an mRNA for only the constant region of the antibody molecule where the allotype marker resides and
perhaps serves as an initiator or regulator. Other
evidence suggests that antigen is part of the transferred molecule (32). If this is true, then macrophages would remain impartial processors of crude
antigen while the lymphocytes specifically respond
to the antigenic portion.

Whether or not the macrophage is required in the
development of immunity may depend on the size and
composition of the antigen. Administered antigen
is easily found in macrophages but not readily
demonstrated in lymphocytes (33). However, Hans and
Johnson (34) have shown that lymphocytes in lymph
nodes can take up antigen within a few minutes of
subcutaneous injection. The eventual resolution of
the relationship will come from continued cellular
or subcellular investigation but even if the macrophage has no direct role in the development of
immunity, several observations point to functional
synergism at some level. Lymphocytes seem to be
able to transform into macrophages and both are
plentiful in a rejecting renal allograft (35).
Moreover, lymphocytes can effectively increase the
number of surrounding macrophages by producing migration inhibitory factor (MIF), a substance that
inhibits the dispersion of macrophages (36). This
enlistment may be important both in sensitization
of additional lymphocytes and graft destruction by
the voracious macrophages.

Whether or not residence in a lymph node is
required for a lymphocyte that has encountered an

antigen is unknown at this time. The lymph node may
be only an efficient waylayer of antigen and structurally advantageous for the interaction of lymphocytes and macrophages, or it may contain immobile
inducing cells necessary for lymphocyte differentiation. In the absence of evidence for the latter, it
is reasonable to consider immunity to be developed
in a number of ways and sites. Certainly, it results
when antigen arrives at the lymph node. Passage
through a transplanted kidney may also be sufficient
for lymphocyte response. Additionally, specific
sensitization may be occurring among the round cells
which infiltrate an allografted kidney. Mitoses are
common in the accumulated cells and in concert with
this proliferation the specific differentiation of
additional lymphocytes is possible.

LYMPHOCYTE RESPONSE

At the subcellular level, little is known about
the events leading to immunity. Scothorne and
McGregor (37) first recognized the lymphocyte
alterations in response to foreign tissue. Lymphocytes are transformed from cells with dense nuclei
and scant cytoplasm to larger cells with more open
nuclei and abundant cytoplasm. This nuclear change
is a morphological indication of increased RNA synthesis and the prominent nucleoli reflect the considerable production or ribosomal RNA. The cytoplasm
of these transformed cells enlarges to contain many
rosettes of free ribosomes with only a modest endoplasmic reticulum. If specialization for the immune
cell requires a well-developed endoplasmic reticulum
with many affixed ribosomes, then the transformed
cell is still immature; an immunoblast. The immunoblast can readily be found in both regional lymph
nodes and the kidney graft and morphologically resembles lymphocytes transformed by antigen in tissue
culture (38-40).

If rejection is divided arbitrarily into afferent and efferent limbs the immunoblast may represent

the crossover point. In this division, the development of immunity has the recognition and processing of antigen on the afferent side while the efferent limb produces the effector molecules. The immunoblast has received antigenic information and begun the tooling up necessary for production of molecules which will bind the antigen. The plasma cell, with its well-developed rough endoplasmic reticulum producing a specific effector, antibody, seems to result from further differentiation of the immunoblast of the B cell line derived from the bone marrow. Other pathways of differentiation are possible and the production of an antibody-like recognition molecule bound to or an integral part of the cellular membrane may result in a population of cells capable of producing cell-mediated immunity, arising from the T cell or thymic cell line.

LYMPHOCYTE PARTICIPATION IN REJECTION

The effector mechanisms in kidney rejection have not been completely defined. Even the basic mode of rejection remains controversial between cellular and humoral mechanisms. Simply, the question is whether the allograft rejection reaction is initiated by circulating antibodies or by the direct contact of specifically sensitized lymphocytes. Its resolution will come with the elucidation of the molecule the sensitized lymphocyte uses for recognition.

Experimentally, allograft immunity has been easily transferred by lymphoid cells, whereas passive transfer with sensitized serum has proven difficult (41-43). These results, although suggestive of a cell requirement, are not conclusive. Proof that the reaction is exclusively cellular is difficult and experimentally requires a restricted system. Govaerts (44) first showed that sensitized lymphoid cells cultured with kidney cells destroyed about 50% of the target cells within 48 hrs. The study has been a prototype for many subsequent experiments

293

that have confirmed the specificity of the reaction
and the apparent lack of antibody participation. In
the presence of target cells, however, the absence
of free antibody is not surprising. The cell inflic-
ting damage is morphologically similar to the immunoblast, although neither the molecule of recognition
nor the mechanism of destruction has been defined
(45).

Recognition by lymphoid cells does occur and in
the allograft kidney a perivascular infiltration is
usually present within 24 hrs and becomes increasingly prominent thereafter. By using our model of dog
allograft rejection, we have provided evidence for
recognition molecules producing this mononuclear cell
infiltration (46). In this experiment, kidneys are
sensitized by passage through a specifically immunized dog rendered severely leukopenic by irradiation. On return to the original dog, the kidneys
were promptly infiltrated by autologous leukocytes.
We interpret this as indicating that antibody-like
molecules in the sensitized dog combined with the
kidney and triggered the mononuclear portion of the
infiltrate after retransplantation. These molecules
may have been cell bound before the x radiation and
only released subsequently. The ability of sensitized plasma from nonirradiated animals to provoke
an infiltration of autologous leukocytes into both
dog and goat kidneys indicates that these factors
can be circulating freely during rejection (47, 48).

The nature of the lymphocyte recognition molecule is unknown. There is evidence that immunoglobulins are present on the cell surface. Antiallo-
typic serum will induce blast transformation in lymphocytes, suggesting that an antigen-antibody reaction has taken place on the cell surface (49). Human
lymphocytes have a decreased electrophoretic mobility
after incubation with antihuman immunoglobulin and
antigen-specific immunoglobulins have been eluted
off lymphocytes from immunized children (50, 51).
However, a portion of lymphoid cells undergoing an
immune response is capable of immunoglobulin

synthesis and may account for these phenomena. In any case, the relevance of these results to the allograft reaction is not yet clear, and the question remains whether rejection sensitization is accomplished by immunoglobulins or whether another kind of recognition molecule is being produced.

The mechanism of transendothelial cell migration by the lymphocytes or the animistic reason for their perivascular accumulation also remains unknown (52). Migration on a lesser scale appears to be a usual process and biopsies of normal kidneys will reveal occasional perivascular round cells. Complement (C) does not appear to be required for this. In our model of kidney allograft rejection, inhibition of serum C levels by 68 to 90% prevented the polymorphonuclear leukocyte (PMN) component of the leukocyte infiltration but did not block round cell accumulation (53). This level of C depletion does not provide a conclusive answer, however.

Mononuclear infiltration of kidneys can also occur without an immunological stimulus and is found in experimental hypertension (54). This suggests that cell damage releases factors chemotactic for mononuclear cells with reparative functions. At this time, although they can show immunological specificity, the inducers of lymphoid infiltration of the allografted kidney are not all defined.

The presence of inflammatory cells at the time and site of graft rejection has always had a strong influence on immunobiological thinking. The earliest and simplest explanation was that sensitized lymphocytes both recognized and destroyed the graft. Now the complexity of the allograft reaction has been recognized, and the fundamental questions concerning it have multiplied. Debate now exists on the relative importance of sensitized cells and antibody in recognition of an allograft. Recognition in both cases may be provided by antibody-like molecules that are attached to the surface of the sensitized cell. The question now centers on the relative importance of antibody from B cells and sensitized cells from the T cell line in initiating allograft rejection. Both immune cells and antibody can recruit immunologically nonspecific cells and molecules to produce damage of the target cells. What remains uncertain, however, is the effectiveness of the immune cell in damaging an allograft alone without the aid of the nonspecific effectors.

Williams and Granger (55, 56) have described a lymphotoxin, produced and released within 3 hrs of PHA stimulation of lymphocytes, that is apparently a single protein of approximately 90,000 molecular weight. Although it has been suggested to act by destruction of target cell membranes, no direct evidence for this is available. Release of lymphotoxin is blocked by puromycin and cyclohexi-mide, and hence it may be newly synthesized in response to PHA.

The release of cytotoxic factors by lymphocytes infiltrating an allograft would be the most direct way these cells could damage foreign tissue but it may not be the most efficient. Several other kinds of molecules have been found to be released by stimulated immune cells. In general, these factors work by initiating immunologically nonspecific mechanisms. These pathways may prove to the most effective means to reject an allograft.

Two factors that are both released by immune lymphoid cells in the presence of the target antigen have similar properties. Under the individual experimental circumstances one is migration inhibitory factor (MIF) for macrophages and the other is a chemotactic factor (CF) for these cells. Although a small difference in molecular weight, together with distinct electrophoretic mobilities, has been reported, it is possible that these two molecules will prove to be either similar or the same (57). The principal consequence of the release of MIF and CF is to increase the number of activated macrophages in the area of the stimulated lymphocytes.

A mitogenic factor has also been found that will stimulate blast cell transformation in normal

lymphocyte cultures. It can be found in the supernatants of mixed lymphocyte cultures and after the
addition of specific antigen to sensitized human or
guinea pig lymphocytes. There may be more than one
mitogenic factor present. This substance, which
stimulates cell division among lymphocytes, is probably immunologically nonspecific and may more
properly belong in the discussion of the afferent
arc of immunity. Its relevance to allograft rejection is unknown.

Lymphocytes, when stimulated by PHA, appear to
produce vascular permeability factors in addition to
cytotoxic agents. This permeability factor can be
found in the supernatant of a PHA-activated lymphocyte culture. On injection to an experimental animal
it will produce the induration characteristic of a
delayed hypersensitivity reaction. At this time,
little else is known about the permeability factor(s)
and no description of the effect, if any, in allograft rejection has been made. However, a prominent
feature of the rejecting kidney is interstitial
edema. A permeability factor may well be released by
the activated lymphoid cells infiltrating a kidney
allograft and thus be of considerable importance to
kidney function and survival.

ANTIBODIES

Antibodies comprise the second category of
specific immunological initiators of the rejection
reaction. One pathway of differentiation for the
immunoblast leads to the plasma cell, an efficient
antibody producer. Plasma cells are found both in
the kidney graft and the lymph node, and this progression may occur in both sites. Although the
plasma cell produces relatively large amounts of
antibody, antibody synthesis begins earlier in the
line of differentiation. Cells that morphologically
resemble the immunoblast can produce immunoglobulins
(58).

Antibodies and antibody-like molecules are now

297

acknowledged contributors to kidney graft rejection. Simonsen (59) made the original observation of an associated antibody response with rejection of dog kidney allografts. Although the antibody response during allograft rejection has been difficult to measure and seemed insufficient, the discrepancy can apparently be resolved.

The allograft would be expected to act as an antigenic sink and remove antibody. Milgrom et al. (60) have demonstrated the appearance of circulating antibody following transplant nephrectomy and its disappearance when the patient was regrafted. A further reason for the difficulty is provided in Nelson's (61) postulate that the antibodies cross react with host tissue. If rejection resembles a classical humoral response, cross reactivity would be expected to increase later in the reaction. Antibodies themselves would evolve during rejection and be synthesized with increasingly greater avidity but less specificity for the allograft. Hager et al. (62) produced support for this theory by finding antibody on host kidney and red blood cells during kidney rejection. Results from the use of newer techniques, such as the antiglobulin consumption method, indicate that antibodies to the graft are present in the serum of virtually all patients after transplantation (63).

The vascular endothelium is the first potentially antigenic site circulating antibody encounters ters. Accordingly, within 2 to 3 days thin layers of IgG line the peritubular capillaries of both rat and dog renal allografts (64, 65).

Several earlier experiments indicated that specific humoral factors were of importance in allograft rejection. The infusion of sensitized serum into kidney grafts converted a primary rejection reaction to one more characteristic of second set reactions (66, 67). Sensitized cells in Millipore chambers were found in some experiments to hasten skin graft rejection, and transferred, labeled, sensitized cells, although accelerating skin

allograft rejection, rarely migrated to the graft
site (68-70). These experiments, however, all superimposed their effects on an existing allogeneic
incompatability and a valid argument was that the
only effect was a hastened migration of specifically
sensitized cells. The experiments discussed in the
previous section using the dog allograft model
eliminated this objection and established the functional importance of humoral factors (46). These
factors were shown to initiate a leukocytic infiltration that rejected the dog's own kidney. Autologous
leukocytes accomplished this; therefore, humoral factors were not merely enhancing an immunological reaction. Renal autograft rejection has now been produced by the passive transfer of sensitized plasma
(47, 48). These reactions have been presumed to be
mediated by antibody but the molecules involved
remain unidentified.

AMPLIFICATION SYSTEMS

Kidney graft rejection, like other immunological
reactions, is initiated by specific antigen-antibody
or antigen-cellular interactions. The specific portion, however, comprises only a small part of the
reaction. Rejection is mainly accomplished by
several amplification systems. These, in turn,
obscure the initiator molecules or cells, making
their identification difficult.

Antibody acts as a specific activator for at
least three nonspecific amplification systems. The
complement system is one of these, although early
experiments did not demonstrate the expected lowering of serum of C levels with renal allograft rejection (59, 73). This result only reveals our lack of
knowledge of C pool size and turnover rates and indicates that efforts aimed at demonstrating lowering of
whole body C levels may be naive. Apparently, when
the rejection reaction is sufficiently active,
decreased C titers are found (74, 75). The demonstration of C consumption may be more easily

accomplished by determining the half-life of infused labeled C components (76).

Evidence for C participation is found within the kidney. Immunofluorescent staining has demonstrated B1C globulin, the third component of the C system, on the walls of peritubular capillaries 2 days after rat kidney transplantation (65). Using our dog allograft model, we have found C uptake by the kidney when renal arterial and venous titers are compared (53).

In keeping with the many biological consequences of C activation, the contribution to rejection will most likely prove to be complex. Amplification of the C sequence is greatest at the reaction of C3 and it is here that biological activity begins (77-79). The presence of the C product on target cells will cause PMN's and platelets, enzymatically potent cells, to adhere to them (79, 80). Factors chemotactic for PMN's are produced with the activation of C_3 and with the interaction of C_5, C_6 and C_7 (81, 82). The C_5 step also produces anaphylotoxin. These properties may reside on the same low molecular weight molecule, but in any case, both the stimulus to PMN infiltration and an aid to migration are provided. Reaction of the entire C sequence on the target cell surface will produce membrane damage. In renal xenografts, considerable endothelial cell lysis can be found, but the extent of cellular disruption caused by C in allograft rejection remains to be determined (83).

We have demonstrated the functional importance of C activation with our dog model. Prior depletion of C with cobra venom factor prevented the PMN infiltration, although not the mononuclear cell accumulation. Thus, the leukocytic infiltration of allografts has at least two mechanisms. One proceeds through complement activation and induces PMN infiltration while the stimulus to mononuclear infiltration does not seem to have this requirement. The importance of platelets and PMN's in both experimental and clinical kidney rejection is gaining recognition. In our dog model, inhibition of PMN infiltration prevented tubular disruption (53). In another dog model, platelet plugging of glomerular loops is rapid and not dependent on fibrin formation, and both cell types have been found in a variety of clinical biopsies (84-88). These findings are consistent with the activation of C and the biological functions of immune adherence, chemotaxis, vascular permeability, and cell membrane damage.

Antibody combined with antigen will trigger clot formation, another cascade system. More than one mechanism may be operating. One entrance is through C activation, resulting in platelet adhesion and release of platelet phospholipids, which promote clotting (89). Another seems to be through the interaction of Hageman factor with antigen-antibody complexes (90). In either case, antigen-antibody complexes trip the coagulation system - the consequences being amplified production of fibrin by thromboplastin. Again, experimental and clinical evidence indicates that fibrin plays a significant part in rejection (65, 85-88, 91, 94).

Antigen-antibody complexes have been shown to activate a third enzyme system, resulting in production of the kinins. The complexes activate Hageman factor and proceed stepwise, finally liberating kinins from kininogen (92, 93). Among their effects, these molecules produce increased capillary permeability and smooth muscle dilation.

These biological activities of the kinins are obviously of potential importance to a transplanted organ. What makes the presence and activity of the kinins likely in an allografted kidney is that the triggers of this system are interrelated with the clotting and fibrinolysin pathway.

Evidence for the activation of the kinin system during the clinical hyperacute rejection reaction has been found (95) in the rapid rejection of a transplanted kidney by a patient with preformed antibodies against the donor. The kallikreinogen levels in blood from the renal vein fell, as did the kallikrein inhibitor. Consumption of both the kallikrein and the inhibitor indicated that activation of the kinin pathway had taken place. Similar results have been found experimentally in hyperacute and xenograft rejection (95, 96).

No assessment has yet been made of the functional consequences of kinin activation to renal allograft function.

This discussion has attempted to isolate and describe each cascade system individually. In a functioning biological system, such as a rejecting kidney allograft, the systems are certain to form a seamless web. Not only are the activators of these systems all interrelated, but the inhibitors are also intertwined. The C_1 esterase inhibitor also decreases the activity of the kinin and plasmin systems. Neither activation nor inhibition of one system can occur without affecting the other pathways.

The property of amplification does not seem to be confined to the molecular cascade system, and analogous mechanisms are available to increase the numbers of cellular participants at the site of immunological reactions. Following immunological recognition, many nonspecific cells, including mononuclear cells, PMN's and platelets, can be enlisted.

Much evidence indicates that the mononuclear cells infiltrating an allograft are not all specifically sensitized to it. When the cells infiltrating one human kidney allograft were electronmicroscopically examined for distinctive ultra structural features, 15% were observed to be macrophages and another 40% were either large lymphocytes or histiocytes (146). This latter group of cells has abundant cytoplasm without significant endoplasmic reticulum, and the cells had many rosettes of ribosomes. These cells could equally well be transformed lymphocytes in the process of specific differentiation against the allograft antigen or immature cells with phagocytic properties.

One mechanism for increasing the number of macrophages, the release of MIF, has been extensively

studied in vitro. MIF is produced by cells sensitized under conditions that will produce delayed
hypersensitivity reactions. If the immunization
schedule is such that both antibodies and delayed
reaction would be produced on challenge, MIF will
also be produced; however, if antibodies alone are
formed, no MIF is synthesized. Sensitized lymphocytes require the same precise antigenic stimulation
to produce MIF as to produce delayed sensitivity
reactions. Thus, carrier specificity was present
when guinea pigs were sensitized to DNP-conjugated
guinea pig albumin. MIF was not released when DNP-
conjugated bovine gamma globulin was used to stimulate the cells (97).

Bloom (57) showed the amplification potential of
MIF and demonstrated much of its significance to the
allograft rejection reaction. With a large preponderance of macrophages only 2% of the cells need to
be lymphocytes to inhibit migration. It was possible
that the macrophages in their study were being
inhibited by a lymphocyte component of only 0.6% of
the cell population. Such an amplification system
would be of obvious advantage. Relatively few cells
would need to specifically differentiate in response
to the antigen and once lymphocytes have defined
the situation immunologically, the destruction may
be carried out principally by indifferent macrophages.
A consistent observation is that only a small percentage of mononuclear cells in a rejecting kidney contain immunoglobulins (65). The nonspecific mononuclear cells are probably drawn from a rapidly repli-
cating bone marrow population and factors released by
tissue damage may recruit additional cells from this
source (71).

Cytophilic antibodies would seem to be another
mechanism by which macrophages are concentrated at a
site of immunological activity. Virtually all of
the work on these antibodies has been done in experimental models unrelated to transplantation; nevertheless, an antibody that has an affinity for macrophages and confers specifically on them has been

found.

Two additional immunologically nonspecific cell types, the polymorphonuclear leukocytes (PMN's) and the platelets, have now been accorded a place in allograft rejection.

PMN's have frequently been found in biopsy specimen allografts, especially during an active rejection reaction, and the greater frequency of their numbers correlates best with an increasing vigor of the reaction. Because the cell is active when stimulated by an immunological reaction in the presence of material to be phagocytized, its life span is rather short. Consequently, probably a significantly larger percentage of PMN's contribute to an allograft rejection reaction than is apparent from any single biopsy.

Antigen-antibody complexes that activate complement produce at least two factors that are attractive to PMN's. The gradient of chemotactic molecules will allow PMN's to actively migrate to the source. The PMN's may also be retained by immune adherence, another function of activated complement. Henson (80) has shown that neutrophils as well as platelets will adhere to a site of antigen-antibody reaction when complement is present and activated (98).

Functional assessments for the potency of PMN's have shown PMN's to be much more effective and more rapidly active in producing allogeneic target cell death than are lymphoid cells. The basis for the potency of PMN's in the allograft rejection reaction is easily demonstrated. The neutrophil is a highly differentiated cell, packed full of lysosomes; cytoplasmic bodies filled with digestive enzymes. The cell fraction containing the cytoplasmic granules has been found to contain acid phosphatase, alkaline phosphatase, lysozyme, collagenase, lipase, ribonucleases, deoxyribonuclease, and -glucuronidase. In addition, proteolytic enzymes have been found of which cathepsins D and E may be an important part in producing immunological damage. At least four

basic proteins from rabbit neutrophil granules, which
can induce both vascular and glomerular basement
membrane permeability, have been isolated (99, 100).
Finally, slow reacting substances or anaphylatoxins
and a kinin generating factor seem to be associated
with neutrophils.

Large immune complexes, greater than 19 S in
density, seem prone to lodge in arterial walls.
PMN's are attracted to these sites, wedge past the
intimal cells, and begin phagocytizing the complexes. This in turn apparently activates the PMN,
causing lysosome degranulation and release of active
enzymes. Damage to the internal elastic membrane and
medical necrosis results (101).

Platelets, like PMN's have only recently been
conceded to be of any significance in allograft
rejection reactions. Identification of platelets in
a histological section requires electron microscopy;
thus, the number of studies are fewer than those
implicating other cells. Platelets are now thought
to be important components of the rejection reaction
and contribute to allograft damage of several mechanisms. Platelets contain many cytoplasmic granules,
at least some of which have been found to contain
acid phosphatase, and glucuronidase (102). This
finding implies that at least some of these granules
are lysosomes and contain various other enzymes
capable of tissue degradation.

The phospholipids found in cell membrane fractions as well as in isolates of platelet granules
are important in both the extrinsic system of blood
coagulation initiated by tissue factors (including
those of platelets) and the intrinsic system that
occurs in the absence of cellular damage (89, 103).
Activation and damage of platelets would release
these factors and engage the clotting pathways.

Another important consequence of platelet function is the release of vasoactive amines. Serotonin
is released by human platelets and both histamine and
serotonin are released by rabbit platelets. It is
not known whether these vasoactive amines are

synthesized or merely stored in the platelets (103).

Platelet activity, which seems to begin with aggregation of these cells, can be initiated by exposed collagen fibers as well as cells coated with immune complexes (104, 105). Consequently, immunological damage may precipitate thrombosis by the uncovering of collagen fibers in basement membrane structures beneath the endothelial cells of capillaries and larger vessels. Platelet aggregation may also be initiated by damage to endothelial cells that exposes ATPases beneath the cellular membranes (106). The formation of ADP by these enzymes would then promote platelet thrombosis. Such aggregation would effectively clog small vessels.

In the allograft rejection reaction, platelets may well congregate secondary to the association of antibody with antigen and the activation of complement. The presence of C_3 products on cell surfaces might be expected to retain the platelets by immune adherence, although this phenomenon did not occur in vitro with sensitized sheep erythrocytes as the target cells (80). In addition, platelets may accumulate by adhering to collagen fibers exposed by other mechanisms, such as PMN-released digestive enzymes or macrophage-induced damage.

The complexity of the allograft reaction is just beginning to be understood. It involves a variety of recognition molecules (antibodies) and presumably a similar variety of specifically sensitized cells. In addition, the main force of the reaction is produced by a bewildering array of amplifying chain reactions that include both molecular and cellular amplification schemes. The activation of complement; the clotting system; kinin formation; and the stimulation of PMN's macrophages, and platelet assault produce a variety of threats to the transplanted kidney. Included are occlusive phenomena within the graft vessels, induced permeability of these same vessels with interstitial edema accumulation, disruption of cellular basement membranes, and the infiltration of the graft with a profusion of cell types.

THE PATHOLOGY OF REJECTION

The pathology of rejection is the product of two groups of events. The first is the direct effect of the host cells and enzymes, as well as the clinical immunosuppressive measures on the kidney cells. The response to this damage forms the second group of events. Insult and response are not always clearly separable, but in general the reaction of the kidney cells themselves produces many of the features seen in rejection pathology. As a consequence of specialization, excessive function or damage affects each cell type in a characteristic way. The basis of this response may derive from an aspect of metabolism that is most labile and revealed by the insult of the rejection reaction. When there is sufficient time for these cellular responses, the pathology of rejection is increasingly formed by them. The more acute the reaction, however, the greater the contribution from the cells and molecules of the rejecting host. This viewpoint will reveal many features of rejection to be nonspecific.

The filtration unit of the kidney, the glomerulus, is composed of at least three cell types; epithelial, endothelial, and mesangial, as well as the apparent filter, the glomerular basement membrane (GBM). Single membranes join the processes of the endothelial and epithelial cells abutting on either side of the GBM and may augment its function. The GMB is not inert and turns over slowly, perhaps requiring a month for replacement by the epithelial cell (107, 108).

Interference with GBM metabolism, surprisingly, is followed most typically by a thickened GBM, rather than an attenuated one. Puromycin aminonucleoside (PA), an inhibitor of RNA synthesis, causes GBM thickening (109-112). Labeled proline has been shown to be taken up and converted to hydroxproline at an increased rate after administration of PA (113).

Collagen metabolism and the proportions of carbohydrate components were not changed. A similar
increase is proline to hydroxyproline conversion and
incorporation into the GBM is produced by giving
nephrotoxic serum (114).

GBM thickening is found in a variety of
circumstances. Radiation nephritis always includes
proteinuria, and when the damage is severe, thickened
GBM's are visible by light microscopy. Many ultra-
structural examinations of the GBM, in both experimental radiation nephritis and following radiation
therapy in many, have confirmed the frequent
occurrence of thickened, tortuous, and fragmented
GBM's (115-118). The frequent finding that GBM
thickness is increased in diabetes mellitus is a
further indication that metabolic factors are
important (108). Hypertension leads to a similar
result and also supports the general nature of the
response.

Why the GBM thickens in these situations is
unknown. Thickening may be compensatory in an
attempt to prevent the proteinuria seen with GBM
damage. The most important consequence of GBM
injury may be the loss of glomerular polyanion postulated to be important in protein filtration (116). A
less likely hypothesis is that the regulation of GBM
production is a particularly vulnerable point of GBM
metabolism. This speculation would have the mRNA's
necessary for GBM production to be stable, whereas
the regulator molecule must frequently be resynthe-
sized. Radiation, PA, and other metabolic derange-
ments would interfere with this synthesis and lead to
overproduction.

In the transplanted kidney, thickened convoluted
GBM's are virtually always seen (85, 86, 119). An
allograft is subjected to a number of damaging
influences that may be responsible for the thickened
GBM's. The most obvious initiator of GBM damage
would be the rejection reaction. The GBM may be
immunogenic and elicit direct immunological injury.
The situation resembles both the experimental model

in which antibodies are directed against the GBM itself and Goodpasture's syndrome.

It was previously felt that the development of anti-GBM antibodies would not be a frequent nor an important finding in clinical kidney transplantation. This view is less tenable following the demonstration of linear immunoglobulin deposition in four patients with apparently well-functioning kidneys (120). These anti-GBM antibodies may represent a continuance of the patient's original renal disease. At this time, the situations that originate or perpetuate GBM immunogenicity are still unknown, and primary stimulation by the GBM following transplantation must be considered.

Alternatively, and probably concurrently with damage initiated by cells and antibodies directed against the GBM, immune complexes arising from other sites of rejection within the kidney may lodge on the GBM. The experimental production of immune complex nephritis requires a rather precise ratio of circulating antigen and antibody. These conditions may be met in the rejecting kidney by a wide variety of antigens in the form of membrane fragments and cellular proteins. This would in turn lead to an inconstant rate and locale of deposition. Some complexes may pass to the epithelial side of the GBM. Although the source and the nature of the antigens are unknown, transplanted kidneys often show a granular fluorescence when tested for the presence of antibody or complement, suggesting that this mechanism is operating.

Immune complexes may form from other sources than the rejection reaction. The use of antilymphocyte serum (ALS) to produce immunosuppression is increasing in frequency and dosage. Immune complexes might be formed with ALS as antigen stimulating antibodies against it, with the ALS as antibody in combination with lymphocyte cell membrane fragments, or by ALS binding directly to the GBM. In any case, activation of complement, attraction of PMN's, and release of vasoactive and proteolytic agents would damage the GBM.

Common viral infections might lead to circulating immune complexes that would have considerable significance in clinical transplantation. Following viremia and antibody production, these complexes could be trapped on the GBM and there initiate immunological damage.

In addition to immunological damage, other mechanisms may lead to GBM thickening. Azathioprine, an RNA inhibitor, is virtually always given in clinical allotransplantation. Actinomycin D, another blocker of RNA synthesis, as well as x-irradiation, is often used to control rejection. These agents, which interfere with the production of RNA molecules, might alter GBM production.

The endothelial cells of the glomerulus are probably representative of these cells throughout the kidney. Whether through antibody, C, and PMN's or through sensitized round cells, the antigens on the endothelial cell surface would likely insure cellular membrane damage. The efforts of these cells to preserve the endothelial lining may account for the proliferation seen in the glomerular tufts of transplanted kidneys (86-90).

The mesangial cell appears to be a special form of the endothelial cell with phagocytic capabilities and the function of sweeping the GBM of nonfilterable particles (110). Steroids and ACTH increase mesangial cell activity. In one study of experimental immune complex disease, treatment with steroids increased the uptake of the complexes and reduced GBM damage (121, 122). The interpretation given was that the steroids decreased GBM permeability and allowed more efficient clearing of the membrane. Steroids may stimulate the mesangial cells directly, however, and have been found experimentally to increase the number of mesangial cell mitoses (123). This effect may either be primary or secondary to enhance phagocytosis.

In transplanted kidneys the mesangium is frequently thickened (86-90). Both clearing the GBM

310

of immunological reactants, as is suggested by the presence of IgG, B_{1C} globulin, and fibrin in the mesangial cells of allografts, and the effect of steroids may contribute to the increased prominence of these cells.

The tubule cells are large differentiated cells whose basal portion is packed with mitochondria. The energy produced is presumable largely utilized in transport functions. As a reflection of high metabolic activity, the total ATP content of the kidney drops to 20% of the control level after 3 min of ischemia. In another study, inability to repair the ATP deficit occurred with 30 min or longer of ischemia and was the best predictor of tubular damage (124, 125). Mitochondrial metabolism recovers, however, and the basis for the irreversibility is not understood.

Even the most facile clinical transplantation tests the respiratory vulnerability of tubule cells. The ischemia produced is sufficient to impair proximal tubular reabsorption of sodium and glucose in the first 24 hrs after transplantation (147). Short increases in ischemia time would lead to acute tubular necrosis and this is relatively commonly seen in clinical transplantation.

With more chronic ischemia, as when arteriolar lesions and tissue edema are produced by rejection, a predictable response is evoked. The cells lose much of their respiratory apparatus and the site of transport exchange, the brush border, diminishes. Flattened tubule cells are common in allograft biopsies and probably represent less a response to direct immunological damage than a reflection of compromised respiration. The tubular cell membrane is antigenic, however, and an immunological reaction could damage the cell directly or impair its high rate of respiration and lead to the described changes (11, 12).

Because tubule cells are highly differentiated, RNA inhibitors (azathioprine) or x-rays would be expected to have relatively little effect on them.

These agents are more disruptive to developing or
transforming cells such as the lymphocyte. Differentiation requires much RNA synthesis and, insofar
as cell division is necessary, DNA synthesis. The
tubule cell, by way of contrast, has many repetitive
functions and the mRNA's needed to produce the participating molecules may be stable. This distinction
between cell types does not preculde an effect on
tubule cells, and clinical proteinuria and blood urea
nitrogen (BUN) elevation with an RNA inhibitor
(mithramycin) suggests both GBM and tubular disruption (126, 127).

There is no information at present about molecular control mechanisms in tubule cells and they may
be susceptible to nucleic acid inhibitors. Certainly these agents would likely be detrimental to
the proliferative potential or repair capacity of
tubule cells. Tubule cell replication occurs at a
low level in normal kidneys (148) and would be of
more importance in the transplanted kidney, which is
doing the work of two in addition to repairing rejection damage.

The vascular system, particularly the endothelial cell, first meets the onslaught of the immunological reaction against the grafted kidney. The
ramifications of this are seen in the endothelial
proliferation in the glomerular capillaries, obli-
terative arterioloitis and, subsequently, the extreme
narrowing of larger vessels as a consequence of
intimal hypertrophy and medial hyperplasia.

A good deal of endothelial cell damage occurs in
the allograft, and the responses of cellular repair,
hypertrophy, and hyperplasia follow. How much of
this injury is because of immunological attack
directed at the endothelial cell histocompatibility
antigens is as yet uncertain. In fact, the accessibility of these antigens has not even been determined. Immunofluorescent studies have detected a
variety of immunoglobulin in the vessels and glomerular loops of transplanted kidneys (87, 88, 128).
The resolving power of these techniques, however, is

not sufficient to localize antibody on the endothelial cell membranes themselves. Consequently,
direct endothelial damage initiated by antibody to
the cell membranes has not yet been proven. Although
it has been presumed that the presence of histocompatibility antigens on the endothelial cell surfaces
would make direct damage likely, a great deal of the
damage may actually result from nearby immunological
reactions. Antibody located on vascular basement
membrane can initiate immunological reactions in the
vicinity of the endothelial cells.

As common as these findings are in transplanted
kidneys, they are also found in such diverse circumstances as clinical essential and experimental hypertension and radiation nephritis (54, 129). Again,
this suggests that the pathology is governed by the
response of the cell involved, the endothelial cell.

Although the endothelial cell does not seem to
be doing the same amount of metabolic work, as judged
by numbers of mitochondria, as the tubule cell, it is
nevertheless active. At least part of this activity
is a low level of proliferation, presumably a constant repair process (130). Certainly, immunological
damage would exacerbate the need for repair and as
will be seen the effectors of immune damage, antibodies, C, PMN's, platelets, and fibrin, are frequently found on the endothelium. When the rejection
reaction is rapid, as in a xenograft, lysis of endothelial cells and disruption of the internal elastic
membrane can be seen (75, 83).

Narrowing of the vessel lumen is also a consequence of the medial thickening. Studies using non-
immunological disease models have shown that most of
the cells proliferating in response to the stimulus
of injury are smooth muscle cells (131, 132). A
reasonable extrapolation is that hyperplasia of these
cells produces much of the lumenal narrowing in allografts. Proliferation of what appears to be smooth
muscle cells can be seen in vessels of all sizes
larger than arterioles.

Although the exposed position of the endothelial

cells and the striking proliferation of the smoother muscle cells argue for their being an important target of the immune reaction, there is evidence that the basement and elastic membranes of the vessel absorb a major portion of the immune-mediated damage. In the experimental production of immune complex disease the antigen-antibody complexes are found trapped on the basement membranes (133).

Why hypertension or x-rays alone should cause this proliferative response is not as clear. The proliferation seems to be an attempt to repair cellular damage caused by hypertension. Fibrin has been found deposited on endothelial cells in pulmonary hypertension and perhaps results from tissue injury and the release of clot activators (134). x-Ray induced proliferation may also be reparative or may indicate that the regulation of cellular division is a vulnerable biological point of this cell.

The interstitium is an area that morphologically becomes increasingly prominent in the transplanted kidney. It is here that the many infiltrating cells from the host gather. Mononuclear cell accumulations are present in virtually all functioning allografts and presumably indicate more subtle incompatabilities in the absence of overt rejection. Antigenic disparity is not the only stimulation to infiltration and although the others are not understood, damage seems to be one.

The interstitial matrix itself also increases. In acute rejection, much of this prominence can be traced to edema formed by the liberation of various vasoactive substances and proteolytic enzymes during the immunological reaction. On a more chronic basis, repair is accomplished by phagocytes and fibrocytes in a way similar to the performance by the mesangial cells in the glomerulus. Replacement of the area formerly occupied by tubule cells results. This portion of the pathological picture is a consequence of normal reparative functions of interstitial cells and incoming macrophages.

CLINICAL REJECTION PATTERNS

A rejection reaction may appear at any time from minutes to years after a kidney is allografted. Although these reactions form a temporal and morphological continuum, clinically useful categories do emerge. A simple classification distinguishes hyperacute, acute, and chronic reactions; however, there can be considerable overlap between them. In general these categories reflect the intensity of the host's immune response.

Occasionally, a fulminant reaction, analogous to xenograft rejection, rejects the kidney within minutes or hours of transplantation (74, 75). Host components completely dominate the pathology. Glomerular loops are plugged with PMN's, platelets, and fibrin. Additional PMN's rapidly disrupt the peritubular capillaries and infiltrate the interstitial spaces (135, 136).

In most cases, preexisting antibodies react with the kidney and trigger the rejection. Activity to the donor antigen has been found in the IgG, IgA, and IgM classes by in vitro techniques (135–138). The relative contributions of these antibody families to the hyperacute reaction has not been established. Presumably, antibodies that fix C would be the most efficient in producing PMN and platelet aggregation. Other pathways, including the production of kinins and clotting, are also probably initiated by the antigen–antibody reaction and may not require C fixation.

Specific immunological recognition is not necessarily required to activate C and deposit fibrin within kidneys (139). These pathways may be tripped fortuitously by endotoxin or antigen–antibody complexes trapped by the transplanted kidney. Only when the initiating reaction is nonspecific do hyperacute rejections belong in this Shwartzman class. Despite this precaution, antigraft antibodies not exposed by standard methods may precipitate the

315

reaction. Histologically, the Shwartzman reaction is virtually indistinguishable from the specific hyperacute rejection and is characterized by heavy deposition of fibrin with varying numbers of enmeshed PMN's in glomerular capillaries and arterioles (135).

Acute rejections can occur within days of transplantation or even after months of function. The relatively abrupt appearance often seen is provocative but unexplained. These reactions are characterized by relatively sudden depressions of kidney function. Both cellular and humoral immunity contribute to these reactions. When the kidneys are biopsied during a rejection crisis, the intravascular triad of PMN's, platelets, and fibrin is frequently found (86-90). Although this was not common in our series, the patchy distribution of allograft rejection coupled with the sampling problems inherent in electronmicroscopy make interpretation of negative biopsies hazardous (90).

Lymphoid infiltration is always present and seems to regress when the reaction is reversed (87-89). The activity of these cells presumably adds to the functional impairment produced by the intravascular lesions. The presence of these cells best distinguishes acute reactions from hyperacute rejection. Their presence implies that immunity was largely or completely acquired subsequent to transplantation. Once immunity has developed, however, many similar effector pathways are used.

The glomerular thrombi seen in these biopsies suggest immunoglobulin participation and C activation but few data are available. In our series, immunoglobulin deposition was unusual but fluorescent antibody staining revealed C (B_{1C}globulin) on vessel walls in more than 70% of cases either in the throes of rejection or with a history of previous crisis (90). Porter and his colleagues (85), however, report that in biopsies of kidneys that had GBM changes but whose relationship to a rejection reaction was not given, 90% contained IgM, 35% had C, and 30% had IgG deposited on the glomerular endothelium.

Acute rejection episodes at any time will superimpose intravascular lesions. In the series of Porter et al. (85), glomerular loops of three kidneys implanted for longer than a year, but in the midst of a rejection reaction, were found to be plugged with platelets, PMN's, lymphocytes, and fibrin.

Kidneys surviving longer than a few days show morphological features characteristic of the response of the kidney cell. Endothelial hypertrophy and proliferation, irregularly thickened basement membranes, fused epithelial foot processes, and mesangial cell proliferation are frequently found in the glomerular tuft (86-90).

Fibrin formation seems to accompany acute rejection and during clinical rejection reactions, fibrinogen degradation products (FDP) appear in the urine (91). The correlation is strengthened by the cessation of FDP production with effective immunosuppressive therapy. Even a thrombus is not a static participant, and severe lesions within capillary loops, which depress kidney function, can be reversible (88, 140). The reversibility of the capillar plugging may contribute to the difficulty in demonstrating occlusion in biopsy specimens.

Another manifestation of a rejection episode may be hypertension, and elevations in circulating renin levels have been demonstrated concomitantly with sudden rises in blood pressure (141, 142). The stimulus for renin release presumably is ischemia secondary to thrombotic vascular obstruction. Transplants of longer duration have arteriolar intimal hypertrophy and occlusion. Hypertension can occur in this situation but here it may not be associated with increased renin levels. These slowly developing blood pressure elevations may reflect decreased prostaglandin production. Ischemia may still be the stimulus and consistent with this, the serum erythropoietin level has risen in association with the blood pressure in three transplantation patients (143). It is a possibility, however, that the loss of antihypertensive capacity of the kidney is a direct consequence of immunological damage.

Chronic rejection is characterized clinically by slow deterioration in renal function. Even so, these symptoms are not always distinguishable from later appearing acute rejections. There is no reason to believe that rejection must manifest itself by a sudden change in function and the decline seen is the product of varying contributions of insidious rejection, antimetabolites, steroids, radiation, and reparative changes.

Both reversible and irreversible chronic rejections have been described and in both may be found features of acute rejection. Glomerular loops plugged with platelets, PMN's and fibrin can be found on biopsy, although the presence of immunoglobulins and C in these kidneys was inconstant (86, 89, 90, 128, 144).

One consequence of chronic rejection is the nephrotic syndrome. By fluorescent antibody techniques, two out of four patients had significant glomerular deposits of IgG, whereas three out of four had heavier staining for IgG in the peritubular areas (96). In three patients, titers of lymphocytotoxic or agglutinating antibody rose following removal of the transplanted kidney. In these studies antibodies eluted from the removed kidneys produced leuko-agglutination, whereas precipitation reactions with GBM preparations were negative (145). This again suggests that GBM damage is not the result of direct injury but rather is due to compromising the epithelial cell producing the GBM.

Much of the morphological change in a chronically rejected kidney is derived from the nonspecific responses of the renal cells. As background of chronic kidney damage and repair increases, the rejection exacerbation intensity needed to produce a clinical crisis decreases. Consequently, immunological spoors may be fewer and the specific evidence of rejection more elusive.

There is reason to believe that completely effective immunosuppression may rarely be attainable and in the absence of complete compatibility, chronic rejection would be the rule. Biopsies of all long-term survivors show definite morphological changes (86-90, 119). Even apparently normally functioning kidneys inevitably show fusion of glomerular epithelial foot processes and frequently have thickened basement membranes. As discussed, these changes are not specific and may result from immunosuppressive therapy or ischemia as well as rejection. The presence of the changes in a biopsy of an autograft confirms their nonspecific nature (88). Progression to convoluted GBM's, proliferation of glomerular endothelial and mesangial cells, and arteriolar intimal hypertrophy can occur without specific indication of etiology and diagnostic interpretations of these kidneys is often difficult.

SUMMARY

In presenting the biology of kidney transplantation, we have discussed both the development of immunity against the allograft and the response of the kidney to it. Many questions remain unanswered, but the portion that is established should apply to other vascular organ grafts.

Although the antigenicity of differentiated cells may vary, the presence of endothelial cells in these organs should insure a similar development and expression of immunity. What will be seen to vary will be the functional and morphological responses of the various cells in the organ. This variation, in turn, will depend upon the limits set by cellular differentiation.

REFERENCES

1. J.-P. Changeux, J. Thiéry, Y. Tung, and C. Kittel, Proc. Nat. Acad. Sci. U.S. 57, 335 (1967).
2. T. Aoki, V. Hammerling, E. DeHarven, E.A. Boyse, and L.J. Old, J. Exp. Med. 130, 979 (1969).
3. B.D. Kahan and R.A. Reisfeld, Transplant. Proc. 1,

483 (1969).

4. B.D. Kahan and R.A. Reisfeld, Science 164, 514 (1969).

5. R. Ceppillini In "Advances in Transplantation", (J. Dausset, J. Hamburger, and G. Mathé, eds.), p. 195. Munksgaard, Copenhagen, 1968.

6. D.B. Amos, M. Zumpft, and P. Armstrong, Transplantation 1, 270 (1963).

7. E.A. Boyse, L.J. Old, E. Stockert and N. Shigeno, Cancer Res. 28, 1280 (1968).

8. J.M. Anderson and K. Benirschke, Ann. N.Y. Acad. Sci. 99, 399 (1962).

9. E.A. Boyse, L.J. Old, and S. Luell, Nat. Cancer Inst., Monogr. 31, 987 (1963).

10. R.D. Guttmann, R.R. Lindquist, and S.A. Ockner, Transplantation 8, 472 (1969).

11. C.A. Krakower and S.A. Greenspoon, AMA Arch. Pathol. 51, 629 (1951).

12. R.W. Steblay, J. Exp. Med. 116, 253 (1962).

13. T.S. Edgington, R.J. Glassock and F.J. Dixon, J. Exp. Med. 127, 555 (1968).

14. J.S. Najarian, J. May, K.C. Cochrum, N. Baronberg, and L.W. Way, Ann. N.Y. Acad. Sci. 129, 76 (1966).

15. K.C. Cochrum and J.S. Najarian, Fed. Proc., Fed. Amer. Soc. Exp. Biol.26, 572 (1967).

16. P. Nathan, Ann. N.Y. Acad. Sci. 120, 458 (1964).

17. J. Hamburger, Transplantation 5, 870 (1967).

18. R.A. Lerner, J.J. McPhaul, Jr., and F.J. Dixon, Ann. Intern. Med. 68, 249 (1968).

19. D.A.L. Davies, Immunology 11, 115 (1966).

20. D.W. Dresser, Immunology 5, 378 (1962).

21. P.B. Medawar, Transplantation 1, 21 (1963).

22. F.P. Stuart, T. Saitoh, and F.W. Fitch, Science 160, 1463 (1968).

23. P.B. Medawar, Proc. Roy. Soc., Ser. B 149, 145 (1958).

24. B.K.H. Semb, G.M. Williams, and D.H. Hume, Transplantation 6, 977 (1968).

25. S. Strober and J.L. Gowans, J. Exp. Med. 122, 347 (1965).

26. G.J.V. Nossal, A. Abbot, J. Mitchell, and Z. Lummus, J. Exp. Med. 127, 277 (1968).
27. G.J.V. Nossal, A. Abbott, and J. Mitchell, J. Exp. Med. 127, 263 (1968).
28. M. Feldman and R. Gallily, Cold Spring Harbor Symp. Quant. Biol. 32, 415 (1967).
29. J.R. Schmidtke and E.R. Unanue, J. Immunol. 107, 331 (1971).
30. M. Fishman and F.L. Adler, J. Exp. Med. 117, 595 (1963).
31. F.L. Adler, M. Fishman and S. Dray, J. Immunol. 97, 554 (1966).
32. B.A. Askonas and J.M. Rhodes, Nature (London) 205, 470 (1965).
33. G.J.V. Nossal, G.L. Ada, and C.M. Austin, J. Exp. Med. 121, 945 (1965).
34. S.S. Han and A.G. Johnson, Science 153, 176 (1966).
35. A.S. Coulson, B.W. Gurner, and R.R.A. Coombs, Int. Arch. Allergy Appl. Immunol. 32, 264 (1967).
36. M. George and J.H. Vaughan, Proc. Soc. Exp. Biol. Med. 111, 514 (1962).
37. R.J. Scothorne and I.A. McGregor, J. Anat. 89, 283 (1955).
38. J.G. Hall, B. Morris, G.D. Moreno and M.C. Bessis, J. Exp. Med. 125, 91 (1967).
39. S.L. Kountz, M.A. Williams, P.L. Williams, C. Kapros, and W.J. Dempster, Nature (London) 199, 257 (1963).
40. G. Pearmain, R.R. Lycette, and P.H. Fitzgerald, Lancet 1, 637 (1963).
41. N.A. Mitchison, Nature (London) 171, 267 (1953).
42. L. Brent and P.B. Medawar, Proc. Roy. Soc. 155, 392 (1962).
43. J.L. Gowans, Ann. N.Y. Acad. Sci. 99, 432 (1962).
44. A. Govaerts, J. Immunol. 85, 516 (1960).
45. H. Ginsburg, W. Ax, and G. Berke, Transplant. Proc. 1, 551 (1969).
46. D.S. Clark, J.E. Foker, R.A. Good, and R.L. Varco, Lancet 1, 8 (1968).

47. K.C. Cochrum, W.C. Davis, S.L. Kountz, and H.H. Fundenberg, Transplant. Proc. 1, 301 (1969).

48. J.M. Dubernard, C.B. Carpenter, G.J. Busch, A.G. Diethelm, and J.E. Murray, Surgery 64, 752 (1968).

49. S. Sell and P.G.H. Gell, J. Exp. Med. 122, 423 (1965).

50. G. Bert, A.L. Massaro, and M. Maja, Nature (London) 218, 1078 (1968).

51. E. Merler and C.A. Janeway, Proc. Nat. Acad. Sci. U.S. 59, 393 (1968).

52. V.T. Marchesi and J.L. Gowans, Proc. Roy. Soc. 159, 283 (1964).

53. J.E. Foker, D.S. Clark, R.J. Pickering, R.A. Good, and R.L. Varco, Transplant. Proc. 1, 296 (1969).

54. C. Wilson and F.B. Bryrom, Lancet 1, 136 (1939).

55. T.W. Williams and G.A. Granger, Nature (London) 219, 1076 (1968).

56. T.W. Williams and G.A. Granger, J. Immunol. 103, 170 (1969).

57. B.R. Bloom In "Mediators of Cellular Immunity", (H.S. Lawrence and M. Landy, eds.), p. 249. Academic Press, New York, 1969.

58. G. Chiappino and B. Pernis, Pathol. Microbiol. 27, 8 (1964).

59. M. Simonsen, Acta Pathol. Microbiol. Scand. 32, 36 (1953).

60. F. Milgrom, B.L. Litvak, K. Kano, and E. Witebsky, J. Amer. Med. Ass. 198, 226 (1966).

61. R.A. Nelson, Jr. In "Proceedings of the Second International Symposium on Immunopathology" (P. Grabar and P. Miescher, eds.), p. 223. Schwabe, Basel, 1961.

62. E.B. Hager, M.P. DuPuy and D.F.H. Wallach, N.Y. Acad. Sci. 120, 447 (1964).

63. Y. Iwasaki, D. Talmage, and T.E. Starzl, Transplantation 5, 191 (1967).

64. R.E. Horowitz, L. Burrows, F. Paronetto, D. Dreiling and A.E. Kark, Transplantation 3, 318 (1965).

65. R.R. Lindquist, R.D. Guttman and J.P. Merrill, Amer. J. Pathol. 52, 531 (1968).
66. J.S. Najarian and R.J. Perper, Surgery 62, 213 (1967).
67. B. Altman, Ann. Roy. Coll.Surg. Engl.33, 79 (1963).
68. J.S. Najarian and J.D. Feldman, J. Exp. Med. 115, 1083 (1962).
69. R.R. Kretschmer and R. Perez-Tamayo, J. Exp. Med. 116, 879 (1962).
70. D.B. Wilson, W.K. Silvers, and R.E. Billingham, Nature (London) 209, 1359 (1966).
71. A. Volkman and J.L. Gowans, Brit. J. Exp. Pathol. 46, 62 (1965).
72. D.C. Dumonde, J. Clin. Pathol. 20, 430 (1967).
73. C.B. Favour, J.E. Murray, C.T. Wemyss, Jr., A. Colodny, and B.F. Miller, Proc. Soc. Exp. Biol. Med. 83, 352 (1953).
74. H. Gewurz, D.S. Clark, J. Finstad, W.D. Kelly, R.L. Varco, R.A. Good, and A.E. Gabrielsen, Ann. N.Y. Acad. Sci. 129, 673 (1966).
75. K.F. Austen and P.S. Russell, Ann. N.Y. Acad. Sci. 129, 657 (1966).
76. C.B. Carpenter, S. Ruddy, I.H. Shehadeh, J.P. Merrill, K.F. Austen, and H.J. Müller-Eberhard, Transplant. Proc. 1, 279 (1969).
77. H.J. Müller-Eberhard, A.P. Calmasso, M.A. Calcott, J. Exp. Med. 123, 33 (1966).
78. M.R. Mardiney, Jr., H.J. Müller-Eberhard, and J.D. Feldman, Amer. J. Pathol. 53, 253 (1968).
79. M. Siqueira and R.A. Nelson, Jr. J. Immunol. 86, 516 (1961).
80. P.M. Henson, Immunology 16, 107 (1969).
81. P.A. Ward, J. Exp. Med. 126, 189 (1967).
82. H.S. Shin, R. Snyderman, E. Friedman, A. Mellors, and M.M. Mayer, Science 162, 361 (1968).
83. D.S. Clark and R.L. Varco, Unpublished observations (1967).
84. R.W. Lowenhaupt, P. Nathan and M.G. Menefee, Fed. Proc., Fed. Amer. Soc. Exp. Biol. 28, 582

(1969).

85. K.A. Porter, J.B. Dossetor, T.L. Marchioro, W.S. Peart, J.M. Rendall, T.E. Starzl, and P.I. Terasaki, Lab. Invest. 16, 153 (1967).

86. P. Kincaid-Smith, P. Lancet 2, 849 (1967).

87. R.R. Lindquist, R.D. Guttmann, J.P. Merrill, and G.J. Dammin, Amer. J. Pathol. 53, 851 (1968).

88. W. Rosenau, J.C. Lee, and J.S. Najarian, Surg. Gynecol. Obstet. 128, 62 (1969).

89. A.J. Marcus and D. Zucker-Franklin, Blood 23, 389 (1964).

90. H.Z. Movat and N.L. DiLorenzo, Lab. Invest. 19, 187 (1968).

91. W.E. Braun and J.P. Merrill, N. Engl. J. Med. 278, 1366 (1968).

92. K.M. Gautvik and H.E. Rugstad, Brit. J. Pharmacol. Chemother. 31, 390 (1967).

93. A.M. Rothchild and A. Castania, J. Pharm. Pharmacol. 20, 77 (1968).

94. J. Hamburger, J. Crosneir, and J. Dormont, Lancet 1, 985 (1965).

95. R.W. Colman, Personal communication (1971).

96. J.E. Foker and R.L. Varco, Unpublished data (1971).

97. J.R. David, H.S. Lawrence, and L. Thomas, J. Immunol. 93, 279 (1964).

98. P.M. Henson, Fed. Proc., Fed. Amer. Soc. Exp. Biol. 28, 1721 (1969).

99. C.G. Cochrane and B.S. Aikin, J. Exp. Med. 124, 733 (1966).

100. Z.A. Cohn and J.G. Hirsch, J. Exp. Med. 112, 983 (1960).

101. W.T. Kniker and C.G. Cochrane, J. Exp. Med. 122, 83 (1965).

102. O. Behnke, J. Ultrastruct. Res. 24, 412 (1968).

103. A.J. Marcus, N. Engl. J. Med. 280, 1213 (1969).

104. T.P. Ashford and D.G. Freiman, Amer. J. Pathol. 50, 257 (1966).

105. E.C. Franklin and B. Frangione, Ann. Rev. Med. 20, 155 (1969).

106. B.D. Jankovic and H.F. Dvorak, J. Immunol. 89

571 (1962).

107. J.M.B. Bloodworth, Jr. and M. Douglass, Lab. Invest. 18, 320 (1968).

108. A. Lazarow and E. Speidel In "Small Blood Vessel Involvement in Diabetes Mellitus", (M.D. Siperstein, A.R. Colwell and K. Meyer, eds.), p. 217. Amer. Inst. Biol. Sci., Washington, D.C., 1964.

109. A.E. Farnham and D.T. Dubin, J. Mol. Biol. 14, 55 (1965).

110. M.G. Farquhar and G.E. Palade, J. Cell Biol. 13, 55 (1962).

111. S.M. Kurtz and J.F.A. McManus, J. Ultrastruct. Res. 4, 81 (1960).

112. J.M. Taylor and C.P. Stanners, Biochim. Biophys. Acta 155, 425 (1968).

113. E. Blau and A.F. Michael, J. Lab. Clin. Med. 77, 97 (1971).

114. A.Y.K. Chow and K.N. Drummond, Lab. Invest. 20, 213 (1969).

115. E.R. Fisher and H.R. Hellstrom, Lab. Invest. 11, 617 (1962).

116. A.F. Michael, E. Blau, and R.L. Vernier, Lab. Invest. 23, 649 (1970).

117. S. Rosen, M.A. Swerdlow, R.C. Muehrcke, and C.L. Pierani, Amer. J. Clin. Pathol. 41, 487 (1964).

118. V.J. Rosen, L.J. Cole, L.W. Wachtel, and R.S. Doggett, Lab. Invest. 18, 260 (1968).

119. A.J. Fish, K.C. Herdman, W.D. Kelly, and R.A. Good, Transplantation 5, 1338 (1967).

120. J.J. McPhail, Jr., F.J. Dixon, L. Brettschneider and T.E. Starzl, N. Engl. J. Med., 282, 412 (1970).

121. O. Vilar and J.J. Christian, Lab. Invest. 17, 645 (1967).

122. F.G. Germuth, A.J. Valdes, L.B. Senterfit, and A.D. Pollacle, Johns Hopkins Med. J. 122, 137 (1968).

123. J.J. Christian, J.A. Lloyd, and D.E. Davis, Recent Progr. Horm. Res. 21, 501 (1965).

124. W. Thorn, F. Liemann, and P.V. Wichert, Pflüegers Arch. Gesamite Physiol. Menschen.

Tiere 273, 528 (1961).

125. M.T. Vogt and E. Farber, Amer. J. Pathol. 53, 1 (1968).

126. J.H. Brown and B.J. Kennedy, N. Engl. J. Med. 272, 111 (1965).

127. B.J. Kennedy, J.F. Van Pilsum, M. Sandberg-Wollheim, and J.W. Yarbro, Proc. Soc. Exp. Biol. Med. 127, 109 (1968).

128. K.A. Porter, G.A. Andres, M.W. Calder, J.B. Dossetor, K.C. Hsu, J.M. Kendall, B.C. Seegal, and T.E. Starzl, Lab. Invest. 18, 159 (1968).

129. T.L. Phillips and G.F. Leong, Cancer Res. 27 286 (1967).

130. R.L. Engerman, D. Pfaffenbach, and M.D. Davis, Lab. Invest. 17, 738 (1967).

131. O. Hassler, Lab. Invest. 22, 286 (1970).

132. H. Imai, S.K. Lee, and S.J. Pastor, Virchows Arch., A 350, 183 (1970).

133. C.G. Cochrane, J. Exp. Med. 118, 489 (1963).

134. Y. Kapanci, Amer. J. Pathol. 47, 665 (1965).

135. T.E. Starzl, R.A. Lerner, F.J. Dixon, D.G. Groth, L. Brettschneider, and P.I. Terasaki, N. Engl. J. Med. 278, 642 (1968).

136. G.M. Williams, D.M. Hume, R.P. Hudson, Jr., P.J. Morris, K. Kano, and F. Milgrom, N. Engl. J. Med. 279, 611 (1968).

137. F. Kissmeyer-Nielsen, S. Olsen, V.P. Peterson, and O. Fjeldborg, Lancet 2, 662 (1966).

138. P.I. Terasaki, D.L. Thrasher, and T.H. Hauber In "Advances in Transplantation" (J. Dausset, J. Hamburger, and G. Mathé, eds.), p. 225. Munksgaard, Copenhagen, 1968.

139. P.F. Hjort and F.T. Rapaport, Annu. Rev. Med. 16, 135 (1970).

140. P. Kincaid-Smith, Austr. Ann. Med. 19, 201 (1970).

141. J.C. Gunnells, Jr., D.L. Stickel, and R.R. Robinson, N. Engl. J. Med. 274, 543 (1966).

142. G. Lundgren, L. Bozovic, and J. Castenfors In "Advances in Transplantation" (J. Dausset, J. Hamburger, and G. Mathé, eds.), p. 627.

Munksgaard, Copenhagen, 1968.

143. P.H. Albrecht and J.A. Greene, Jr., Ann. Intern. Med. 65, 908 (1966).

144. G.M. Williams, H.M. Lee, R.F. Weymouth, W.R. Harlan, Jr., K.R. Holden, C.M. Stanley, G.A. Millington, and D.M. Hume, Surgery 62, 204 (1967).

145. G.M. Williams, P.J. Morris, W.R. Harlan, and D.M. Hume In "Advances in Transplantation" (J. Dausset, J. Hamburger, and G. Mathé, eds.) p. 373, Munksgaard, Copenhagen, 1968.

146. P. Galle and H. de Montera, Rev. Franc. Etud. Clin. Biol. 7, 40 (1962).

147. L.W. Henderson, K.D. Nolph, J.B. Puschett, and M. Goldberg, N. Engl. J. Med. 278, 467 (1968).

148. G. Threfall, D.M. Taylor, and A.T. Buck, Amer. J. Pathol. 50, 1 (1967).

PATHOLOGY IN ALLOGRAFT RECIPIENTS

David T. Rowlands, Jr.
School of Medicine
University of Pennsylvania
Philadelphia, Pennsylvania

Peter M. Burkholder
University of Wisconsin Medical School
Madison, Wisconsin

The purpose of this discussion is to review the
pathologic alterations that may be encountered in
allograft recipients. Particular emphasis will be
placed on human renal transplants and many of the
histologic changes seen in these patients will be
compared with those in certain experimental organ
grafts. The complexity of the pathologic picture
and the contribution of nonspecific factors to these
changes will be described but those features that
are directly related to allografts and immunosuppression will be emphasized. The principle determinants
of the pathology in graft recipients are the genetic
relationship of the donor and recipient, immunosuppressive therapy, host disease, and factors related
to the mechanics of transplantation.

MORPHOLOGY OF GRAFT REJECTION

Two general pathologic processes have been identified in graft rejection (27). The first is cellular immunity, which has been classically regarded as
a form of delayed hypersensitivity. The second,
humoral immunity has long been known to be significant in rejection of xenografts (5, 17, 18, 25, 29,
32) and certain allografts (13, 14, 34). The determinants of the relative degree of participation of

one or the other of these pathologic processes include the genetic relationships of the hosts and donors, the previous immunologic history of the recipient (e.g., sensitization to donor antigens), and the type and amount of immunosuppressive agents used.

Ordinarily, the earliest demonstrable change in renal graft rejection is adherence of inflammatory cells and platelets to the vascular endothelium (19). This is followed by the rapid extension of cells and fluid through damaged capillary endothelium forming on interstital cellular exudate associated with edema. The cellular exudate is most heavily concentrated in the cortex and tends to localize about tubules, glomeruli, and smaller blood vessels. The inflammatory cells are largely mononuclear. In this respect they resemble delayed hypersensitivity but the cellular exudates are more heterogeneous in graft rejection than in delayed hypersensitivity and consist of small and medium lymphocytes, eosinophils, and plasma cells (Fig. 1).

The mononuclear cell aggregates about tubules differ from those surrounding renal glomeruli and arterioles in that these inflammatory cells infiltrate and disrupt the renal tubular epithelium. Figure 2 is an electronmicrograph showing disruption of peritubular capillaries and injury to the basement membranes of a renal tubule. In contrast to these tubular lesions, Bowman's glomerular capsule remains intact and there is no mononuclear cellular infiltrate within the walls of arterioles during rejection of renal grafts.

The initial studies of the morphology and physiology of graft rejection were almost exclusively concerned with the role of these cellular exudates in graft rejection. More interest has been generated in recent years by the vascular injuries in organ grafts (3, 4, 12, 19, 23). The first vascular lesions to be thought of as participating in graft rejection were, curiously, those in longer standing renal allografts. Figure 3 is a photomicrograph of

330

such a lesion with marked thickening of the vascular intima and a narrowed lumen. The media in these arteries is severely scarred and the elastica is distorted and duplicated. It is obvious that there is nothing intrinsic in these healed vascular lesions to suggest that they are of immunologic origin. However, the frequent association of these lesions with previous episodes of graft rejection and the absence of factors, such as hypertension, that may be responsible for identical lesions suggested that immunologic graft rejection might be responsible for these changes in arterial walls.

It was reasoned that if these vascular lesions were, in fact, part of graft rejection, a more acute form of vascular damage should be evident early on in the rejection process. Such lesions, appearing as fibrinoid necrosis in renal arterioles, were then identified in both experimental animals (21) and man (3, 12, 24). This evidence taken together suggests that the acute lesions result from antigen-antibody mediated injury. However, only a few authors (3, 10, 15) have demonstrated the presence of immune reagents in the vasculature of rejecting allografts.

The lesions that have been discussed and demonstrated to this point have been taken from biopsies of human renal allografts when the patients were treated with immunosuppressive agents. These examples serve to emphasize the point that rejection can take place even in the face of immunosuppression. However, it is reasonable to inquire as to whether these changes are similar to those seen in untreated organ grafts and in organs other than the kidney. In order to show the general nature of the lesions already described, we have selected some illustrations from recent experiments utilizing canine renal and cardiac heterotopic transplants (16, 30). Both kidneys and hearts were placed in the necks of recipients so that they could be readily biopsied.

The kidneys were placed so that the renal artery was anastomosed to the carotid artery and jugular vein received the renal vein. The average survival of these untreated renal allografts was 6 days. An interstitial cellular exudate similar in every respect to that seen in human renal allografts, appeared by the second posttransplant day. The inflammatory exudate increased rapidly and associated vascular lesions were common. Figure 4 is a photomicrograph of a canine renal allograft biopsied 4 days after transplantation, showing interstitial edema and abundant mononuclear cells.

Canine cardiac transplants were placed in the same way as the kidneys with the aorta being attached to the carotid artery and the pulmonary artery to the jugular vein. A significant portion of the aortic blood flow was therefore directed into the coronary arteries. Defects were created in the atrial septa of these transplants to reduce the chance of intracardiac thrombosis. The average survival of heterotopic canine cardiac grafts was 7.5 days. The morphologic differences between the cardiac grafts and the renal transplants were minor, being easily accounted for by the anatomic differences between these organs. The earliest changes in the cardiac grafts were perivascular cellular exudates appearing on the second day. Later in the course of rejection, the inflammatory reactions became more severe (Fig. 5), with extensive myocardial necrosis being evident. Although such regions of myocardial necrosis were often associated with inflammatory cellular exudates, there were other areas in which the necrotic myocardium lacked inflammatory cells. Because acute vascular lesions similar to those already described in human and canine renal allografts were frequent, it was tempting to speculate that these might account for the inflammatory cell-free zones of myocardial necrosis. Studies of renal and cardiac graft blood flow were made to evaluate this more thoroughly (16). In each case, measurements were made using an implantable sine-wave electromagnetic flow probe positioned at the carotid arteries and jugular veins. The blood flow in the grafts increased during the initial 4 posttransplant days of both the cardiac

and renal grafts and, as might have been anticipated,
declined later until graft rejection was complete.
It would be premature to attribute this response to
the small vessel changes discussed earlier, because
these vascular alterations appeared at a time when
blood flow was increased above that immediately
following transplantation. However, it is entirely
possible that these overall hemodynamic measurements
do not accurately reflect redistribution of the blood
flow in the graft bed during rejection.

HYPERACUTE GRAFT REJECTION

The cellular and vascular lesions described thus
far make up most of the pathologic changes encountered in conventional rejection of organ grafts.
Clearly, these types of graft rejection can be
classified as acute or chronic, depending on the
degree of development of the vascular lesions with
thickened scarred walls and narrowed lumens. As
indicated earlier both the acute and chronic changes
probably rely on the same pathogenetic mechanisms
and seem to differ principally because of variation
in the ability of immunosuppressive agents to prevent
immunologic graft rejection.

Hyperacute graft rejection may be separated from
these more usual types of acute or chronic responses.
The onset of hyperacute graft rejections may occur
only a few minutes after the blood flow is reestab-
lished or they may be delayed in onset (3). They
are often accounted for by preexisting humoral antibodies in the recipient that are specific for donor
antigens.

In those cases in which there were major blood
group mismatches between the donor and recipient
(31, 33), graft rejection became apparent almost
immediately after blood flow was begun in the graft.
The kidneys enlarged rapidly and became discolored.
Microscopically, the glomeruli were enlarged because
of masses of red cells lodged in glomerular capillaries.

The pathologic picture of hyperacute rejection, which depends on preexisting antibodies directed at donor antigens other than red cell antigens, differs from this pattern. The physiologic changes due to such antibodies are rapid and are associated with decreased vascular flow and marked cortical necrosis. Microscopically, polymorphonuclear leukocytes are abundant in these kidneys as are platelet and fibrin thrombi.

Figures 6 and 7 illustrate the changes that may be seen in hyperacute graft rejection. In this case, the patient had a renal graft from his HL-A identical brother. However, renal failure began after the first posttransplant week and an arteriogram carried out on the fourteenth day (Fig. 6) revealed irregular cortical margins, a pattern consistent with diffuse small vessel occlusion. Microscopic sections taken at this time confirmed the fact that there were multiple areas of cortical necrosis and that this was associated with fibrin thrombi in glomerular capillaries and in arterioles (Fig. 7). Although anti-kidney antibodies were not detected in this patient, it can be suggested that this episode of hyperacute rejection resulted from prior sensitization of the graft recipient to non-HL-A antigens. Of additional interest is the fact that the patient retained his transplant with the use of increased levels of steroids. When a second renal biopsy was carried out 5 months later, hyalinization of small numbers of vessels and glomeruli were the only residual changes of the earlier rejection episode.

COMPLICATIONS OF RENAL ALLOGRAFTS

Many of the clinical problems and pathologic changes seen in organ graft recipients are determined by factors other than immunologic graft rejection. These changes can be conveniently divided between those resulting from the overall effects of immuno-suppression and those appearing as glomerular alterations in the graft.

The complications arising directly from the use of immunosuppressive agents will only be touched on briefly here because these have been covered more extensively in other portions of this volume. One general consequence of immunosuppressive therapy has been depression of the patients' inflammatory and immunologic responses leading to overwhelming and often fatal infections (9, 26).

The causative organisms seen in these infections are often fungal or viral, although bacterial infections are not uncommon. Pneumocystis carinii and cytomegalic inclusion disease are frequently seen. The clinical and pathologic depression of response to infection is well illustrated by a transplant patient who presented with an abscess of a finger soon after steroids were begun for graft rejection. The patient then developed and recovered from septic pulmonary infarcts. His final episode was acute shock with no localizing signs or symptoms. At necropsy, the patient was found to have died of an unsuspected intraperitoneal hemorrhage resulting from erosion of an artery in a large, partially healed pancreatic abscess. In addition to such overwhelming relatively asymptomatic infections, these patients have more than their share of malignant neoplasms. These lesions have been attributed to immunologic deficiencies resulting in diminished natural immunologic surveillance. However, in this regard it is curious that the neoplasms mostly arise in the reticuloendothelial system.

There is now considerable evidence that glomerular abnormalities are frequent in both renal isografts and allografts. These changes include both frank recurrence of the host disease and less well-understood alterations of the glomerular basement membrane and glomerular mesangium. Some may reflect healed lesions of graft rejection (3). Recurrence of glomerulonephritis has been well documented in renal isografts (6, 7, 20, 24). More recently there has been increasing concern regarding glomerular lesions in renal allografts (6, 8, 20, 22, 28).

Glomerulopathy has, in fact, been recognized in 74% of renal allografts in one series (20, 22) but most of these changes were not felt to represent frank recurrence of host disease. The glomerular basement membranes were altered in these patients with sub-endothelial electron dense deposits being frequently seen. IgM immunoglobulins were identified in linear or finely granular patterns and these deposits were often associated with fixed complement. Such changes were usually interpreted as resulting from host antibodies reacting with glomerular basement membranes rather than necessarily representing true recurrence of the host disease. Other investigators (6, 28) have explicitly compared host disease with glomerular changes in renal allografts with particular attention being given to similarities in both mechanisms and morphology. When two groups of patients having either antiglomerular basement membrane nephritis or antigen-antibody complex nephritis as the host disease (6) were evaluated, 7 of 13 patients who had antiglomerular basement membrane nephritis had apparent recurrence of their original host disease. Six of 26 patients whose original renal disease was of the immune complex type also developed recurrent disease. Our own experience has been previously reported in detail (28) but will be summarized in the section immediately following.

TRANSPLANTATION IN HL-A IDENTICAL PATIENTS

In recent years tissue typing of donors and recipients has been used extensively in the hope that fewer genetic differences between hosts and donors will permit maintainence of organ grafts with use of less immunosuppression. An initial study (28) of biopsies of 12 such recipients 2 to 42 months after transplantation has shown that graft rejection is relatively minor and that these grafts can usually be maintained with azathioprine alone. One patient, in fact, was taken off all immunosuppressive therapy with no apparent adverse results as long as one full

336

year later. An additional patient, not included in this group of 12, experienced hyperacute graft rejection as illustrated earlier (Figs. 6 and 7).

Eleven of the 12 cases displayed some degree of glomerulopathy at the time of biopsy. However, these were, for the most part, of minor degree consisting of local fusion of epithelial foot processes, electron-dense membrane deposits, and increases in mesangial cells and membrane matrix (Figs. 8 and 9). The lack of resemblence of the pathologic changes in these grafts and in the hosts' own kidneys suggests that the glomerular lesions are complex pathogenetically. They may be accounted for by factors such as the host's original renal disease, graft rejection, the mechanics of transplantation, drug therapy, or new hypersensitivity responses affecting the kidney graft either singly or in combination.

Recurrence of the host disease was apparent in two of our patients. One showed a widened basement membrane and electron-dense deposits in the mesangium and both immunoglobulins (IgG, IgM) and complement could be demonstrated in small segments of the glomerular capillary walls. The second patient was of more interest. In this case the host had lobular glomerulonephritis (Fig. 10) necessitating a renal allograft from his HL-A identical brother. Only minimal amounts of azathioprine were required to maintain the graft without clinically apparent rejection. However, graft function decreased after 2 years at which time a biopsy (Fig. 11) showed frank recurrence of the host's lobular glomerulonephritis in the transplanted kidney.

DIAGNOSIS OF GRAFT REJECTION

It is obviously of the utmost importance to understand the extent to which the pathologic information described above may be used in the diagnosis and direction of management in organ transplantation (3, 28). It is important to point out that the correlation between the morphologic observations and

clinical evidences of graft rejection are imperfect.
In many instances biopsies will show minimal to
moderate evidence of graft rejection before the
signs and symptoms have reached a clinically apparent level. The overall result of this is that
neither clinical criteria nor structural studies can
be relied upon exclusively for the diagnosis of
graft rejection.

It is also of obvious importance in the diagnosis of graft rejection by renal biopsy to draw a
sharp distinction between those lymphoid infiltrates
of graft rejection and those that are less specific.
Subcapsular infiltrates can present particular problems. These are frequently a result of perirenal
disease and can only be interpreted as graft rejection if the diagnosis of perirenal disease can be
excluded and if the pattern of the exudate shows
peritubular concentrations of heterogeneous lymphoid
cells associated with basement membranes and tubular
cell injury. Similarly, vascular lesions of the
types described and illustrated earlier (Fig. 3)
can only be considered as part of chronic graft
rejection if hypertension can be excluded in both
donor and recipient.

Renal biopsies can also be used to make the
diagnosis of causes of renal failure other than
graft rejection. The importance of this with respect to recurrent host disease has already been
described in detail. In one other case renal biopsy
was used to distinguish failure due to ureteral obstruction from that due to graft rejection. The
diagnosis of obstruction was made on the basis of
greatly dilated renal tubules and the absence of
lymphoid infiltrates.

There has, of course, been considerable interest
in devising means of distinguishing graft rejection
from other forms of renal failure by laboratory means
other than renal biopsy. In this regard, attention
has recently been directed at examination of the
urinary sediment in renal allograft recipients (1, 2,
11). The chief premise of this work was that graft

rejection might be associated with qualitative differences in the composition of the urinary sediment.
The technique selected for preparation of the sedi-
ments was collection on Millipore filters which were
stained with the Papanicolau technique. The advantages of this method are that small quantities of
urine can be used, the mechanics of preparation are
simple, and mechanical trauma to cellular elements
is minimized. The characteristics of the urinary
sediment from patients undergoing graft rejection
included nuclear Saterations, casts, red blood cells,
a dirty background of the preparations, mixed cell
clusters, lymphocytes, and tubular cells. It was
discovered that five or more of these seven types of
abnormalities could be recognized consistently in the
urinary sediment of patients undergoing frank graft
rejection. The pattern of changes seen was significantly different from that in patients with pyelonephritis or other forms of renal disease. The sensitivity of this technique was demonstrated by the
fact that recognition of a urinary rejection pattern
could often be made several days before rejection
became clinically apparent. The specificity of the
urinary rejection pattern is shown by the observation
that treatment of recipients undergoing graft rejection resulted in prompt reversal of the abnormal
urinary findings. As a spin off of this investigation, it was found that the Millipore technique per-
mitted easy identification of viral infections of the
urinary tract including cytomegalic inclusion disease (1).

SUMMARY

Morphologic studies of allografts support the
concept that both cellular and humoral factors participate in graft rejection. The importance of cellular immunity is suggested by aggregates of lymphoid
cells that superficially resemble a type of delayed
hypersensitivity. However, the lymphoid cells in
graft rejection are more heterogeneous than in

339

delayed hypersensitivity and the most obvious lesions in graft rejection are those in which renal tubular cells are injured following disruption of the tubular basement membranes. Vascular lesions observed in graft rejection include disruption of peritubular capillaries, fibrinoid necrosis of renal arterioles, and more chronic changes, including the appearance of thick walled arterioles with narrow lumens. The arteriolar lesions are believed to result from humoral antibodies directed against donor transplantation antigens. In some cases, such antibodies can result in hyperacute graft rejection manifested by multiple fibrin thrombi.

Complications in graft recipients include infections often with unusual organisms and an increased incidence of malignant neoplasms due to immunosuppression as well as various sorts of glomerulopathies. In some instances these glomerular lesions undoubtedly represent recurrence of the host disease but in other cases they are less specific.

The total pathologic picture in graft recipients is complex and depends on the genetic relationship between the donor and recipient, immunosuppressive therapy, duration of the graft, the host's original disease, and factors related to the mechanics of transplantation surgery.

Acknowledgements

Supported in part by USPHS grants AM-14372, HE-13931 and AM-11092.

REFERENCES

1. Bossen, E.H., Johnston, W.W., Amatulli, J., and Rowlands, D.T., Jr. Exfoliative cytopathologic studies in organ transplantation. I. The cytologic diagnosis of cytomegalic inclusion disease in the urine of renal allograft recipients. Amer. J. Clin. Pathol. 52, 340-344 (1969).
2. Bossen, E.H., Johnston, W.W., Amatulli, J.,

and Rowlands, D.T., Jr. Exfoliative cytopathologic studies in organ transplantation. III. The
cytologic profile of urine during acute renal
allograft rejection. Acta Cytol. 14, 176-181
(1970).

3. Busch, G.J., Reynolds, E.S., Galvenek, E.G.
    Braun, W.E., and Dammin, G.J. Human renal allo-
    grafts. The role of vascular injury in early
    graft failure. Medicine (Baltimore)50, 29-83
    (1971).

4. Darmady, E.M., Offer, J.M., and Stranack, F.
    Study of renal vessels by microdissection in
    human transplantation. Brit. Med. J. 2, 976-
    978 (1964).

5. Dewitt, C.W. Serologic response of humans to
    chimpanzee tissue. Fed. Proc., Fed. Amer. Soc.
    Exp. Biol. 24, 573 (1965) (abstr.).

6. Dixon, F.J., McPhaul, J.J., Jr., and Lerner, R.
    Recurrence of glomerulonephritis in the trans-
    planted kidneys. Arch. Intern. Med. 123, 554-
    557 (1969).

7. Glassock, R.J., Feldman, D., Reynolds, E.S.,
    Dammin, G.J., and Merrill, J.P. Human renal
    isografts: A clinical and pathologic analysis.
    Medicine (Baltimore) 47, 411-454 (1968).

8. Hamburger, J. Observations in patients with a
    well tolerated homotransplanted kidney: Pos-
    sibility of a new secondary disease. Ann. N.Y.
    Acad. Sci. 120, 558-577 (1964).

9. Hill, R.B., Jr., Rowlands, D.T., Jr., and Rif-
    kind, D. Infectious pulmonary disease in
    patients receiving immunosuppressive therapy for
    organ transplantation. N. Engl. J. Med. 271,
    1021-1027 (1964).

10. Horowitz, R.E., Burrows, L., Paronetto, F.,
    Dreiling, D., and Kark, A.E. Immunologic obser-
    vations on homografts. II. The canine kidney.
    Transplantation 3, 318-325 (1965).

11. Johnston, W.W., Bossen, E.H., Amatulli, J., and
    Rowlands, D.T., Jr. Exfoliative cytopathologic
    studies in organ transplantation. II. Factors

in the diagnosis of cytomegalic inclusion disease in urine of renal allograft recipients. Acta Cytol. 13, 605–610 (1969).

12. Kincaid-Smith, P. Vascular changes in homotransplants. Brit. Med. J. 1, 178–179 (1964).

13. Kissmeyer-Nielsen, F. Humoral antibodies in human kidney allotransplantation In "Advances in Transplantation" (J. Dausset, J. Hamburger, and G. Mathé, eds.), p. 415. Williams & Wilkins, Baltimore, Maryland, 1967.

14. Kissmeyer-Nielsen, F., Olsen, S., Petersen, U.P., and Fieldberg, O. Hyperacute rejection of kidney allografts, associated with preexisting humoral antibodies against donor cells. Lancet 2, 662–665 (1966).

15. Najarian, J.S., and Foker, J.E. Interpretations of transplanted kidney morphology. Transplant. Proc. 1, 1022–1031 (1969).

16. Osteen, R.T., Ebert, P.A., and Rowlands, D.T., Jr. Relationship between rejection and organ blood flow in sensitized and non-sensitized cardiac and renal grafts. J. Surg. Oncol. 2, 399–405 (1970).

17. Perper, R.J., and Najarian, J.S. Experimental renal heterotransplantation. I. In widely divergent species. Transplantation 4, 377–388 (1966).

18. Perper, R.J., and Najarian, J.S. Experimental renal heterotransplantation. II. Closely related species. Transplantation 4, 700–712 (1966).

19. Porter, K.A. Morphological aspects of renal homograft rejection. Brit. Med. Bull. 21, 171–175 (1965).

20. Porter, K.A., Andres, G.A., Calder, M.W., Dossetor, J.B., Hsu, K.C., Rendall, J.M., Seegal, B.C., and Starzl, T.E. Human renal transplantation II. Immunofluorescent and immunoferritin studies. Lab. Invest. 18, 159–171 (1968).

21. Porter, K.A., Calne, R.Y., and Zukoski, C.F. Vascular and other changes in 200 canine renal homotransplants treated with immunosuppressive

drugs. Lab. Invest. 13, 810–824 (1964).

22. Porter, K.A., Dossetor, J.B., Marchioro, T.L., Peart, W.S., Rendall, J.M., Starzl, T.E., and Terasaki, P.I. Human renal transplants. I. Glomerular changes. Lab. Invest. 16, 153–181 (1967).

23. Porter, K.A., Peart, W.S., Kenyon, J.R., Joseph, N.H., Hoehn, R.J., and Calne, R.Y. Rejection of kidney homotransplants. Ann. N.Y. Acad. Sci. 120, 472–495 (1964).

24. Porter, K.A., Rendall, J.M., Stolinski, C., Terasaki, P.I., Marchioro, T.L., and Starzl, T.E. Light and electron microscopic study of biopsies from 33 human renal allografts and an isograft 1 3/4–2½ years after transplantation. Ann. N.Y. Acad. Sci. 129, 615–636 (1966).

25. Reemtsma, K., McCracken, B.H., and Sehlegel, U. Reversal of early graft rejection after renal heterotransplantation in man. J. Amer. Med. Ass. 187, 691–696 (1964).

26. Rifkind, D., Starzl, T.E., Marchioro, T.L., Waddell, W.R., Rowlands, D.T., Jr., and Hill, R.B., Jr. Transplantation pneumonia. J. Amer. Med. Ass. 189, 808–812 (1964).

27. Rowlands, D.T., Jr., and Bossen, E.H. Immunological mechanisms of allograft rejection. Arch. Intern. Med. 123, 491–500 (1969).

28. Rowlands, D.T., Jr., Burkholder, P.M., Bossen, E.H., and Lin, H.H. Renal allografts in HL-A matched recipients. Light, immunofluorescence, and electron microscopic studies. Amer. J. Pathol. 61, 177–198 (1970).

29. Rowlands, D.T., Jr., Kirkpatrick, C.H., Vatter, A.E., and Wilson, W.E.C. Immunologic studies in human organ transplantation IV. Serologic and pathologic studies following heterotransplantation of the kidney. Amer. J. Pathol. 50, 605–622 (1967).

30. Rowlands, D.T., Jr., Vanderbeek, R.B., Seigler, H.F., and Ebert, P.A. Rejection of canine cardiac allografts. Amer. J. Pathol. 53, 617–

629 (1968).

31. Starzl, T.E., Marchioro, T.L., and Holmes, J.H. The incidence, cause and significance of immediate and delayed oliguia or anuria after human renal transplantation. Surg. Gynecol. Obstet. 118, 819–827 (1964).

32. Starzl, T.E., Marchioro, T.L., Peters, B.N., Kirkpatrick, C.H., Wilson, W.E.C., Porter, K.A., Rifkind, D., Ogden, D.A., Hitchcock, C.R., and Waddell, W.R. Renal heterotransplantation from baboon to man: Experience with six cases. Transplantation 2, 752–776 (1964).

33. Starzl, T.E,, Marchioro, T.L., Rifkind, D., Holmes, J.H., Rowlands, D.T., Jr., and Waddell, W.R. Factors in successful renal transplantation. Surgery 56, 296–318 (1964).

34. Terasaki, P.I., Trasher, D.L., and Hauber, T.H. Serotyping for homotransplantation. XIII. Immediate transplantation rejection and associated preformed antibodies. In "Advances in Transplantation" (J. Dausset, J. Hamburger, and G. Mathé, eds.), pp. 225–229. Williams & Wilkins, Baltimore, Maryland, 1967.

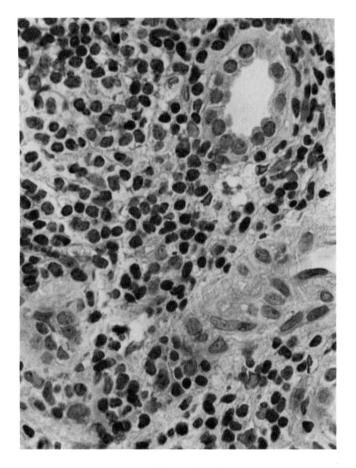

Fig. 1

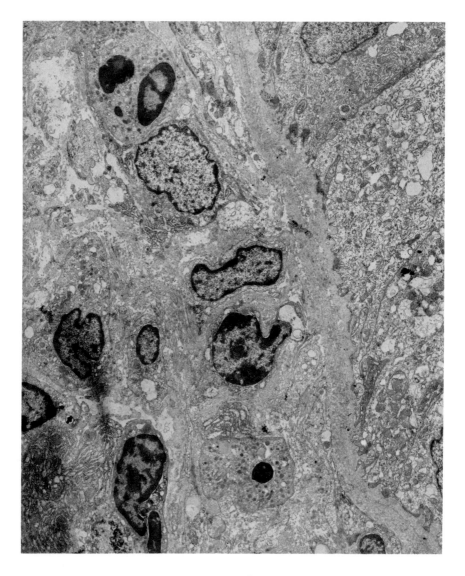

Fig. 2

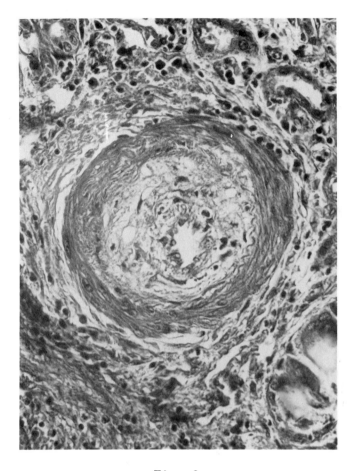

Fig. 3

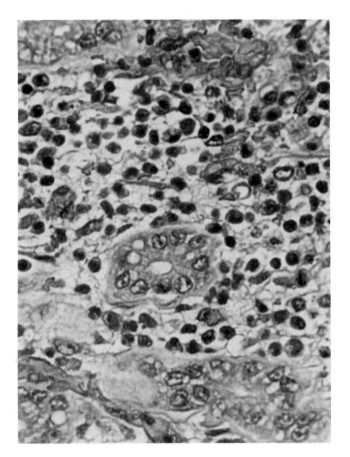

Fig. 4

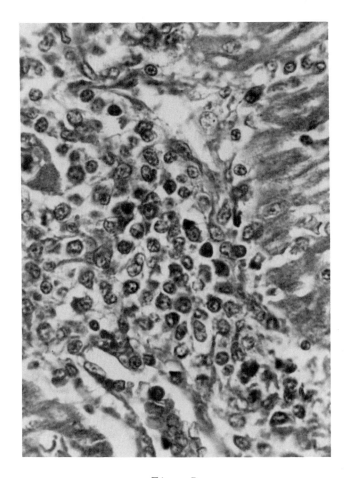

Fig. 5

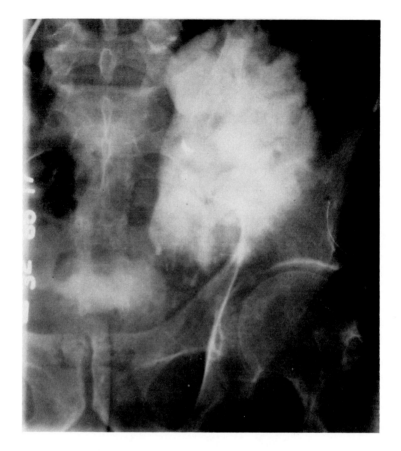

Fig. 6

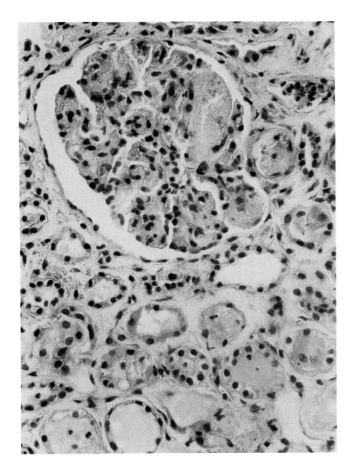

Fig. 7

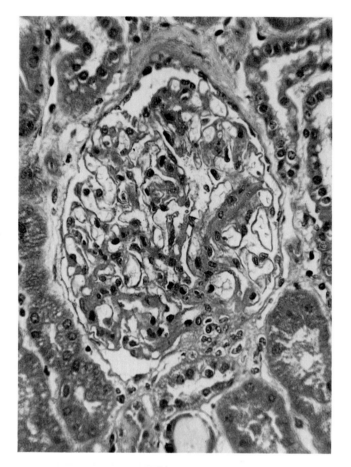

Fig. 8

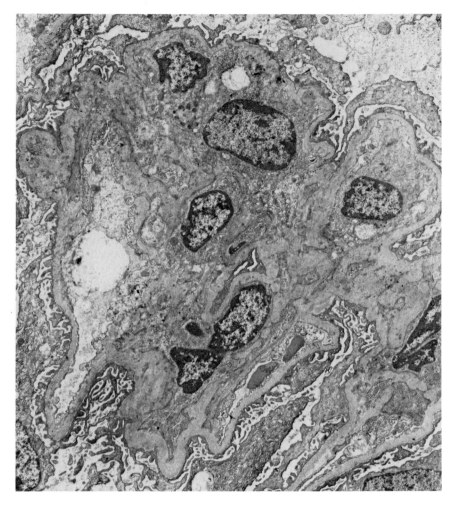

Fig. 9

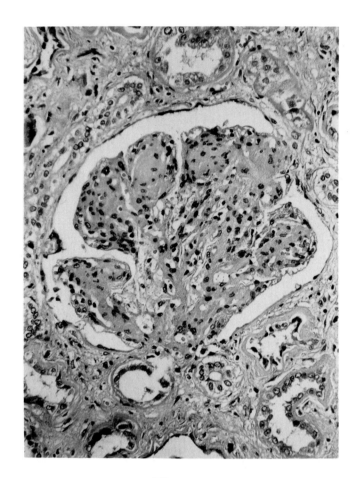

Fig. 10

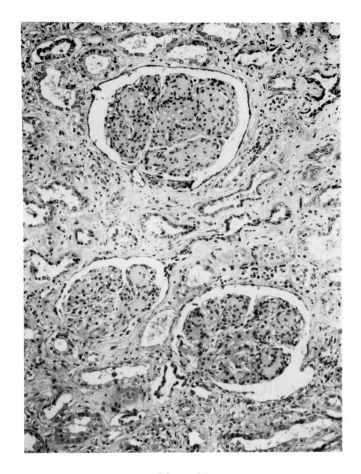

Fig. 11

A SEARCH FOR CHEMICAL TAGS ON TRANSPLANTATION ANTIGENS

R. A. Popp, Mary W. Francis, and Diana M. Popp

Biology Division, Oak Ridge National Laboratory,
Oak Ridge, Tennessee

INTRODUCTION

Transplantation of a tissue from one noninbred animal into another of the same species causes immunologically competent cells in the recipient's body to produce humoral and cellular immunities directed against specific antigens in the transplanted tissue. These antigens are gene controlled and are natural constituents of tissues; they are usually identified by serological means. The immune response leads to cell destruction and rejection of the transplanted tissue. The period of survival of the grafted tissue depends on the quantity and quality of the antigenic differences between the donor and recipient (48). The number of reported blood group systems in laboratory and domestic animals ranges from five to eight for rat, rabbit, horse, and sheep; from 12 to 14 for chickens, swine, and cattle; and 15 or more for mice and man (47). However, only one or two loci determine the major histoincompatibility barrier for each species. Tissue transplantation across a single major incompatibility system results in more rapid tissue rejection than transplantation across multiple minor incompatibility groups (12, 19). Structural factors that determine whether an antigen is a major or a minor transplantation antigen are as yet unknown; however, the primary structures of the individual antigens are implicated because these differences are genetically controlled

357

by multiple alleles at several loci. To establish
that unique structural determinants are involved,
the chemical and physical characteristics of major
versus minor antigens must be studied. In addition,
the chemical compositions of transplantation antigens
must be known before intelligent approaches can be
suggested to control the ultimate association of
antibodies with tissue antigens. It is necessary to
understand the chemistry of specificity in order to
control selectively the immune response to specific
transplantation antigens in ways that do not impair
the normal immune response to pathogens. Evidence
to date suggests that once the immune response to the
major transplantation antigens can be controlled by
directed chemical or immunological intervention,
then the immune response to the minor transplantation
antigens will be controllable by moderate doses of
immunosuppressant drugs (46).

The major transplantation antigens in mice are
controlled by the H-2 locus (17). The major transplantation antigens in man are controlled by the
HL-A locus (5, 8, 14). The genetics of both H-2
and HL-A are quite well defined (1). Both H-2 and
HL-A are complex, highly polymorphic systems and
their respective antigens are present in relatively
large amounts on most tissues (6); therefore, it is
assumed that studies on the chemistry of the H-2
antigens in mice should provide a good model for
future chemical studies on HL-A in man. The fact
that several inbred strains of mice are available,
whereas human populations are very heterogeneous,
makes the mouse a more suitable animal in which to do
initial studies on the chemistry of transplantation
antigens.

This paper describes a combination of genetic
and biochemical methods that are being used to search
for genetically controlled, chemically unique segments of transplantation antigens in mice, which will
then be used as chemical tags to identify transplantation antigens and to judge their degree of purity
after each step in their isolation.

ANTIGEN ISOLATION AND CHEMISTRY

Transplantation antigens are either integral parts of or intimately associated with plasma membranes (20-22, 40). The basic function of these antigens in the plasma membrane is unknown but it may be only indirectly associated with their known immunological roles. Different tissues in the mouse have quite different quantities or expressivity of H-2 antigens (6); e.g., spleen, lymph nodes, and liver will induce and adsorb H-2 antibodies much more readily than erythrocytes or brain. The dissimilar tissue distribution of these antigens may be closely correlated with their principal physiological roles but it provides little direct information on exactly what their more specialized functions might be. Additional information on this point may be obtained through studies on the comparative chemistry of these antigens and other constituents in membranes.

A number of investigators have attempted to isolate H-2 antigens to study their chemical compositions and structures (27). Plasma membranes must be solubilized in order to isolate their antigenic and nonantigenic components. Organic and inorganic reagents, enzymes, and sonication have been used to solubilize membranes. The measure of success of any of these methods depends on the fidelity of the assay used to measure the antigen in the solute. Methods presently used - antibody inhibition or antibody induction - to identify soluble H-2 antigens require that the molecules retain their capacity to combine with or to induce antibody (28, 30, 40, 50). The experience of most investigators is that the soluble form of H-2 antigens is more labile than the membrane-bound form. Assessment of the quantity of the antigen solubilized really reflects the combined effectiveness of the agents used to solubilize membranes and the stability of the antigens under the conditions used. Methods such as 90% phenol extraction used to recover carbohydrate ABH determinants (35) denature H-2 antigens (6). Therefore, any H-2

antigen that might be released by such treatment
would be undetectable by present methods of assay.
The requirement that the immunological activity of
transplantation antigens be maintained in order to
identify them at successive steps during their
isolation severely limits procedures that might be
used to purify the labile form of the soluble antigens further. Therefore, we have begun to examine
other methods to identify transplantation antigens.

We believe that transplantation antigens are
basically proteins, but they probably also contain
some carbohydrate prosthetic groups. Genetic experiments have shown that the serological specificities
of H-2 antigens are controlled by a linear arrangement of genetic material at the H-2 locus, which is
in the ninth linkage group of the mouse genome (17).
The H-2 locus is compound and the specific antigenic
determinants are controlled by limited regions of
the H-2 locus, as shown by serological analyses of
the gene products in H-2 crossover lines of mice
(49). There is still some question about whether the
five segments that have been separated by crossing
over really represent five subloci; however,
proximal genetic determinants within the H-2 locus
that have not been separated by crossing over are
correlated with a concomitant elution of these antigenic specificities in single fractions during
column chromatography (15). A similar observation
has been made from analyses of solubilized HL-A
antigens (11). Such close relationships between
genetic and serological specificity, which are controlled by a defined chromosomal region, are consistent with our premise that H-2 antigens have a polypeptide backbone to which carbohydrates and lipids
may be covalently linked.

Because H-2 antigens are basically proteins, it
is logical to apply methods to the study of antigens
that are commonly used to study the chemistry and
structure of proteins. Several types of human and
mouse hemoglobins can be classified by the uniqueness
of a segment of their polypeptide chains. For

example, an analysis of a single peptide such as
βT-1 of human hemoglobin, in which the amino acid in
the sixth position is valine rather than glutamic
acid (24), immediately characterizes the polypeptide
as β6val derived from sickle-cell hemoglobin rather
than normal A hemoglobin. Similarly, an analysis of
αT-9 of mouse hemoglobin can be used to identify the
five chemically distinguishable classes of α-chain
polypeptides in mice (23). Some mouse and human
hemoglobin chains can be classified by the characteristic chromatographic and electrophoretic properties of one of their tryptic peptides. Such observations suggested to us that it might be possible to
identify some unique tryptic peptides in digests of
plasma membranes that contain different H-2 antigens.
Some of these peptides should be derived from the H-2
antigens and should show genetic association in a
segregating population or in congenic lines.

Several methods could be used to separate and
characterize tryptic, chymotryptic, methionyl,
aspartyl, or other peptide fragments of plasma membranes. In general, tryptic peptides are fragments
of convenient size for separation and characterization. Once different peptides from plasma membranes
of mice are observed, genetic and biochemical methods
can be used to determine whether the variant peptides
are a part of H-2 or non-H-2 molecules. Unique peptides found in enzymic digests of plasma membranes
from parental strains of mice would be expected to
segregate with the H-2 serotypes of F2 progeny when
the peptides are derived from the H-2 antigens, but
such an association should be lacking when the unique
stromal peptides are not a product of the H-2 locus.
Of course, products of genes closely linked to H-2
would have to be taken into consideration before a
positive association between H-2 and a peptide
variant could be made. There are several genes near
the H-2 region that affect plasma membrane function,
such as TL antigen (7), the IR locus of McDevitt and
Tyan (32), and susceptibility to viruses (29).

Because of its homogeneity, mouse red cell

stroma is being used in the initial studies, even
though erythrocytes may have a lower concentration
of H-2 antigen than nucleated cells or whole tissue
such as lymphocytes or spleen (2). It has been
shown recently that red cells have a substantial
quantity of H-2 antigen, although the antigen on red
cells appears to have a lower affinity for antibody
than H-2 antigen on lymphocytes (37). In addition,
the constituents of the red cell stroma are likely
to become the basis for comparison of membrane constituents in other mouse tissues.

Stroma was prepared (37) from the erythrocytes
of eight strains of mice. The strains and their H-2
types are A/Sn (H-2a), C57BL/6 (H-2b), C57.F-H-14
(H-2b), B10.D2 (H-2d), DBA/2 (H-2d), A.CA (H-2f),
RFM/Un (H-2f), and C3H (H-2k).

The sulfhydryl groups in stroma were aminoethylated to add a basic group to the proteins and
to provide an additional site for peptide bond
cleavage by trypsin (41). Proteins in stroma contain a large number of acidic residues (Table 1);
such proteins usually are not digested easily by
trypsin. Approximately 100 mg of lyophilized stroma
was dissolved in 7.5 ml of a solution containing 8M
urea, 0.2% EDTA, and 0.2M Tris-HCl buffered at pH
8.6. Nitrogen was bubbled through the solution for
2 hrs at room temperature, 0.1 ml of β-mercapto-
ethanol was added, nitrogen stirring was continued
for 30 min before 0.2 ml of ethylenimine was added,
and the reaction mixture was stirred by nitrogen
bubbling for an additional 30 min. The sample was
diluted with distilled water and dialyzed overnight
against cold distilled water. The insoluble phase
was pelleted by centrifugation, and the aqueous
supernatant was also saved. The pellet was washed
in 10 to 15 ml of cold acetone, and the supernatant
of the acetone wash was added to the aqueous supernatant, which caused some of the soluble material in
the aqueous supernatant to precipitate. This precipitate was sedimented by centrifugation and added
to the acetone-washed pellet. The acetone-insoluble

pellet was suspended in 10 ml of 0.2M NH_4HCO_3 and lyophilized. The acetone-soluble fraction was dialyzed against cold distilled water to remove acetone and then lyophilized. About half of the original stroma by weight was found in the acetone-insoluble pellet and half in the acetone-soluble fraction.

Fifty milligrams of the aminoethylated acetone-insoluble pellet and 50 mg of the acetone-soluble fraction were separately dissolved in 10 ml of 0.2M NH_4HCO_3 buffered at pH 8.3. Four milligrams of dry trypsin was added, and digestion was carried out at $37°C$ for 4 hrs and continued overnight at room temperature. The quantity of trypsin was higher than commonly used, but poor digestion was obtained when only 1 mg of trypsin was used for each 50 mg of sample. Aliquots of the trypsin digests were placed on 18 X 22 in. sheets of Whatman No. 3 chromatography paper, and the tryptic peptides were separated (9) by descending chromatography in butanol, acetic acid, and water (4:1:5) for 18 hrs at room temperature and by high-voltage electrophoresis in pyridine, acetic acid, and water (1:10:289) at pH 3.5 for 75 min at 2000 V and 100 mA. Five chromatograms of the tryptic digests of stroma from each strain of mice were prepared. The tryptic peptides were located on a fingerprint by reaction with ninhydrin, and special stains were used on the remaining four chromatograms to detect peptides containing arginine, histidine, tyrosine, and tryptophan (38).

Fingerprints of the ninhydrin-positive peptides in the tryptic digests of the acetone-insoluble pellet of C3H and A/Sn stroma are shown in Fig. 1. A few unique tryptic peptides were seen on fingerprints of stroma from each of the eight strains tested. Additional differences were observed when special stains were used but there still were no obvious correlations between unique peptides and H-2 genotypes. The fingerprint patterns were very complex; i.e., there were too many peptides for good resolution of most of the peptides, and it seemed likely that any variant H-2 peptides could easily be masked by other peptides on the fingerprints. Some separation of peptides into various classes by size and charge would be required in order to detect the variant H-2 peptides in these stromal digests.

At this point it also became necessary to select two strains of mice to be used for a comparative study of stromal peptides and for a study of the association of variant peptides with H-2 and non-H-2 proteins. The choice lay between using H-2 congenic lines of mice, which differ at H-2 and closely linked loci, and using two inbred strains of mice, which differ at H-2 and many non-H-2 loci. We chose to begin with two inbred strains. C57BL and C3H were chosen because their H-2 antigenic specificities are very different and because the two strains were readily available. Also, the crossover lines H-2H and H-2I (18) could be used to show that certain H-2 peptides were nearer the D or K region of the H-2 antigen.

A population of (C57BL X C3H)F2 mice was serotyped and the tryptic peptides from the stroma of the H-2b/b and H-2k/k segregants were compared with the tryptic peptides from the stroma of C57BL and C3H mice. The tryptic peptides were initially separated by size using gel filtration over Sephadex G-25. Figure 2 shows the elution profile for C3H stromal peptides. Fractions I and II contained large peptides; peptides ranging from three to ten amino acids in length were found in fraction III; fraction IV contained several dipeptides and the free amino acids arginine and lysine; and fraction V contained ammonium salts that were discarded. For practical purposes, fractions III and IV were combined, because the dipeptides and lysine and arginine are quite well resolved from other peptides during the subsequent isolation procedures. The smaller peptides, i.e., Sephadex G25 fractions III and IV, were analyzed first because the smaller peptides are better resolved both by fingerprinting and by column chromatography and because detection of a small peptide derived from the H-2 molecule by fingerprinting rather than by more elaborate methods would greatly facilitate the progress of this research, even though the small peptide itself may not constitute an antigenic site.

The tryptic peptides in each Sephadex fraction were further separated by ion-exchange chromatography (44) over Dowex 50-X2 resin (Fig. 3) using the standard stream divider assembly (25) on a Spinco Model 120C automatic amino acid analyzer. Each major peak in the elution profile from the Dowex 50-X2 column coincided with the elution of one or two major peptides seen on the fingerprints. Most of the fractions contained several peptides that were separated by high-voltage electrophoresis (39) on Whatman No. 3 chromatography paper (Fig. 4). The electrophoretic patterns of the tryptic peptides in each fraction from the Dowex 50-X2 column of C57BL and C3H stroma were compared to locate possible peptide differences that would require chemical analysis. The electrophoretic profiles suggested that most of the peptides from the two stromal digests are alike. One difference that has been observed is shown in Fig. 5; a peptide (C) is present in Dowex 50-X2 fraction IX of C57BL stroma that is absent in the corresponding fraction from C3H. These electrophoretically separable components must be recovered for further chemical analysis. At the present time the peptides are being separated by high-voltage paper electrophoresis because only small quantities of material are being used. Later, chromatography over Dowex 1-X2 resin will be used to give cleaner separations and higher yields.

Some aliquots of the Dowex 50-X2 fractions were used to locate the positions of each peptide after electrophoresis, and the remainder of each sample was streaked along an 8 cm line located 5 in. from the shorter edge of the chromatography paper. Amino acid standards were placed on the lateral edges for reference. After electrophoresis, the paper was cut into strips that corresponded to the positions of each peptide, and the peptides were eluted from the paper strips by descending chromatography, using 10% acetic acid as eluant (23). Acetic acid in the eluate was removed by evaporation, and the peptides were hydrolyzed in 2 ml of redistilled 6N HCl for 21 hrs at 110°C in vials sealed under vacuum. HCl was removed by evaporation and the amino acid content of each peptide was determined by a Spinco Model 120C automatic amino acid analyzer. Only a few of the fractions have been analyzed to date but eventually all fractions will be analyzed.

Amino acid analysis of the electrophoretically separable peptides in fraction IX (Fig. 4) from C57BL and C3H mice revealed that there was a ValProLys peptide present in the C region of C57BL stromal digests (Fig. 5) that was not present in C3H stromal digests. As shown in region G of Fig. 5, a (GlxLeuLeu)Arg peptide was present in tryptic digests of C57BL stroma but was lacking in similar digests of C3H stroma. In contrast, there was a (GlxProValTyr)Lys peptide in region G of C3H stromal digests that was not present in C57BL samples. The amino acid compositions of some peptides are given in the legend of Fig. 5. Some regions contain more than one peptide. When two or more peptides are present in unequal quantities, it is sometimes possible to determine the amino acid composition of each peptide. In region D of Fig. 5 there are two peptides; an arginine and a lysine peptide are present in nearly equal quantities but the amino acid content of each peptide is not clear.

The comparable fraction of (C57BL X C3H)F2 segregants was examined to determine whether the ValProLys, (GlxLeuLeu)Arg, and (GlxProValTyr)Lys peptide differences between C57BL and C3H mice were in the H-2 molecule. If the ValProLys and (GlxLeuLeu)Arg peptides were a part of the H-2 molecule they would be expected to segregate with the H-2b serotype of the F2 progeny; if not, then they should be present in both the H-2b/b and H-2k/k segregants. The electrophoretic patterns of the tryptic peptides in fraction IX from the Dowex 50-X2 separation of both the H-2b/b and H-2k/k segregants suggest that the ValProLys peptide is not a part of the H-2 molecule (Fig. 5). The amino acid compositions of the electrophoretically separable regions indicate that both of the H-2 segregant classes contained the unique C57BL ValProLys and (GlxLeuLeu)Arg peptides, as would be expected for peptides that are not derived from the H-2 molecule. The unique C3H (GlxProValTry)Lys peptide found in stromal preparations of the H-2k/k segregants apparently was not present in digest of the H-2b/b stroma. This peptide satisfies the criterion of genetic segregation with the appropriate H-2 allele but the observation requires confirmation. The peptides should be separated more cleanly to establish specifically that this peptide is a part of the H-2 molecule.

To date we have found two tryptic peptides that are positively not associated with H-2 antigen and one that may be an H-2 peptide. The results certainly establish the credibility of this approach. When the identification of an H-2 peptide is confirmed - and others are likely to be found - we will have chemical markers that can be used to identify H-2 molecules, even those that are no longer immunologically active. Then a number of chromatographic and physical methods will be available to purify H-2 molecules more rigorously for complete chemical studies.

DISCUSSION

Now I should like to discuss our evaluation of this approach and to state our general plans. It was clear to us at the outset that this project would be a major task. Nevertheless, the project was undertaken, with the expectation that some of the data we would obtain on tryptic peptides of stroma would correspond to the type of information that we expect to obtain in the future, when and if intact H-2 molecules are purified. The data we

gather should be directly applicable to elucidation
of the structure of the H-2 molecule, which, if done
by classical methods, will include structural analyses of tryptic peptides and other peptide derivatives
of the H-2 molecule. It was also evident that data
on the molar yields of individual tryptic peptides
would indicate that certain peptides could possibly
be derived from the same polypeptide chain in plasma
membranes. Moreover, data on the molar yields of
peptides derived from H-2 antigens should give a
rough estimation of the quantity of H-2 protein in
the plasma membranes used as starting material.
Determinations of the purity of an antigen that
are based on chemical data are likely to be more
accurate than estimations based on immunological
assays; this is particularly true for antigens that
are readily denatured during isolation.

　　We are presently testing zonal centrifuge (40)
and chromatographic systems for their potential usefulness in separating membrane constituents. Zonal
centrifugation of erythrocyte stroma gives five
poorly resolved peaks (Fig. 6), but the H-2 antigens
are located in a limited region (cuts 14 and 15) of
the zonal centrifuge profile. One chromatographic
system has been used to separate at least ten fractions with different amino acid and amino sugar contents. Once the separation systems become better
developed, the tryptic peptides in each of these
fractions will be examined. Some fractions will
contain unique tryptic peptides derived from non-
H-2 proteins, such as the ValProLys peptide discussed above. One or more of the fractions will
contain the H-2 constituents of plasma membranes,
which will be detected by an association of unique
peptides and H-2 genotype, as we have discussed
earlier. Once the variant H-2 peptides are identified, the plasma membranes of the H-2 crossover
lines will be examined to determine which variants
are controlled by the D and K regions of the H-2
locus. Identification of a few variants that are
positively controlled by the D and K regions should

enable us to establish that all of these peptides are located in a single polypeptide chain or that the H-2 locus is really a cluster of 2 to 5 or more subloci.

Studies on the antigenic nature of globular proteins, such as myoglobin (13) and tobacco mosaic virus (3), suggest that transplantation antigens may be large molecules that contain several antigenic sites along their polypeptide chains. A small alteration in amino acid sequences may alter regions in the polypeptide chains that are exposed to act as antigens on the surfaces of plasma membranes.

We hope to conjugate the variant peptides to proteins or to polyamino acids (45). These conjugates will be tested for their ability to inhibit or induce antibodies and for the possible correlation of peptide variants with specific H-2 antigenic sites. Not all amino acid substitutions will be expected to be immunogenic and some of the variant peptides may be incomplete segments of antigenic sites. In such cases, larger fragments more likely to contain the entire antigenic site will be obtained by chemical cleavage (51). Larger fragments that contain the H-2 variant peptides of interest will be recognized by the presence of unique tryptic peptides within them. Even though the antigenic site may be small, structural integrity of the site is also important. The size of the antigenic sites of carbohydrates (26) and proteins (43) have been calculated to be about 34 X 12 X 7 Å and 25 X 11 X 6.5 Å, respectively, which is the size of a pentapeptide. An octapeptide is the smallest peptide able to form a stable αhelix (16). Antibodies to globular proteins are not only directed to determinants consisting of linear sequences of amino acids (10, 42) but are also directed to determinants whose configurations result from the folding of polypeptides (4, 36). Thus, amino acid sequences that are widely separated in the unfolded chains may be adjacent in the native protein, and as a consequence the larger fragments are usually more antigenically active. Two possible approaches to successful tissue transplantation are interference with

369

antigen-antibody complexes and induction of specific
antigenic sites represent only limited segments of
the antigen, and that these limited regions might be
used as specific toleragens. If attempts are to be
made to use specific antigenic sites as toleragens,
perhaps it will be more practical to synthesize these
small molecules than to extract them. Protein syn-
thesizing equipment, such as the Merrifield system
(33), can synthesize reasonable quantities of chemically pure peptides. Variations in the peptide
sequence can be programed to differ at any preset
position in order to produce peptides that differ at
a single amino acid residue. Comparative assays with
such peptides can establish whether certain amino
acids singularly are important in a specific antigenic site. Such information may correlate with
recent findings that certain strains of mice respond
quite differently to synthetic polypeptides with
different amino acid residues in the short peptides
added to the amino termini of the branched poly-DL-
alanine side chains attached to poly-L-lysine.
Strains of mice differ in their capacity to respond
immunologically to poly(Tyr,Glu)poly-DL-Ala - poly-
L-Lys, poly(His,Glu)poly-DL-Ala - poly-L-Lys, or
poly(Phe,Glu)poly-DL-Ala - poly-L-Lys (32). C57BL
mice respond well to (Tyr,Glu-Ala-L and (Phe,Glu)-
Ala-L but not to (His,Glu)-Ala-L; C3H mice respond to
(His,Glu)-Ala-L and (Phe,Glu)-Ala-L but not to
(Tyr,Glu)-Ala-L. The difference in the ability of
these strains of mice to respond to these particular
synthetic polypeptides is controlled by the H-2
locus or a closely linked locus (31). Two amino
acids in these synthetic polypeptides that induce
different immune responses in different strains of
mice are tyrosine and histidine; peptides that contain these amino acids can be detected on fingerprints (38). A few tyrosine peptide variants have
been observed on fingerprints of stroma from different strains of mice, and we are presently attempting to determine the possible relationship of these
peptides to H-2 antigens.

Knowledge of the chemistry of antigenic sites is also necessary in order to know what types of agents are likely to interfere with the formation of specific antigen-antibody complexes or with lymphocyte-antigen interactions (34). Means to interfere with the degree of interaction between specific antigens and antibodies would effectively regulate the immune response, which would have considerable importance in medicine not only for tissue transplantation but also for treatment of the Arthus reaction, serum sickness reaction, and poststreptococcal glomerulonephritis.

ACKNOWLEDGEMENT

Research supported by the U.S. Atomic Energy Commission under contract with the Union Carbide Corporation.

REFERENCES

1. D.B. Amos, Advan. Immunol. 10, 251 (1969).
2. D.B. Amos, M. Zumpft, and P. Armstrong, Transplantation 1, 270 (1963).
3. F.A. Anderer, Z. Naturforsch B18, 1010 (1963).
4. M.Z. Atassi, and A.V. Thomas, Biochemistry 8, 3385 (1969).
5. F.H. Bach, and D.B. Amos, Science 156, 1506 (1967).
6. R.S. Basch, and C.A. Stetson, Ann. N.Y. Acad. Sci. 97, 83 (1962).
7. E.A. Boyse, E. Stockert, and L.J. Old, Proc. Nat. Acad. Sci. U.S. 58, 954 (1967).
8. R. Ceppellini, E.S. Curtoni, P.L. Mattiuz, V. Miggiano, G. Scudeller, and A. Serra, In "Histocompatibility Testing 1967" (E.S. curtoni, P.L. Mattiuz, and R.M. Tosi, eds.), p. 149. Munksgaard, Copenhagen, 1967.
9. A.I. Chernoff, J.C. Liu, Blood 17, 54 (1961).
10. G.T. Cocks, and A.C. Wilson, Science 164, 188

11. J. Colombani, M. Colombani, D.C. Viza, O. Degani-Bernard, J. Dausset, and D.A L. Davies, Transplantation 9, 228 (1970).

12. S.P. Counce, P. Smith, R. Barth, and G.D. Snell, Ann. Surg. 144, 198 (1956).

13. M.J. Crumpton, and J.M. Wilkinson, Biochem. J. 94, 545 (1965).

14. J. Dausset, R. Walford, J. Colombani, L. Legrand, N. Feingold, A. Barge, and F.T. Rapaport, Transplant. Proc. 1, 331 (1969).

15. D.A.L. Davies, Transplantation 8, 51 (1969).

16. P. Doty, and R.D. Lundberg, J. Amer. Chem. Soc. 78, 4810 (1965).

17. P.A. Gorer, S. Lyman, and G.D. Snell, Proc. Roy. Soc., Ser. B 135, 499 (1948).

18. P.A. Gorer, and Z.B. Mikulska, Proc. Roy. Soc., Ser. B 151, 57 (1959).

19. R.J. Graff, W.K. Silvers, R.E. Billingham, W.H. Hildemann, and Snell, G.D. Transplantation 4, 605 (1966).

20. G. Haughton, Transplantation 3, 238 (1966).

21. R. Herberman, and C.A. Stetson, J. Exp. Med. 121, 533 (1965).

22. L.A. Herzenberg, and L.A. Herzenberg, Proc. Nat. Acad. Sci. U.S. 47, 762 (1961).

23. K. Hilse and R.A. Popp, Proc. Nat. Acad. Sci. U.S. 61, 930 (1968).

24. V.M. Ingram, Nature 180, 326 (1957).

25. R.T. Jones, Cold Spring Harbor Symp. Quant. Biol. 29, 279 (1964).

26. E.A. Kabat, J. Cell. Comp. Physiol. 50 Suppl. 1, 79 (1957).

27. B. Kahan and R.A. Reisfeld, Science 164, 514 (1969).

28. A.A. Kandutsch and J.H. Stimpfling, Transplantation 1, 201 (1963).

29. F. Lilly, Genetics 53, 529 (1966).

30. L.A. Manson and J. Palm, J. Cell. Comp. Physiol. 68, 207 (1966).

31. H.O. McDevitt and A. Chinitz, Science 163, 1207 (1969).

32. H.O. McDevitt and M.L. Tyan, *J. Exp. Med.* 128, 1 (1968).
33. R.B. Merrifield, *Biochemistry* 3, 1385 (1964).
34. H.J. Meuwissen, O. Stutman, and R.A. Good, *Semin. Hematol.* 6, 28 (1961).
35. W.T.J. Morgan, *Proc. Roy. Soc., Ser. B* 151, 308 (1960).
36. Z. Ovary, *Immunochemistry* 1, 241 (1964).
37. D.M. Popp and R.D. Brown, *Transplantation* 9, 151 (1970).
38. R.A. Popp, *J. Hered.* 53, 142 (1962).
39. R.A. Popp, *J. Biol. Chem.* 240, 2863 (1965).
40. R.A. Popp, D.M. Popp, N.G. Anderson, and L.H. Elrod, *Biochim. Biophys. Acta* 184, 625 (1969).
41. M.A. Raftery and R.D. Cole, *Biochem. Biophys. Res. Commun.* 10, 467 (1963).
42. M. Reichlin, M. Hay, and L. Levin, *Immunochemistry* 1, 21 (1964).
43. H.J. Sage, G.F. Dutsch, G.D. Fasman, and L. Levin, *Immunochemistry* 1, 133 (1964).
44. W.A. Schroeder, R.T. Jones, J. Cormick, and K. McCalla, *Anal. Chem.* 34, 1570 (1962).
45. M. Sela, *Science* 166, 1365 (1969).
46. W.K. Silvers, D.B. Wilson, and J. Palm, *Science* 155, 703 (1967).
47. G.D. Snell, *Folia Biol.* 14, 335 (1968).
48. G.D. Snell,and J.H. Stimpfling *In* "Biology of the Laboratory Mouse" (E.L. Green, ed.), p. 457. McGraw-Hill, New York, 1966.
49. J.H. Stimpfling and A. Richardson, *Genetics* 51, 831 (1965).
50. H. Wigzell, *Transplantation* 3, 423 (1965).
51. B. Witkop, *Science* 162, 318 (1968).

Table 1

Amino Acid Content of Erythrocyte Stroma from RFM Mice

Amino acids	Residues/100 amino acid residues	Amino acids	Residues/100 amino acid residues
Lysine	4.75	Alanine	8.19
Histidine	2.13	Cystine/2	0.53
Arginine	5.12	Valine	6.14
Aspartic acid	9.03	Methionine	2.24
Threonine	6.27	Isoleucine	4.40
Serine	8.83	Leucine	11.77
Glutamic acid	11.95	Tyrosine	2.39
Proline	6.16	Phenylalanine	3.98
Glycine	8.19		

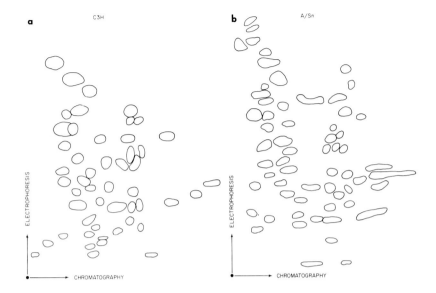

Fig. 1. Fingerprints of tryptic digests of (a) C3H
and (b) A/Sn red cell stroma. The tryptic
peptides were separated by chromatography
and electrophoresis and the peptides were
developed by reaction with ninhydrin (9).

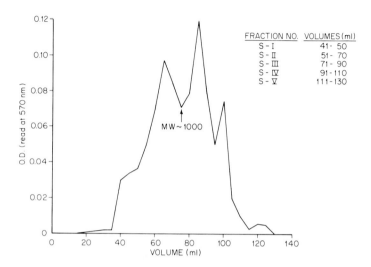

Fig. 2.   Sephadex G-25 separation of tryptic digests
of C3H stroma.   The peptides were dissolved
in 0.2M pyridine-acetate buffer at pH 3.1
(44) and eluted with the same buffer from a
1.9 x 45 cm column of Sephadex.   Five milliliter samples were collected; aliquots of
0.1 ml were reacted with ninhydrin (39) and
the color that developed was read at 570 nm.

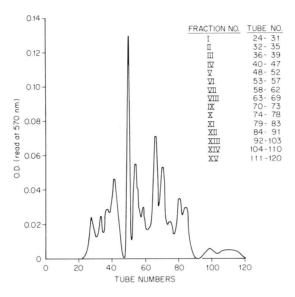

Fig. 3. Dowex 50-X2 separation of tryptic peptides in Sephadex G-25; fractions III and IV from C3H stroma. The tryptic peptides from 150 mg of stroma were dissolved in 5 ml of 0.2M pyridine-acetate and applied to a 1.9 x 57 cm column of Dowex 50-X2 resin. The peptides were eluted with a 0.2 to 2.0M and pH 3.1 to 5.0 gradient of pyridine-acetate (44).

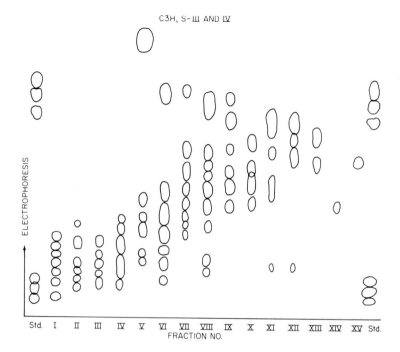

Fig. 4. Electrophoretic separation of the tryptic peptides in Dowex 50-X2 fractions I to XV. The peptides were separated by high-voltage electrophoresis in pyridine-acetate buffer (39). The peptides were developed by reaction with ninhydrin.

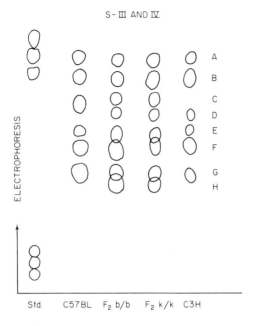

Fig. 5.   Comparison of the electrophoretically separable tryptic peptides in Dowex 50-X2;
fraction IX of stroma from C57BL, C3H, and
the (C57BL x C3H)F2 segregants of H-2b/b and
H-2k/k genotypes. See Fig. 4 for methods.
The tryptic peptides found in each region
are as follows: (A) AlaLys, (B) ThrLys,
(C) ValProLys, (D) uncertain, (E) LeuLeuLys
and (GlxGlyAla)Arg, (F) (GlxProGlyValLeu)Arg
and (AsxThrTyr)Lys, (G) (GlxLeuLeu)Arg for
C57BL and (GlxProValTyr)Lys for C3H, and
(H) uncertain.

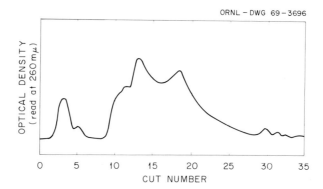

Fig. 6. Zonal centrifuge profile of a homogenate of C57BL erythrocyte stroma. Centrifugation was performed in B–XIV rotor using a 25 to 55% sucrose gradient and a total force of $8600 \times 10^6\, \omega^2 t$ (40). Cuts 14 and 15 contained most of the H–2 antigen.

THE SOLUBILIZATION AND CHARACTERIZATION
OF THE HL-A TRANSPLANTATION ANTIGENS

Edward E. Etheredge

Department of Surgery
University of Minnesota Health Sciences Center
Minneapolis, Minnesota

INTRODUCTION

A major histocompatibility locus has been demonstrated in every well-studied species. In man, the
HL-A antigens are the products of a histocompatibility locus (HL-A) and, with the ABO antigens, comprise
the major human transplantation antigen systems (1).
Clinical transplantation gave impetus to the study of
the HL-A system and there has been increasing interest in solubilization and characterization of HL-A
alloantigens. Not only will characterization of
soluble antigens provide information concerning an
important human genetic locus, but the purified antigens hold clinical promise as immunogens, for the
production of HL-A typing sera, and as tolerogens,
for the induction of immune tolerance. This chapter
reviews the current knowledge of the biochemistry of
soluble HL-A alloantigens.

DISTRIBUTION OF HL-A ALLOANTIGENS

With the known possible exceptions of the erythrocyte (2, 3) and trophoblastic syncytia (4), the HL-A
alloantigens are thought to be present on most human
cells, including such diverse cell types as fibroblasts (5), human tissue culture cells (6), and in
human spermatozoa in haploid expression (7). While
there is considerable controversy concerning the

381

intracellular distribution of HL-A substances, the
bulk of evidence favors their localization at the
surface membrane of cells (8, 9). The ubiquity of
distribution and cell-surface location suggest that
these antigens are involved in some important cellular function, such as cell contact and recognition
phenomena. HL-A alloantigens seem to appear early in
ontogeny. Seigler and Metzgar (4) grew human fetal
cells in monolayer cultures and, using the technique
of mixed agglutination, demonstrated the presence of
some HL-A alloantigens on cells at as early as 6
weeks gestation. These workers were unable to demonstrate the presence of HL-A alloantigens on trophoblastic syncytia. Pellegrino and co-workers (10)
were able to solubilize HL-A alloantigens by sonication of spleen, lung, liver, and kidney of 3, 4, and
$5\frac{1}{2}$ month old fetuses. There were significant differences in yield of soluble antigen from various
tissues, with fetal kidney appearing to be the richest source. The absence of HL-A activity in sonicates of spleen and liver when activity was present
in sonicates of kidney and lung from the same fetus
requires further investigation.

The apparent lack of HL-A alloantigens on the
erythrocyte is especially interesting in view of the
indirect demonstration by absorption studies of
Harris and Zervas (2) that some HL-A alloantigens are
present on the reticulocyte and are subsequently lost
with maturation. However, Morton et al. (11) cast
doubt on the absence of HL-A alloantigens on erythrocytes by their demonstration of the correlation of
the Bga blood group with the HL-A7 leucocyte group.
Based on the demonstration of both hemagglutinating
and cytotoxic activity in the antisera showing Bga
and HL-A7 specificity, they state that the HL-A7
antigen is present on the erythrocyte and that Bga is
the surviving remnant of the compound antigen HL-A7
following maturation.

While attempts to isolate soluble HL-A alloantigen from milk and urine have been unsuccessful, there
has been a recent demonstration of soluble HL-A

alloantigen in normal human serum. Suggestive evidence came from the reports of Zmijewski et al. (12), showing that a substance in human serum could inhibit the detection of HL-A alloantigens by the defibrinated leukocyte agglutination technique, and from Berg et al. (13), showing that a significant correlation exists between survival of skin allografts and lipoprotein allotypes. Charlton and Zmijewski (14) reported the presence of soluble HL-A7 alloantigen in the low-density B-lipoprotein fraction of human serum obtained from HL-A7-positive donors; its presence in high concentration may inhibit direct leukocyte grouping, leading to erroneous results. In addition, van Rood et al. (15, 16) have reported that the antibody activity of HL-A2 and 7b antisera can be neutralized with whole serum from donors carrying these alloantigens. Further, van Rood (15) has been able to sensitize skin graft recipients by injecting plasma from donors positive for the 7b antigen. Clear demonstration of the other HL-A alloantigens in soluble form in normal serum has not been achieved. The biologic significance of soluble alloantigens in normal serum is yet to be explained.

There have been several attempts to quantitate both the alloantigen content of human tissue as well as the immunogenic potential of the specificities. In general, this may be done by quantitative extraction methods, indirect quantitation by absorption studies, or transplantation.

Berah et al. (17) studied the capacity of homogenates of fresh tissue to absorb lymphocytotoxic antibody detecting HL-A2. On a unit weight basis, spleen was the richest in the alloantigen, followed by lung, liver, intestine, kidney, and heart; aorta tissue had little antigen and fat and brain had practically none. Attempting to relate total antigen content to total weight of the individual normal organ, they found liver to have the greatest antigen content, followed by lung, intestine, spleen, heart, kidney, and brain. Using the technique of parental crossimmunization, followed by allografting

of skin obtained from children bearing different
maternal or paternal haplotypes, Rapaport et al. (18)
studied the comparative immunogenicity of human HL-A
alloantigens. They concluded that most, if not all,
HL-A alloantigens functioned as strong transplantation antigens, but within the conditions of their
experiments they concluded that HL-A9 appeared to be
a stronger immunogen than antigens Da-15 and HL-A12.
Dausset and Rapaport (19) correlated the rejection
times of skin allografts from children to their
father with the incompatible HL-A alloantigens and
found that HL-A2, Da-15, and Lc-17 were frequently
incompatible in the shorter surviving grafts. Ward
et al. (20) studied intrafamilial skin allografting
and found that HL-A1, HL-A2, HL-A3, HL-A5, HL-A8,
HL-A12, and groups 24, 65, and 4C* were significantly
associated with rapid rejection.

ASSAY SYSTEMS

In vivo, transplantation alloantigens are
capable of the induction of allograft immunity of
allograft tolerance, the stimulation of alloantibody
formation, and the induction of specific cutaneous
hypersensitivity. Attempts to solubilize and purify
HL-A alloantigens are predicated on the assumption
that these substances will retain in the soluble form
some measurable aspect of their biologic activity
and specific identity. As emphasized by Kahan and
Reisfeld (8), a putative transplantation antigen
must influence the fate of a subsequent donor-speci-
fic graft, either by accelerating its rejection or
through induction of immune tolerance. Such rigorous
definition of a transplantation antigen requires
lengthy procedures that are neither easily quanti-
tated nor necessarily discriminating among individual
antigenic specificities. They are also impractical
in routine human HL-A testing. Other techniques have
been developed based on immunologic responses to
transplantation alloantigens and presumably related
to histocompatibility. Kahan and Reisfeld (8, 9)

have written excellent discussions of these techniques, which include: (a) delayed hypersensitivity
reactions, including the direct reaction (21),
the transfer reaction (22), the irradiated hamster
test (23), and the blast transformation phenomenon
(24); and (b) in vitro inhibition of alloantibody
activity.

Several serological techniques have been
developed to detect transplantation alloantigens (or
histocompatibility substances if their effect on
graft survival has not been shown). Immunization
with allogeneic tissue can lead to the production of
alloantibodies with capacities for hemagglutination,
leucoagglutination, and leucocytotoxicity. Each of
these alloantibody functions has been the basis of
assays for putative alloantigen that, if incubated
with antibody, blocks the respective alloantibody
activity. Hemagglutination inhibition has not been
possible in humans because the erythrocyte seems to
lack the HL-A alloantigens (2); and leucoagglutination, although not complement dependent, lacks the
sensitivity of leucocytotoxicity.

Inhibition of lymphocytotoxicity is the technique most commonly employed for the detection of
soluble HL-A alloantigens, although there are
numerous methodological variations. Phase-contrast
microscopy (25), trypan blue dye exclusion (26), and
release of isotipic markers from labeled lymphocytes
(27) are most frequently used to measure cytotoxicity. A radioimmune assay has been described for
transplantation antigens (28). Etheredge and associates (29) have recently studied the variables in
the detection of soluble HL-A alloantigens, using
inhibition of a two-stage lymphocytotoxicity assay.
It was demonstrated that this assay is (a) less
sensitive when there is platelet contamination of the
target lymphocytes; (b) more sensitive to low antigen
concentration if antisera are diluted to titer using
AB serum; (c) responsive to the solvent of the protein solution; (e) markedly affected by the concentration of the protein solution being tested; (f)

more sensitive with rabbit complement than with an
equal mixture of rabbit and human complement, for the
sera studied; and (g) dependent on optimal incubation
times (which were determined). The data suggest that
the conditions of each variation of lymphocytotoxicity assay must be optimized to assure maximal sensitivity and specificity. Using phase-contrast
microscopy to detect cytotoxicity, Kahan et al. (30)
reported that 6 x 10^{-14} mole of antigen specifically
inhibited a lymphocytotoxicity assay. While inhibition of lymphocytotoxicity is an extremely sensitive
technique, its specificity must be assured through
appropriate controls. Monospecific antisera are the
sine qua non for specificity of lymphocytotoxicity
reactions and their antigen-specific inhibition;
aspects of this requirement are discussed elsewhere
in this volume.

Limited success has been achieved using
xenogeneic sera to detect specific human alloantigens
but there is a recent renewal of interest in this
approach. Albert and his co-workers (31) have
demonstrated that rabbit homotransplantation sera can
detect some human lymphocyte isoantigens. Such cross
reactivity of HL-A alloantigens with proteins from
other species was confirmed by the demonstration that
streptococcal M proteins inhibited anti-HL-A cytotoxic antisera (32). Metzgar and co-workers (33)
demonstrated that chimpanzee sera, following immunization of the animals with human buffy coat, could
detect human isoantigen but also an antigen seemingly
present on all human leukocytes. Similarly, Balner
et al. (34) have been able to detect some human alloantigens with chimpanzee sera. However, Batchelor
(35) and Batchelor and Sanderson (36) studied the
capacity of rabbit sera, following immunization of
rabbits with partially purified HL-A2 substance, to
detect differences in human phenotype. On the basis
of absorption experiments, he concluded that rabbits
so immunized were not able to discriminate by phenotype and that either the HL-A2 substance specificity
is part of the rabbit antihuman species determinant,

or it is in very close proximity on the macromole-
cule. Einstein et al. (37) reported the preparation
of HL-A specific heterologous antiserum, prepared in
rabbits by immunization with partially purified,
papain-solubilized HL-A alloantigens. Following
extensive absorptions with human lymphoid cells not
sharing HL-A specificities with the immunizing cells,
there was residual cytotoxic activity against the
immunizing cells. The specificity demonstrated after
absorption indicated that rabbits could recognize and
produce antisera to individual HL-A alloantigenic
determinants. However, following these absorptions
to narrow the specificities of this heterolous antisera, the residual cytotoxic activity was very low.
These data indicate the need for more studies of production of HL-A specific heterologous antisera in
large quantities. In order for the antisera to be
practically useful, they must have restricted specificity of high titer.

SOLUBILIZATION AND PURIFICATION OF HL-A ALLOANTIGENS

Solubilization of the HL-A alloantigens has
been achieved by a wide variety of nonspecific techniques for membrane disruption, including autolysis,
papain proteolysis, sonication, neutral salt extraction, and detergent treatment. Widely variable
molecular weights and chemical constituents, notably
carbohydrate content, have been reported for the
soluble products of these several techniques, suggesting a degree of association of the HL-A substances
with membrane fragments that may be unnecessary for
the conformation required for biologic activity.
Whereas complex genetic theories and discussions of
intraspecific molecular heterogeneity have been
advanced, the nonspecificity of the solubilization
techniques suggested that differences in products
might be attributed, in part, to the differences in
techniques. Etheredge and Najarian (38) demonstrated
that the single specificity HL-A2, solubilized from
the spleen of a single donor bearing the specificity,

had a variable biochemical character according to the
technique of solubilization. Autolysis released
HL-A2 activity that eluted from calibrated gel filtration columns at positions indicating an apparent
molecular weight of greater than 800,000 to below
50,000. Papain proteolysis released HL-A2 from the
same spleen, with a molecular weight of 32,000.
Hypertonic KCl extraction released HL-A2 from the
same spleen with apparent molecular weights of 45,000
and about 10,000. While these data do not disprove
the theory of intraspecific molecular heterogeneity,
they are highly suggestive that the solubilization
technique and preparative procedures determine the
molecular class of HL-A to be studied. Simple
preparative maneuvers such as high-speed or extended
ultracentrifugation may clear a heterogenous mixture
of its larger insoluble fragments or soluble, but
relatively dense, components. A low yield of a class
of HL-A molecules may cause them to be overlooked
during the preparative stages.

Because of this procedure-related variability,
both for a single HL-A specificity and among the
several HL-A specificities, the following discussion
of soluble human HL-A alloantigens is grouped according to the method of solubilization used.

Solubilization of HL-A Alloantigens by Autolysis

Autolysis has been extensively studied by
Davies and his co-workers (39-43). Using as
starting material a crude lipoprotein suspension prepared by hypotonic NaCl elution from human spleen
cells (40), this group studied the autolytic release
of HL-A alloantigens. The yield of crude lipoprotein
was found to average about 8% of the spleen dry
weight. After storage at 2°C for days to weeks, an
aqueous suspension of the crude lipoprotein was centrifuged at 120,000g for 90 min and the supernatant
was tested for HL-A activity. Whereas this "unassis-
ted" autolysis released HL-A substances from some
spleen preparations, its effectiveness was not

uniform and its yield was low. Incubation of the sedimented lipoprotein with 0.05M Tris, pH 8, for 150 min at 37°C solubilized with regularity HL-A substances that were not sedimented at 120,000g for 90 min and were representative of the donor HL-A mosaics. These substances eluted in a reasonably characteristic fashion from gel filtration columns. Hl-A activity could be found in material eluting in the void volumes of G-200 Sephadex, although this was an inconstant finding; most activity eluted in the "partially included" pool and subsequently eluted from calibrated gel filtration columns at a position indicating an apparent molecular weight of about 50,000. Using an autolytically solubilized preparation, Davies and co-workers (41) partially purified this gel filtration and, by ion-exchange chromatography, separated molecules carrying different immunological specificities determined by a single genotype. This resolution did not suggest separation separation of alloantigens determined by the two main subloci of HL-A and there was considerable overlap of the elution profiles, depending on the antisera used to detect the specificities. Colombani and co-workers (44) studied the behavior of HL-A alloantigens on DEAE Sephadex A-50 following solubilization by autolysis from spleen cells. Based on elution patterns of the different specificities, they concluded that the specificities of the first sublocus of HL-A had no family relationship; data was insufficient to draw conclusions concerning the second sublocus. Alloantigen HL-A2 from spleen 20 eluted early in the salt gradient elution, whereas HL-A9 and HL-A1, from spleens 18 and 22, respectively, eluted much later. These authors did not report the ability to separate the first sublocus specificities solubilized from a single spleen with more that one well-defined specificity of the first sublocus represented. Studies in our laboratory (38) confirmed the effectiveness of autolysis in releasing the major HL-A specificities tested; however, substances with HL-A activity eluted from calibrated

G-200 Sephadex columns in positions indicating a
range of apparent molecular weights from greater than
800,000 to less than 50,000. Sedimentation of the
autolyzate for 60 min at 250,000g cleared the larger
fragments and most activity eluted in the molecular
weight range of 48,000, although low yields of alloantigen were detected at lower molecular weights.
This finding corroborated those of Sanderson (45),
which indicated a wide range of molecular weights
for HL-A substances derived by autolysis. He
attributed this phenomenon to denaturation induced by
a lyophilization step used in his procedure. Such
instability of the autolysis-derived protein was
suggested by his finding that DEAE-separated HL-A
substances following autolysis tended to precipitate,
with a reduction of activity, upon storage at $4^{\circ}C$.
It is curious that denaturation to the extent postulated could occur without loss of biologic activity.
Presumably, autolytic membrane structural dissolution
occurs as a result of the activity of endogenous
proteolytic enzymes. The technique's major disadvantage seems to be the lack of predictable response and
the relatively low yields.

HL-A Alloantigen Extraction by Papain

Davies (39) and Summerell and Davies (43)
extracted HL-A alloantigens from crude lipoprotein
prepared from spleen cells, using 1 part papain to
150 parts lipoprotein in Tris buffer, 0.05M, pH 8,
with 0.35mM cysteine at $37^{\circ}C$. Incubation for 180
min was most effective for solubilization and the
reaction was terminated by the addition of sodium
iodoacetate. There was considerable variation in
yield from the different spleens studied. Papain
was removed by passage of the digest through G-75
Sephadex columns that excluded the alloantigen fraction. This solubilized material was partially purified with ion-exchange chromatography and gel filtration; elution from calibrated gel filtration indicated an apparent molecular weight of about 45,000.

It is curious that alloantigen having a molecular
weight of 45,000 would have been excluded from G-75
Sephadex, because the fractionation range of this gel
is 3000 to 70,000 for peptides and globular proteins.

Insoluble papain was used by Sanderson and
Batchelor (46) and Sanderson (45) to solubilize HL-A
alloantigens because soluble papain was shown to have
considerable inhibitory action on the cytotoxic
assay. Digestion was for 4 hrs at 37°C, using 300 mg
protein to 15 mg papain with 5mM cysteine. It was
noted that there was substantial variation in the
amounts of alloantigen released from different
spleens and that there was always a large amount of
nonspecific inhibitory substances released. These
authors described a useful index of specificy, a
specificity ratio:

$$SR = \frac{\text{Inhibition of donor-positive antiserum}}{\text{Inhibition of donor-negative antiserum}}$$

They emphasized that in some soluble preparations as
much as 30% of the total inhibition measured was
nonspecific. Following ultracentrifugation of the
digest, partial purification was achieved using a
concave gradient elution from DEAE-cellulose. The
elution positions for the HL-A specificities were
said to be characteristic and highly reproducible,
and separation of two specificities was achieved.
Subsequent calibrated gel filtration of the two
separated specificities revealed quite similar
behavior, with each specificity eluting in the void
volume of G-200 Sephadex but demonstrating a low SR
and also eluting with an apparent molecular weight of
45,000 and a high SR of more than 100. Some specificities were destroyed by papain.

Sanderson and Cresswell (47) further studied
DEAE-cellulose purified HL-A substances solubilized
by papain digestion. These substances eluted from
calibrated gel filtration columns in the apparent
molecular weight range of 40,000 to 50,000 were heat
labile above 50°C and essentially stable from pH 4 to
pH 10 for 30 min at 20°C. The different specifici-

391

ties tested demonstrated differential sensitivity to sodium metaperiodate treatment, with destruction of specific inhibitory activity ranging from 11 to 70% in 1 hr. It is interesting to note that, under the identical conditions of metaperiodate treatment, about 50% of the nonspecific inhibitor activity was destroyed. Periodate sensitivity of the HL-A specificities is understood in this paper and others to implicate carbohydrate participation in the antigenic determinant, although it is likely that proteins are also sensitive to this agent and the conclusions are therefore only inferential.

Mann and co-workers have studied papain-solubilized HL-A alloantigens (48-54). Crude membranes were prepared from human tissue culture lines RAJI and RPMI-4265 and subject to hypotonic NaCl elution. The crude protein so eluted was centrifuged and the pellet treated with crude papain. With 2 mg papain to 1 mg membrane protein, the maximal solubilization occurred with 60 min incubation at 37°C, after which there was a loss of activity. Recovery of isoantigenic activity in the soluble form was found to be 45 to 50% of the total membrane activity. Ammonium sulfate precipitation of the solubilized material resulted in an average 67% recovery of the isoantigenic activity. Gel filtration on calibrated G-150 Sephadex columns indicated apparent molecular weights of 60,000 to 70,000, although some activity was found in the void volume (48). Based on elution patterns from G-150 Sephadex columns, Mann et al. (50) concluded that soluble HL-A alloantigens, prepared from papain extractions of crude protein from the cell line RPMI-4265, exhibited molecular heterogeneity demonstrable by separation of components having either the LA or 4 series of alloantigenic determinants. However, specificities of both series eluted in the void volume as well as in the included volume, where separation of the alloantigen LA and 4 series was demonstrated using polyspecific antisera. Mann and Nathenson (51) reported the carbohydrate composition of purified HL-A alloantigenic materials

derived from the RAJI and R-4265 cell lines. Neutral
sugars constituted 7.33% in RAJI, 6.14% in R-4265;
sialic acid, 0.9% in RAJI and 0.75% in R-4265; and
amino sugars were 0.5% in both. Because neither the
exact specificities tested nor criteria of purity
were reported, these data are difficult to analyze.
In an extension of their use of gel filtration to
separate specificities of the two series, Mann,
Fahey, and Nathenson (53) report two classes of
papain-solubilized alloantigens: class I, molecular
weight 60,000, and class II, molecular weight 40,000.
The specificity A17 was found to be class I, while
specificities A2 and A9 were found to be class II in
the experiment reported. No mention is made of the
presence or absence of activity eluting in the void
volume as these authors have reported. In a previous
paper (50) it was reported that most HL-A2 activity
eluted in the void volume of G-150 Sephadex columns,
and the antigen source in both studies was papain-
solubilized material from R-4265 cells.

Using papain (0.5 units enzyme activity to 1 mg
membrane protein) to solubilize HL-A alloantigens
from the RAJI, RPMI-4265, and 1M-1 human lymphoid
cell lines, Mann et al. (52) confirmed their previously reported kinetics of solubilization but
demonstrated marked differences in percentage solubilization of different specificities, ranging from
7.0 to 67.0%.of the alloantigenic activity of the
membranes before digestion. Heat lability and pH
stability were reported, as was storage stability.
The HL-A alloantigens were stable at 4°C for 24 hrs
and after freezing to -10°C; at room temperature
(24°C) about half of the activity is lost after 24
hrs. The carbohydrate composition was similar to
that from their previous report; overall amino acid
composition of alloantigenic material from RAJI and
RPMI-4265 was quite similar, though small differences
of serine and possibly histidine were postulated to
be responsible for the gross differences in alloantigenic phenotypes of the two cell lines.

Nathenson et al. (55) reported that class I

fragments obtained after papain digestion are glycoproteins with a molecular weight of about 57,000,
having a protein content of around 85 to 90% and a
carbohydrate content of about 10 to 15% including
neutral sugar, glucosamine, and sialic acid; class II
fragments have a molecular weight of about 35,000
and are glycoproteins similar to the class I fragments in composition.

Boyle (56) achieved limited separation of
papain-solubilized HL-A specificities using DEAE-
cellulose and demonstrated that the molecules carrying the specificities were similar in size (approximately 60,000 to 70,000 molecular weight) and had
identical or very similar electrophoretic mobilities
both in free solution and in acrylamide gel.

Using papain proteolysis as described by Mann et
al. (48), we solubilized HL-A2 substance from human
spleen cell-derived crude protein (38). Based on the
elution position from calibrated gel-filtration
columns, its apparent molecular weight was 32,000,
a value in close agreement with that of the class II
glycoprotein of Nathenson et al. (55). Class I
type alloantigenic molecules were not seen (for the
specificities tested) although differences in preparative technique could account for this.

Solubilization of HL-A Alloantigens by Sonication

Low-intensity, low-frequency sound releases
water-soluble transplantation antigens from a variety
of tissues. Sonic energy has a variety of effects,
including generation of heat, oxidative effects,
mechanical effects, frictional effects, and gaseous
cavitation. Thus, the mode of distribution, intensity, and frequency of sonic energy are important
variables to control, as are temperature and cell
concentration for unit time of sonication (9). Kahan
et al. (30) solubilized HL-A alloantigens from human
spleen cells by exposing about 10^9 cells in 50 ml
volumes to a 3 to 5 min burst of 15.5 w/cm^2 sonic
energy generated over 4.7 cm diameter diaphragm.

Following ultracentrifugation and gel filtration of
the concentrated ultracentrifugal supernatant, the
active fraction that appeared at the front of the
inner volume was further purified by discontinuous
polyacrylamide gel electrophoresis. The purified
HL-A substances inhibited cytotoxic reactions and
elicited specific Arthus-type cutaneous hypersensitivity reactions in those individuals producing
antibodies directed against the specificities present
in the spleen donors. Substances with both properties were present on the same band on gel electrophoresis. Further studies (57) of this sonication-
solubilized, purified product showed it to be electrophoretically homogeneous (Rf = 0.80). Molecular
weight determinations by sedimentation equilibrium
methods showed a component that was 94% monodisperse
with a molecular weight of 34,000 and a 6% aggregated
moiety with a molecular weight of 150,000. Calculation of the molecular weight from the amino acid
composition of the alloantigen gave a value of
33,000. No carbohydrate or lipid could be detected
within the limitation (1%) of the methods employed.
Of interest is the finding of the specificities HL-A3
and HL-A5 in the same electrophoretically homogeneous
band from gel electrophoresis; note that these are
the products of the two major HL-A subloci. It
would be interesting to subject this electrophoretically homogeneous substance to isoelectric focusing.
Reisfeld et al. (58-60) extended the use of sonication to solubilization of HL-A alloantigens from
human lymphocytic cell lines (RPMI-1788, RPMI-7249,
and RPMI-4098) maintained in continuous culture.
Essentially the same technique was used for sonication of tissue culture cells as was used for spleen
cells (30). All specificities detected on the peripheral blood lymphocytes of the cell-line donor were
solubilized from the cultured cells. This crude
alloantigen preparation had a specificity ratio
higher than that of a partially purified, papain-
solubilized preparation. Optimal yields of HL-A
alloantigens released by sonication from lymphoid

395

cell lines was 10,000 ID_{50} Units/mg protein or 400,000 ID_{50} Units/10^9 cells. (ID_{50} Unit is the dose of antigen that causes 50% inhibition of an alloantiserum). Purification of the alloantigens was achieved with preparative acrylamide gel electrophoresis and a 25-fold increase in ID_{50} Unit activity/mg of antigen was achieved. Purified alloantigen bearing the HL-A2 and HL-A7 determinants from one cell line differed significantly in content of aspartic acid, serine, proline, alanine, and tyrosine compared to purified HL-A3 alloantigen from another cell line. Pellegrino et al. (61) reports that the HL-A alloantigens solubilized by sonication of lymphoid cell lines have a molecular weight of 31,000 and are a single polypeptide chain with two intrachain disulfide bridges.

Solubilization of HL-A Alloantigens by Hypertonic Potassium Chloride

Reisfeld and Kahan (58) reported the use of 3M KCl to extract soluble HL-A alloantigens from human lymphoblast cell lines maintained in continuous culture. The cells were washed with Hank's balanced salt solution, adjusted to a count of 10^9 in 10 ml of Hank's solution containing 3M KCl, and stirred at $4^{\circ}C$ for 16 hrs. Following ultracentrifugation of the extract for 2 hrs at 130,000g, the supernatant was dialyzed against Hank's solution. The crude preparations had specificity ratios ranging from 50 to 100 and represented 10 to 15% of the antigenic activity of the crude cell particulate fraction. The preparation contained 15,000 ID_{50} Units/mg protein, giving a total yield of 525,000 ID_{50} Units/10^9 cells. These authors reported that the pellet remaining after ultracentrifugation of the sonicate could be treated with 3M KCl with an additional yield of 132,000 ID_{50} Units from the original 10^9 cells. No distinction is made between the products of sonication and 3M KCl, implying no difference in the biochemical characteristics of alloantigens solubilized by these differing techniques.

Etheredge and Najarian (38) reported the use of
3M KCl to extract soluble HL-A alloantigens from
human spleen. Crude spleen cell membrane lipoprotein
was prepared by the method of Davies (40) and suspended in distilled water at 50 mg/ml. Aliquots of
this suspension were adjusted to 3M KCl, homogenized
with a tight-fitting mortar and pestle, and stirred
on a magnetic stirrer for 1 hr at 4°C. Following
ultracentrifugation at 250,000g for 60 min, the
supernatant was desalted by passage through a G-25
Medium Sephadex column equilibrated with 0.1M Tris-
HCl, pH 7.4. The concentrated protein was partially
purified on calibrated columns of G-200 and G-75
Sephadex. This extraction procedure releases in
soluble form all major alloantigens tested, including
HL-A1, 2, 3, 5, 7, 8, 9, 12, 4a, and 4b. Alloantigen
HL-A2 was studied primarily and the activity of this
alloantigen eluted from calibrated columns at positions indicating an apparent molecular weight of
45,000 and about 10,000. The yield of the low
molecular weight species was quite small and specific
blocking was demonstrated. The small species can
be demonstrated in preparations from each spleen. It
is dialyzable, heat labile, and unstable in storage
at 4°C.

Mann (54) reported the use of 3M KCl to solubilize HL-A alloantigens from cell membranes of tissue
culture cells. The soluble HL-A alloantigens were
excluded from G-200 Sephadex columns, tended to
aggregate on concentration, and were not effectively
purified by gel filtration. It is difficult to
resolve the differences among these findings and
those of Reisfeld and our group.

Miscellaneous Methods for Solubilization of HL-A
Alloantigens

Detergent extraction has had limited use for
solubilization of the HL-A alloantigens. Metzgar
et al. (6) solubilized 4a and 4b alloantigens from

tissue culture cells using deoxycholate. The
soluble product was used to induce accelerated rejection of skin grafts. Reisfeld and Kahan (58) used
the cationic detergent sodium lauryl sarcosinate to
solubilize HL-A2 and HL-A7 alloantigens from lymphoid
tissue culture cells. The detergent (0.7% w/v)
releases 7000 ID_{50} Units/mg protein and 168,000 ID_{50}
Units/10^9 cells. The molecular species solubilized
is identical to that solubilized by these investigators using sonication or 3M KCl.

Mann and Levy (62) reported the solubilization
of HL-A alloantigens using the detergent sodium
dodecyl sulfate (SDS), using human lymphoid tissue
culture cells as the source material. Cell membranes
were washed repeatedly with 2M NaCl and 0.01M EDTA;
the washed membranes were treated with 2.5% SDS.
Following ultracentrifugation at 100,000g for 1 hr,
the supernatant contained alloantigenic activity that
approximated 90% of that found in the washed cell
membranes. SDS in concentrations greater than 0.1%
inhibited the cytotoxic assay system and dialysis
for 72 hrs against 0.01M sodium bicarbonate solution
was required to remove this nonspecific inhibitory
activity of the detergent.

DISCUSSION AND SUMMARY

The data reported in this review demonstrate
the extreme difficulties encountered in solubilization and purification of membrane-associated proteins. Each technique for solubilization releases a
complex array of protein species, only a small
fraction of which is HL-A alloantigen. In subsequent purification procedures following solubilization, there appears to be a preparative selection of
classes of alloantigens and the final products tend
to be dissimilar. The finding by Reisfeld and Kahan
(9, 58) that the products of sonication, 3M KCl and
sodium lauryl sarcosinate extraction are biochemi-
cally identical is appealing since purification procedures following initial solubilization were

essentially identical. However, there are significant unresolved contradictions concerning molecular
size, carbohydrate components, and molecular distribution of specificities. Glycoproteins with about
10% carbohydrate composition and molecular weights
of 58,000 are clearly different from proteins of
molecular weights of 31,000 and less than 1% carbohydrate. Before meaningful analysis of biochemical
structure is made, it seems desirable to isolate the
smallest molecular weight species with biological
activity as a transplantation antigen or histocompatibility substance. Our findings (38) of a
histocompatibility substance with an apparent
molecular weight of 10,000 led us to the theory that
this class of molecule may be a hapten, the sole
product of the HL-A locus, and that there is a
common association with a carrier molecule, perhaps
identical in all humans. This species is obtained
in extremely small yield, is labile, and obviously
requires confirmation by more rigorous methods of
molecular weight determination. This small species
has not been tested for transplantation antigen
activity. Molecular heterogeneity of individual
HL-A alloantigenic specificities has not been dis-
proved despite the attribution of molecular diversity to the nonspecific techniques for the cell
membrane disruption. The failure of each technique
to solubilize more than a small percentage of alloantigenic activity from membrane fragments implies,
perhaps, a heterogeneity of antigen-membrane interaction. To this may be attributed the adjuvant
effect of membrane in association with alloantigenic
determinants.

There is conflicting data concerning the ability
to separate individual HL-A specificities solubilized
from cell membranes carrying an HL-A mosaic.
Reisfeld and Kahan have demonstrated an electrophoretically homogeneous substance with HL-A2, HL-A7
activity, solubilized from cell lines bearing HL-A2,
HL-A7 mosaic; an HL-A3 substance was solubilized
from cell lines bearing the HL-A3 type. In a recent

report, Einstein et al. (37) describes the gel
electrophoretic separation of individual specificities of a mosaic, a unique observation. Certainly,
this question of more than one specificity (haplotype expression) per molecule is interesting in
light of theoretical discussions (63, 64) of the
nature of the HL-A antigenic sites and attendant
implications for serological studies. Obvious per-
tinence exists for the application of soluble HL-A
alloantigens as immunogens and tolerogens.

REFERENCES

1. Curtoni, E.S., Mattiuz, P.L., and Tosi, R.M.,
   eds. "Histocompatibility Testing 1967."
   Munksgaard, Copenhagen, 1967.
2. Harris, R., and Zervas, J.D. Reticulocyte HL-A
   antigens. Nature (London) 221, 1062 (1969).
3. Dausset, J., and Rapaport, F.T., eds. "Human
   Transplantation," p. 367. Grune & Stratton,
   New York, 1968.
4. Seigler, H.F., and Metzgar, R.S. Embryonic
   development of human transplantation antigens.
   Transplantation 9, 478 (1970).
5. Engelfriet, C.P., Heersche, J.N.M., Eijsvoogel,
   V.P., and Van Loghem, J.J. Demonstration of
   leucocyte iso-antigens on skin fibroblasts by
   means of the cytotoxic antibody test. Vox
   Sang. 11, 625 (1966).
6. Metzgar, R.S., Flanagan, J.F., and Mendes, N.F.
   Serological studies of extracted human tissue
   isoantigens. In "Histocompatibility Testing
   1967" (E.S. Curtoni, P.L. Mattiuz, and R.M. Tosi,
   eds.), p. 307. Munksgaard, Copenhagen, 1967.
7. Fellous, M., and Dausset, J. Probably haploid
   expression HL-A antigens on human spermatozoon.
   Nature (London) 225, 191 (1970).
8. Kahan, B.D., and Reisfeld, R.A. Transplantation
   antigens: Solubilized antigens provide chemical
   markers of biologic individuality. Science 164,
   514 (1969).

9. Reisfeld, R.A., and Kahan, B.D. Transplantation antigens. Advan. Immunol. 12, (1970).
10. Pellegrino, M.A., Pellegrino, A., and Kahan, B.D. Solubilization of fetal HL-A antigens. Transplantation 10, 425 (1970).
11. Morton, J.A., Pickles, M.M., and Sutton, L. The correlation of the Bg^a blood group with the HL-A7 leucocyte group: Demonstration of antigenic sites on red cells and leucocytes. Vox Sang. 17, 536 (1969).
12. Zmijewski, C.M., McCloskey, R.V., and St. Pierre, R.L. The effect of environmental extremes on the detectibility of leukocyte iso-antigens in normal humans with inference to tissue typing of prospective donors. In "Histocompatibility Testing 1967" (E.S. Curtoni, P.L. Mattiuz, and R.M. Tosi, eds.), p. 397. Munksgaard, Copenhagen, 1967.
13. Berg, K., Ceppellini, R., Curtoni, E.S., Mattiuz, P.L., and Bearn, A.G. The genetic antigenic polymorphisms of human serum B-lipo-protein and survival of skin grafts. In "Advances in Transplantation" (J. Dausset, J. Hamburger, and G. Mathé, eds.), p. 253. Munksgaard, Copenhagen, 1968.
14. Charlton, R.K., and Zmijewski, C.M. Soluble HL-A7 antigens: Localization in the B-lipo-protein fraction of human serum. Science 170, 636 (1970).
15. van Rood, J.J., van Leeuwen, A., Koch, C.T., and Frederiks, E. HL-A inhibiting activity in serum serum. In "Histocompatibility Testing 1970" P.I. Terasaki, ed.), p. 483. Munksgaard, Copenhagen, 1970.
16. van Rood, J.J., van Leeuwen, A., and Santen, M.C.T. Anti HL-A2 inhibitor in normal human serum. Nature (London) 226, 366 (1970).
17. Berah, M., Hors, J., and Dausset, J. A study of HL-A antigens in human organs. Transplanta-tion 9, 185 (1970).
18. Rapaport, F.T., Casson, P.R., Converse, J.M.,

Legrand, L., Colombani, J., and Dausset, J. Approach to the study of the comparative immunogenicity of human transplantation (HL-A) antigens. In "Histocompatibility Testing 1970" (P.I. Terasaki, ed.), p. 411. Munksgaard, Copenhagen, 1970.

19. Dausset, J., and Rapaport, F.T. Histocompatibility studies in haplo-identical genetic combinations. Transplant. Proc. 1, 649 (1969).

20. Ward, F.E., Seigler, H.R., Southworth, J.G., Andrus, C.H., and Amos, D.B. Immunogenicity of HL-A antigens. In "Histocompatibility Testing 1970" (P.I. Terasaki, ed.), p. 399. Munksgaard, Copenhagen, 1970.

21. Merrill, J.P., Friedman, E.A., Wilson, R.E., and Marshall, D.C. The production of "delayed type" cutaneous hypersensitivity to human donor leukocytes as a result of the rejection of skin homografts. J. Clin. Invest. 40, 631 (1961).

22. Brent, L., Brown, J.B., and Medawar, P.B. Quantitative studies on tissue transplantation immunity. VI. Hypersensitivity reactions associated with the rejection of homografts. Proc. Roy. Soc., Ser. B 156, 187 (1962).

23. Ramseier, H., and Streilein, J.W. Homograft sensitivity reactions in irradiated hamsters. Lancet 1, 622 (1965).

24. Viza, D.C., Degani, O., Dausset, J., and Davies, D.A.L. Lymphocyte stimulation by soluble human HL-A transplantation antigens. Nature (London) 219, 704 (1968).

25. Terasaki, P.I., and McClelland, J.D. Microdroplet assay of human serum cytotoxins. Nature (London) 204, 998 (1964).

26. Boyse, E.A., Olds, L.J., and Stockert, E. Some further data on cytotoxic isoantibodies in the mouse. Ann. N.Y. Acad. Sci. 99, 574 (1962).

27. Rogentine, G.N., and Plocinik, B.A. Application of the ^{51}Cr cytotoxicity technique to the analysis of human lymphocyte isoantigens. Transplantation 5, 1323 (1967).

28. Manson, L.A. A radioimmune assay for transplantation antigens. In "Histocompatibility Testing 1970" (P.I. Terasaki, ed.), p. 469. Munksgaard, Copenhagen, 1970.

29. Etheredge, E.E., Franecki, B.H., and Najarian, J.S. Variables in an assay of soluble human transplantation antigens. Tissue Antigens 1, 109 (1971).

30. Kahan, B.D., Reisfeld,R.A., Pellegrino, M.A., Curtoni, E.S., Mattius, P.L., and Ceppellini, R. Water-soluble human transplantation antigen. Proc. Nat. Acad. Sci. U.S. 61, 897 (1968).

31. Albert, E., Kano, K., Abeyounis, C.J., and Milgrom, F. Detection of human lymphocyte isoantigens by rabbit homotransplantation sera. Transplantation 8, 466 (1969).

32. Hirata, A.A., Armstrong, A.S., Kay, J.W.D., and Terasaki, P.I. Specificity of inhibition of HL-A antisera by streptococcal M proteins. In "Histocompatibility Testing 1970" (P.I. Terasaki, ed.), p. 475. Munksgaard, Copenhagen, 1970.

33. Metzgar, R.S., Zmijewski, C.M., and Amos, D.B. Serological activity of human and chimpanzee antisera to human leukocyte isoantigens. In "Histocompatibility Testing, 1965" (D.B. Amos and J.J. van Rood, eds.), p. 45. Munksgaard, Copenhagen, 1965.

34. Balner, H., van Leeuwen, A., Dersjant, H., and van Rood, J.J. Chimpanzee isoantisera in relation to human leukocyte antigens. In "Histocompatibility Testing 1967" (E.S. Curtoni, P.L. Mattiuz, and R.M. Tosi, eds.), p. 257. Munksgaard, Copenhagen, 1967.

35. Batchelor, J.R. The relationship between HL-A specificity and a human species antigen. Transplantation 7, 554 (1969).

36. Batchelor, J.R., and Sanderson, A.R. HL-A substances: Properties and immunization of rabbits. Transplant. Proc. 1, 489 (1969).

37. Einstein, A.B., Jr., Mann, D.L., Fahey, J.L., Gordon, H., and Trapani, R.J. HL-A specific

heterologous antisera prepared against solubilized HL-A antigen. Fed. Proc., Fed. Amer. Soc. Exp. Biol. 30, 523 (1971).

38. Etheredge, E.E., and Najarian, J.S. Solubilization of human histocompatibility substances. Transplant. Proc. 3, 224 (1971).

39. Davies, D.A.L. Transplantation antigens. In "Human Transplantation" (F.T. Rapaport and J. Dausset, eds.), Chapter 38, p. . Grune & Stratton, New York, 1968.

40. Davies, D.A.L., Manstone, A.J., Viza, D.C., Colombani, J., and Dausset, J. Human transplantation antigens: The HL-A (Hu-1) system and its homology with the mouse H-2 system. Transplantation 6, 571 (1968).

41. Davies, D.A.L., Colombani, J., Viza, D.C., and Dausset, J. Human HL-A transplantation antigens: Separation of molecules carrying different immunological specificities determined by a single genotype. Biochem. Biophys. Res. Commun. 33, 88 (1968).

42. Davies, D.A.L., Colombani, J., Viza, D.C., and Dausset, J. Isoantigens of mice and their human homologues. In "Histocompatibility Testing 1967" (E.S. Curtoni, P.L. Mattiuz, and R.M. Tosi, eds.), p. 287. Munksgaard, Copenhagen, 1967.

43. Summerell, J.M., and Davies, D.A.L. Further characterization of soluble mouse and human transplantation antigens. Transplant. Proc. 1, 479 (1969).

44. Colombani, J., Colombani, M., Viza, D.C., Degani-Bernard, O., Dausset, J., and Davies, D.A.L. Separation of HL-A transplantation antigen specificities. Transplantation 9, 228 (1970).

45. Sanderson, A.R. HL-A substances from human spleens. Nature (London) 220, 192 (1968).

46. Sanderson, A.R., and Batchelor, J.R. Transplantation antigens from human spleens. Nature (London) 219, 184 (1968).

47. Sanderson, A.R., and Cresswell, P. HL-A substances. In "Symposium on Transplantation Antigens and Tissue Typing" (N.W. Nisbett and M.W. Elves, eds.), p. 87. Oswestry, England, 1968).

48. Mann, D.L., Rogentine, G.N., Jr., Fahey, J.L., and Nathenson, S.G. Solubilization of human leucocyte membrane isoantigens. Nature (London) 217, 1180 (1968).

49. Mann, D.L., Rogentine, G.N., Fahey, J.L., and Nathenson, S.G. Solubilization, properties and molecular separation of HL-A alloantigens. Transplant. Proc. 1, 494 (1969).

50. Mann, D.L., Rogentine, G.N., Jr., Fahey, J.L., and Nathenson, S.G. Molecular heterogeneity of human lymphoid (HL-A) alloantigens. Science 163, 1460 (1969).

51. Mann, D.L., and Nathenson, S.G. Comparison of soluble human and mouse transplantation antigens. Proc. Nat. Acad. Sci. U.S. 64, 1380 (1969).

52. Mann, D.L., Rogentine, G.N., Fahey, J.L., and Nathenson, S.G. Human lymphocyte membrane (HL-A) alloantigens: ˙Isolation, purification and properties. J. Immunol. 103, 282 (1969).

53. Mann, D.L., Fahey, J.L., and Nathenson, S.G. Molecular comparisons of papain solubilized H-2 and HL-A alloantigens. In "Histocompatibility Testing 1970" (P.I. Terasaki, ed.), p. 461. Munksgaard, Copenhagen, 1970.

54. Mann, D.L. The use of gel filtration chromatography to partially purify solubilized HL-A alloantigens. "Soluble Antigen Conference Abstracts." National Institute of Allergy and Infectious Diseases, Transplantation Immunology Branch, Bethesda, Maryland, 1970.

55. Nathenson, S.G., Shimada, A., Yamene, K., Muramatsu, T., Cullen, S., Mann, D.N.L., Fahey, J.L., and Graff, R. Biochemical properties of papain-solubilized murine and human histocompatibility alloantigens. Fed. Proc., Fed. Amer.

Soc. Exp. Biol. 29, 2026 (1970)

56. Boyle, W. Soluble HL-A iso-antigen preparations. Transplant. Proc. 1, 491 (1969).

57. Kahan, B.D., and Reisfeld, R.A. Advances in the chemistry of transplantation antigens. Transplant Proc. 1, 483 (1969).

58. Reisfeld, R.A., and Kahan, B.D. Biological and chemical characterization of human histocompatibility antigens. Fed. Proc., Fed. Amer. Soc. Exp. Biol. 29, 2034 (1970).

59. Reisfeld, R.A., Pellegrino, M., Papermaster, B.W., and Kahan, B.D. HL-A antigens from a continuous lymphoid cell line derived from a normal donor. J. Immunol. 104, 560 (1970).

60. Reisfeld, R.A., Pellegrino, M., Papermaster, B.W., and Kahan, B.D. Serologic characterization of soluble HL-A antigens from continuous lymphoid cell lines derived from normal donors. In "Histocompatibility Testing 1970" (P.I. Terasaki, ed.), p. 455. Munksgaard, Copenhagen, 1970.

61. Pellegrino, M.A., Pellegrino, A., and Reisfeld, R.A. Biochemical characterization of HL-A antigens. Fed. Proc., Fed. Amer. Soc. Exp. Biol Biol. 30, 691 (1971).

62. Mann, D.L., and Levy, R. Solubilization of HL-A alloantigens with SDS. Fed. Proc., Fed. Amer. Soc. Exp. Biol. 30, 691 (1971).

63. Amos, D.B. Genetic aspects of human HL-A transplantation antigens. Fed. Proc., Fed. Amer. Soc. Exp. Biol. 29, 2108 (1970).

64. Batchelor, J.R., and Sanderson, A.R. Implications of cross-reactivity in the HL-A system. Transplant. Proc. 2, 133 (1970).

BONE MARROW TRANSPLANTATION
THE MINNESOTA EXPERIENCE UP TO 1970

H. J. Meuwissen[1]

Pediatric Research Laboratories
Variety Club Heart Hospital
University of Minnesota
Minneapolis, Minnesota

Our first transplantation (TP) of HL-A identical marrow was very encouraging (1,2). Our group had visions of being able to transplant marrow and cure a variety of patients with previously incurable disorders of hemopoietic and reticuloendothelial systems. This optimism was modified by our subsequent experience which has been published elsewhere (3) and which I will briefly summarize here.

The next patient we transplanted had non-lymphopenic hypogammaglobulinemia, with normal delayed hypersensitivity, and normal skin rejection time. HL-A-identical lymph node and bone marrow cells were given but were rejected. It should be noted here that complete rejection was not established until six weeks after TP. This is longer than one would expect from a transfusion with HL-A-non-identical cells. Our next patient had, as did our first patient, a strong family history of lymphopenic immune deficiency. He had numerous infections, no demonstrable cell-mediated immune function (CMIF) and received cells from an HL-A identical sister. Although her bone marrow graft took well, and the patient appeared to be immunologically reconstituted to our satisfac-

---

[1]Present address: Department of Pediatrics, Albany Medical College of Union University, Albany New York.

tion, serious problems nevertheless developed, all
related to the graft-versus-host disease. This
disease develops when the injected cells attack host
tissues due to tissue incompatibilities. Although
our patient was matched at HL-A, this was apparently
not sufficient to completely prevent GVH disease.
Two marrow transplants were given. After the first
transplantation, which was given with probably an
insufficient number of cells, her skin rash which had
antedated her transplant disappeared. A second
transplant was done because of our concern that she
might contract a fatal virus disease. The second
transplant contained a greater number of cells: 10^9
per kilogram. Her immunological reconstitution
seemed to accelerate very rapidly following this
second transplant but at the same time she developed
an increase of her previous rash, which finally
resembled a chronic exfoliative dermatitis. Approximately eighteen months after transplant this rash is
still present, although much improved as compared to
previously. During the GVH disease, her body weight
dropped but subsequently she has started gaining
weight and growing. It seems that she has overcome
whatever was holding her back and we have good hopes
that she may yet overcome the chronic graft-versus-
host disease.

The next patient had Hodgkin's disease; he had
received much irradiation and chemotherapy, and
ended up with decreased cell-mediated immune functions; he was transplanted with HL-A identical marrow
after a dose of 100 milligrams/KG of cyclophosphamide. Shortly after TP, the white count dropped and
we saw a rise in leucocytes, associated with development of fever, and a rash. These three criteria we
considered indicative of graft-versus-host disease.
The initial rash subsided, but a few days later GVH
disease recurred and his bone marrow graft started
to fail. He was treated with antibiotics but at
this time, denudation of the intestinal mucosa
occurred. He died of superinfection of Pseudomonas
of the gut. It had become obvious that the intestinal

flora was important for success or failure of the
transplant.

   In our next patient we faced a different problem.
She was infected chronically with Candidiasis and had
incomplete cell-mediated immune functions. She
could not be immunosuppressed because the risk of
widespread Candidiasis would have been overwhelming.
Therefore, we decided to give this patient a try with
bone marrow cells without prior immunosuppression.
Dr. Buckley had obtained recovery in a similar case
by transfusion of paternal cells to the patient (4).
We had only RBC markers, but no white cell markers.
The marrow we gave was from a non HL-A identical
sister. Our data indicate that cells of donor type
were present in the patient's blood, maximally at
approximately three and a half months after transplantation. At the same time, there was great
improvement in her mucocutaneous candidiasis. However, already two weeks after transplant there was
diarrhea which had not been present before. This
diarrhea was not very bothersome at this time, but
later the patient came back to the hospital with
severe enteritis, hypokalemia, hypoalbuminemia,
having lost approximately five of her fifteen
kilograms or thirty per cent (30%) of her body
weight. She was in desperate condition. After long
and hard work by all involved, the patient finally
seemed to get over her diarrhea, but at this point we
noticed that the percentage of donor type RBC's was
decreasing and her Candida was returning. So it
seemed that what we had accomplished was an about-
face. We made her sick with graft-versus-host
disease and got rid of her Candida. Then when the
cells finally seemed to be rejected or leave the
circulation, she got her Candida back (which was in
any case somewhat better than her graft-versus-host
disease) and we ended up with very little improvement
after a harrowing experience. This result has given
us a great deal of information on how cells act and
how Candida responds and what really constitutes a
anti-Candida defense.

The last patient I will present, was a cousin of
our first, successful patient. He had the same diagnosis of lymphopenic immunologic deficiency and had
no siblings so there was no chance of obtaining an
HL-A identical marrow. We wanted to keep this
patient free of infections as much as possible and to
this end we used a laminar air flow room in which a
high degree of protection from bacteria and viruses
can be obtained. He was treated with ALG before bone
marrow transplantation. In animal systems ALS has
been one of the most effective ways of modifying or
diminishing the graft-versus-host disease. In addition, the patient was treated with albumin gradient
separated bone marrow stem cells, in the hope of
reducing graft-versus-host disease. The albumin
gradient separation was performed by Drs. Van Bekkum
and Dicke in our lab. A total number of 5 x 10^6
cells was given. Finally, following BMTP, he was
treated with methotrexate, half a milligram per
kilogram after transplantation. Following TP, we
obtained some evidence of immunological reconstitution. The number of PHA responsive cells in the
circulation rose to approximately forty per cent
which is markedly different from what it was before.
Approximately nineteen days after transplant patient
developed mild but recurrent GVH disease with fever,
and bone marrow hypoplasia. Lymphocytes had
decreased and small lymphocytes had completely
disappeared. About one week before death the patient
had an apparent recovery of the marrow. We were
very pleased with his progress at this point. Unfortunately, approximately four weeks past TP, the
patient went into shock with massive gram-negative
pneumonia and septicemia and died within three hours.
At postmortem he had graft-versus-host disease, but
above all, he had the same organisms in his lungs
and in his blood which he had had in his stool. And
we were sure those organisms were not introduced
during the course of the hospitalization, but were
his own bacteria which had gained entry to the circulation through the gut.

410

In summary, we have had eleven BMTP patients so far. Of the eleven transplants two did not take and eight were HL-A-identical. We have obtained a cure of the original disease in two patients and transient improvement in two. Two patients have died from cyclophosphamide alone, indicating that cyclophosphamide therapy should not be undertaken lightly. Those latter patients died with severe sepsis caused by their own gut organisms.

The conclusions we have drawn from our experience are as follows: 1) The recipient's cell-mediated immune functions must be repressed before there is any chance of getting a permanent take or a long term take of bone marrow. If there is insufficient suppression of recipient immune function, a partial take or no take of the donor marrow may be expected. 2) Although donor marrow should be HL-A-identical for good results, even under these conditions GVH disease may occur and end in sepsis. 3) With HL-A-non-identical marrow TP, no improvement or reconstitution can at present be obtained even by the concomitant use of ALS, stem cell separation and post transplant immunosuppression.

ACKNOWLEDGEMENT

Supported by grants from the American Heart Association, American Cancer Society, Minnesota Division of the American Cancer Society, The National Foundation-March of Dimes and the U.S. Public Health Service (CA-11505, AI-08677 and HE-06314).

REFERENCES

1. R.A. Gatti, H.J. Meuwissen, H.D. Allen, R. Hong, and R.A. Good, Lancet 2, 1366 (1968).
2. H.J. Meuwissen, R.A. Gatti, P.I. Terasaki, R. Hong, and R.A. Good, N. Engl. J. Med. 281, 691 1969.
3. H.J. Meuwissen, G. Rodey, J. McArthur, H. Pabst, R. Gatti, R. Chilgren, R. Hong, D. Frommel,

R. Coifman, and R.A. Good, Amer. J. Med. 51,513
(1971).

4. R.H. Buckley, Z.J. Lucas, B.G. Hattler, C.M.
Zmijewski, and D.B. Amos, Exp. Immunol. 3, 153
(1968).

BONE MARROW TRANSPLANTATION IN COMBINED IMMUNODEFICIENCY DISEASE

W. D. Biggar, B. Park, P. Niosi,*
E. J. Yunis and R. A. Good

Pediatric Research Laboratories, Variety Club
Heart Hospital and the Dept. of Laboratory Medicine
University of Minnesota, Minneapolis, Minnesota

Allogenic bone marrow transplants have been used for many years in attempting to treat a variety of diseases (1). Prior to 1968, successful bone marrow chimeras had been established in patients with aplastic anemia (2), lymphoreticular malignancy (3, 4), and bone marrow aplasia secondary to total body irradiation (5). Since the first successful immunologic reconstitution of a patient with severe combined immunodeficiency disease in 1968 (6,7), more than a dozen additional successful transplants have been reported throughout the world. Today, bone marrow transplantation is being used primarily to treat patients with immunodeficiency diseases, lymphoreticular malignancies and leukemia, and various forms of bone marrow aplasia. It is the purpose of this chapter to briefly review the patients who have received bone marrow transplants at the University since 1968. Some of these patients have been reviewed previously (8) and these cases will not be detailed in this report.

MATERIALS AND METHODS

The immunologic methods

Quantitation of serum immunoglobulins was done by radial immunodiffusion (9). Quantitative serum

---

*Deceased

IgE determinations were made by Dr. K. Ishizaka, using a double antibody technique. The capacity to produce antibodies was determined by the serologic responses to diphtheria, tetanus, and pneumococcal immunization and the presence of serum isohemagglutinins. Cellular immunity was assayed by the in vivo responses to an intradermal challenge of the following test antigens: tuberculin (PPD) (1 and 5 μg), Candida albicans (Hollister-Stier) (10 to 50 units), mumps (Eli Lilly), streptokinase-streptodornase (Lederle), and dinitrochlorobenzene or dinitrofluorobenzene (30%, 1%, and 0.5%)(8,10). In addition, the in vitro lymphocytic responses to phytohemagglutinin-M (PHA) (11), allogenic cells (12), and antigens to which the patient had previously been sensitized were assayed.

Method of Bone Marrow Transplantation

Details of the protocol have been published (8). Since 1970, we have modified the technique of marrow aspiration to reduce contamination of the marrow aspirate by peripheral blood (13). Small aliquots of marrow (0.2 to 0.3 ml) are aspirated at four or five sites along each iliac crest. The marrow is aspirated in a heparinized plastic syringe (6 ml capacity) by withdrawing the plunger to 3 ml and allowing only 0.2 to 0.3 ml to enter the syringe. Cell counts are made on each aliquot and those aliquots with the highest cell counts are pooled to provide the desired number of nucleated cells. The marrow is administered intraperitoneally, using a small catheter.

PATIENTS

All the patients were treated at the University of Minnesota. The diagnosis in every case was combined immunodeficiency disease. Patients 1 to 4 in Table 1 have been described previously (8) and these cases are not detailed in this summary.

Case 5

The patient, JP, had a family history of autosomal recessive combined immunodeficiency disease
(14). The child presented at 4 months of age with
severe lymphopenia, no in vitro response to lymphocyte stimulation by PHA and allogenic cells, agammaglobulinemia (IgG ＜ 90 mg/100 ml, IgA ＜ 3 mg/100 ml,
IgM ＜ 3 mg/100 ml), no thymic shadow or palpable
lymph nodes, and negative skin tests for delayed
hypersensitivity. A total of 0.35 ml of bone marrow
from an HL-A identical, ABO compatible female sibling
donor containing 45×10^6 nucleated cells (9×10^6
cells/kg body weight) was transplanted intraperitoneally (IP). A graft versus host (GVH) reaction, which
was characterized by fever, hepatosplenomegaly,
eosinophilia, and the characteristic skin rash, began
12 days after transplantation. Twenty-four days
after transplantation, a second febrile episode
occurred, which lasted 6 days. This was associated
with irritability, neck stiffness, and eosinophilia.
A roentgenogram of the chest revealed bilateral diffuse pulmonary infiltrates. Microscopic examination
of lung tissue obtained by open lung biopsy showed
thickened alveolar septa and a chronic mononuclear
cell inflammatory reaction. Examination of the
cerebral spinal fluid (CSF) revealed 126 mononuclear
cells and normal concentrations of sugar and protein.
Cultures of CSF and lung tissues were negative. The
nitroblue tetrazolium dye test (15) was generally
negative for these reactions.

The patient remained well until 47 days after
transplant, when a third mild febrile episode
occurred. The rash and pulmonary infiltrates were
subsiding and repeat examinations of the CSF showed
a gradual return to normal.

The patient was discharged 53 days after transplantation at a time when the quantitative immunoglobulins and the in vitro responses to PHA stimulation showed clear evidence of immunologic reconstitution. Granulocytes with drumsticks were seen in the

peripheral blood, demonstrating donor-derived cells to be present in this male child.

Six weeks after discharge (13 weeks after transplantation), at a time when the quantitative immunoglobulins and the lymphocyte responses to PHA were normal, the patient developed infectious diarrhea and required intravenous therapy. Congestive heart failure and severe aspiration pneumonia ensued. During the heart failure, the patient aspirated and developed severe aspiration pneumonia. He was then referred back to the University of Minnesota and died 4 days later as a complication of massive aspiration pneumonia. Details of this report have been published (13).

Case 6

The patient, CMa, had suffered from recurrent sinopulmonary infections and chronic otitis media since 3 months of age. At 11 months of age, he developed a chronic, scaling, hyperkeratotic eczematoid skin rash. The patient was admitted to the University of Minnesota at 12 months of age with diffuse chronic, irregular, raised erythematous scaling skin lesions and severe malnutrition. The liver was enlarged. Liver enzymes were normal and microscopic examination of liver tissue obtained by a percutaneous liver biopsy showed mild fatty metamorphosis of hepatic cells. The blood smear showed 5% neutrophils, 15% lymphocytes (no small lymphocytes), 66% monocytes, and 11% eosinophils. The bone marrow was hypocellular, with decreased numbers of mature neutrophils and neutrophil precursors. The blood monocytosis subsided but lymphopenia persisted. Quantitative immunoglobulins were (mg%) IgG, 100 to 150; IgA, 10 to 20; IgM, 17 to 35; and no detectable IgE. Repeated in vitro analysis of cellular immunity (PHA and MLC) showed it to be severely depressed with only an occasional positive lymphocyte response to PHA stimulation. No leukoagglutinins, cytotoxic antibodies, or inhibitors of

in vitro lymphocyte responses to stimulation by PHA
or allogenic cells could be demonstrated in the
patient's serum. A diagnosis of combined immunodeficiency was made and bone marrow transplantation
was attempted from an ABO and HL-A identical male
sibling donor. Despite three attempts at bone marrow
transplantation, no successful immunologic reconstitution was apparent. During this time, the patient
had several episodes of pneumonia characterized by
diffuse bilateral pulmonary infiltrates. Microscopic
examination of lung tissues obtained by an open lung
biopsy showed thickened alveolar septa with a mononuclear cell infiltrate predominating. Cultures of
lung tissue were sterile and no evidence of pneumocystis carinii was found. However, polio virus type
2 (vaccine type) was isolated from the lung tissue.
The skin eruption varied considerably in severity.
On several occasions 75 to 80% of the skin surface
was acutely inflamed, with marked confluent and
splotchy erythema plus desquamation, a picture similar to that seen in severe GVH disease. Repeated
skin biopsies were not diagnostic of GVH disease and
no female karyotypic cells were found in the skin or
peripheral blood.

The child died suddenly of overwhelming
Escherichia coli sepsis 70 days after the first
effort at transplantation. Autopsy findings were
compatible with severe combined immunodeficiency
disease. In summary, this patient, with clinical,
laboratory, and autopsy findings of combined immunodeficiency disease, died with no discernible evidence
of GVH disease or evidence of immunologic reconstitution, despite three bone marrow transplants.

Case 7

This patient, TT, a 10 month old female, had
suffered from severe and recurrent pulmonary infections since 10 weeks of age. At the time of admission to the University of Minnesota, she was small
and emaciated. Roentgenograms of the chest showed a

417

collapsed right upper lobe. Quantitative immunoglobulins (in mg/100 ml) were IgG, 150 to 200; IgA, 5 to
13; and IgM, 21 to 58. The patient was of blood
group O but had no isohemagglutinins. The child had
received oral polio immunization at 3, 4, and 5
months of age and polio virus types II and III could
be regularly isolated from stool. Blood lymphopenia
was present. No delayed hypersensitivity skin reactions were seen foIowing intradermal challenge with
Candida albicans, histoplasmin, streptokinase-streptodornase, and PPD antigens. Peripheral lymph nodes
were very small; no thymus shadow was visible on
roentgenograms of the chest. The response of blood
lymphocytes to in vitro stimulation by phytohema-
glutinin and by allogenic cells was absent or very
minimal. HL-A typing (Table 2) showed the only
sibling, a female, to be identical with the exception of HL-A5, which was present in the patient but
absent in the donor. Further studies of the HL-A
typing of this family are to be reported in detail.
The sister's lymphocytes did not respond to the
patient's lymphocytes in mixed culture.

The patient was given a total of five bone marrow transplants over a 6 month period from the
matched sibling donor. Details of the clinical
course and parameters of immunologic reconstitution
are to be published. Approximately 1 month after
the fifth attempted transplant (220 x 10^6 cells/kg
body weight intravenously, IV) early evidence of
immunologic reconstitution was seen. At the time of
this writing (60 days after the fifth transplant)
the child was well and gaining weight. The quantitative immunoblobulins and the in vitro lymphocyte
responses to phytohemagglutinin showed clear
evidence of immunologic reconstitution. Antibody
responses to diphtheria and tetanus were normal.
Furthermore, polio virus types II and III were no
longer cultured from the stool. A mild skin rash
was seen, which on microscopic examination was compatible with, but not diagnostic of, GVH disease.
No evidence of liver or bowel involvement with the

GVH disease was seen. Eosinophilia was minimal. HL-A5 no longer could be demonstrated on the patient's lymphocytes. This change in leukocyte HL-A antigens suggests that the donor lymphoid cells are established in the patient.

Case 8

This patient, CMo, an only child, was well until 10 days of age, when severe oral candidiasis and weight loss began. This was soon followed by severe respiratory infections and diarrhea. At 7 months of age, the child was referred to the University of Minnesota, where severe combined immunodeficiency disease was diagnosed. Profound malnutrition was evident. The patient's HL-A type was 1, 2, 8, and 12, and there were no siblings. Bone marrow transplantation was attempted from an unrelated, HL-A identical, ABO compatible, but MLC unidentical donor. Three transplants were attempted. Initially, 7×10^5 marrow cells/kg obtained from continuous albumin gradient (16) were infused intraperitoneally. No GVH was seen, nor was there evidence of a marrow take. Forty-two days later, a second, unfractionated marrow graft of 1×10^6 cells/kg was given intraperitoneally. Since no evidence of GVH disease or immunological reconstitution was seen 30 days after the second transplant, a third unfractionated marrow graft of 5×10^6 cells/kg was given. A mild GVH reaction occurred 14 days later, with some return of in vitro lymphocyte responses to stimulation by PHA. Four weeks after the third transplant, when the GVH reaction was minimal and the child was clinically well, severe bilateral pneumonia and respiratory arrest suddenly occurred and the child expired. Extensive Pneumocystis carinii pneumonia was found at autopsy.

Case 9

The patient, LH, a 9 month old female, had

419

suffered from severe diarrhea, oral candidiasis, and
respiratory tract infections since 3 months of age.
On admission to the University of Minnesota Hospitals
at 9 months of age, the child was severely emaciated,
febrile, dehydrated, and in marked respiratory dis-
tress. A diagnosis of severe combined immunodeficiency was established. No matched sibling donors
were available. The child died of severe pneumonia
6 days after 350 x 10^6 bone marrow cells from the
mother were given. There was no evidence of GVH
disease at autopsy. A heavy growth of parainfluenza
virus type III and Pseudomonas aeruginosa was isolated from the lungs. The pulmonary inflammation
contained giant cells with no intranuclear or cytoplasmic inclusions.

Case 10

The patient, BH, was referred at 9 months of age
because of chronic diarrhea, weight loss, and recurrent pulmonary infections since 6 months of age.
Severe combined immunodeficiency disease was diagnosed. HL-A typing of the donor and the recipient is
shown on Table 2. The patient was placed in a
laminar air flow room and nursed in a sterile environment with sterile supplies and sterile food.
Elimination of his bacterial flora was attempted by
oral and topical antibiotics. After 14 days of antibiotic administration, cultures of the skin and stool
failed to grow any bacteria. At this time, 700 x 10^6
bone marrow cells from the mother were administered
intraperitoneally. In addition, large amounts
(5 to 10 ml /kg) of maternal plasma and anti-HL-A 1
and -8 serum from an unrelated donor were given
amost daily after transplantation. Fulminating GVH
disease began 7 days after transplantation. Sixteen
days later, disseminated intravascular coagulopathy
and severe electrolytic imbalance occurred.
Cultures of the stool remained sterile to the tests
administered. Death occurred 23 days after transplantation. The same strain of Pseudomonas aeruginosa that had been cultured from the stool prior to

the initiation of antibiotics was cultured from the
blood prior to death. Autopsy revealed evidence of
severe generalized GVH disease but little evidence of
immunologic reconstitution. Pseudomonas sepsis was
widespread.

Case 11

This patient, KR, the first child of healthy
parents with no family history of immunologic
disease, was referred to the University of Minnesota
at 7 months of age with a history of recurrent severe
pulmonary infections and failure to thrive since 2
months of age. At 6 months of age, she had severe
bilateral pneumonia that was unresponsive to broad
spectrum antibiotic therapy. She was given 12 days
of pentamidine and showed significant clinical and
radiological improvement.

A diagnosis of severe combined immunodeficiency
disease was established. HL-A and ABO typing of the
family was as follows: patient: blood group A,
HL-Al, W17, W32, 4a and 4b; father: blood group A,
HL-A 1, -8, W14, W17, 4a and 4b; and mother: blood
group O, HL-Al, W14, W15, W32, Maki & 4b. The father
chosen as the marrow donor and 1×10^6 (2×10^5
cells/kg) total nucleated cells contained in 0.01 ml
of aspirated bone marrow were given intraperitoneally. Twenty-two days after transplantation, a moderate GVH reaction began. This was characterized by
a mild but typical skin rash, fever, hepatosplenomegaly, and marked blood eosinophilia. The absolute
lymphocyte counts increased and, 48 days after
transplant, the in vitro lymphocyte response to PHA
was normal and evidence of humoral immunity was
found. Cytogenetic studies 70 days after transplantation revealed that all the dividing cells in the
peripheral blood were XY, clearly demonstrating
chimerism. Furthermore, the patient's HL-A type was
now -1, -8, and W17, 4a., and 4b . At 75 days after
transplant, because the lymphocyte responses to PHA
and the serum immunoglobulins were again deficient,

a second and larger graft (5 x 10^6 total cells) was given. A mild exacerbation of the GVH was seen. Chronic diarrhea and malnutrition became severe problems. Intravenous hyperalimentation was attempted. Despite caloric intakes in excess of 200 cal/kg/day, no appreciable weight gain occurred.

One hundred days after the first transplant, bone marrow aplasia developed. This was followed by sepsis and death 4 days later. The principal findings at autopsy were a rudimentary thymus; extensive bilateral pneumonia caused by Cytomegalovirus and Pseudomonas aeruginosa; and GVH lesions in the gut, skin, and liver. The lymph nodes were numerous and large and, on microscopic examination, were found to contain numerous plasma cells and small lymphocytes. The lungs contained many large cells with intranuclear and cytoplasmic inclusions, characteristic of cytomegalic inclusion virus disease. Clinical and postmortem findings are presented in detail elsewhere (17).

COMMENTS

Since 1970, our efforts to improve allogenic bone marrow transplantation as a therapeutic tool for a variety of clinical diseases have been focused on children with severe combined immunodeficiency diseases. Each of these patients has provided unique clinical experience that deserves specific comment.

Case 5 represents the autosomal recessive form of severe combined immunodeficiency disease. To date, bone marrow transplantation affords the only effective method of achieving immunologic reconstitution in these children. The ideal marrow graft is one that will establish within the host a population of immunocompetent cells with minimal or no GVH disease.

In this child, the apparent rapid and successful immunologic reconstitution was achieved with only minimal GVH reaction, because of some modifications of our previous method of bone marrow transplantation.

When HL-A identical sibling marrow cells are grafted, the severity of the GVH reaction varies, in part, with the number of cells grafted and the number of immunocompetent cells contributed by peripheral blood contamination of the aspirated marrow. Small aspirations (0.2 to 0.3 ml) of marrow yield a more standardized specimen (18) with minimal contamination by peripheral blood. Precautionary measures are essential because peripheral blood contains immuno-competent lymphocytes capable of enhancing the GVH reaction, whereas the marrow itself contains few, if any, such cells. In support of this is the finding that marrow cells aspirated in small aliquots have a much lower in vitro response to PHA than do marrow cells aspirated in larger volumes (19). The nucleated cells of marrow with minimal peripheral blood contamination would contain higher numbers of marrow lymphoid precursor cells. This may have been important for the apparently successful immunologic reconstitution of this patient utilizing a small number of marrow cells. In this patient, antagonism by autologous serum of the cytotoxicity of donor-derived lymphocytes on the host's fibroblasts was demonstrated (20).

Case 6 had combined immunodeficiency disease as defined by present day methods for immunologic evaluation. Prior to transplantation, this child had a chronic generalized skin rash that was very similar clinically to the rash of GVH disease. We postulated that a placental transfer of immunocompetent lympho-cytes of maternal origin had initiated a chronic GVH reaction in the patient. Failure to thrive, chronic diarrhea, hepatomegaly, and the skin rash were all compatible with this diagnosis. However, repeated skin biopsies, although compatible, were not diagnostic of GVH disease. Furthermore, no female cells could be found either in the peripheral blood or in the skin. The failure to find female cells in the patient does not exclude a maternally induced GVH reaction; in mice an early but short-lived burst of donor cell activity occurs, after which these donor cells are difficult to demonstrate (21).

The failure to achieve immunologic reconstitution with HL-A identical sibling marrow in a patient
with combined immunodeficiency disease remains unexplained. The patient may have had sufficient, but
undetectable, cellular immunity that enabled him to
reject the marrow graft; moreover, the presence of
an on-going maternally induced GVH reaction may have
precluded immunologic reconstitution at the cell
dosages used.

In a given patient, the optimal number of marrow
cells required to achieve immunologic reconstitution
is a critical question that must await further
experience to be answered. In addition to the number
of cells grafted, it is probable that additional factors, present in the host and/or the donor, are
important in achieving successful reconstitution.
Quantitative analysis of the immune function in these
children, by present methodology, is not adequate.
It is possible that, with more sensitive techniques
for analyzing cellular and humoral immunity, significant qualitative and/or quantitative differences in
the severity of the immune deficiency will be found.
Therefore, it seems likely that the optimal number of
marrow cells may vary significantly for individual
patients. If minimal residual immunity exists, for
example, it may take more marrow cells and/or multiple transplantations to achieve reconstitution
than if the patient has an absolute deficiency.

The fact that patients with combined immunodeficiency disease have been reconstituted immunologically by bone marrow transplantation does not
exclude the possibility that other patients will be
found who, in addition to having stem cell deficiencies, may lack the normal microchemical environment
of the thymus and/or bursal equivalent necessary for
the complete reconstitution of their central and
peripheral lymphoid organs. These children may
require replacement of the microchemical environment
essential for cellular differentiation (fetal thymus,
lymph nodes, spleen) in addition to marrow grafts.

In such patients, an alternative hypothesis might be that large transplants can establish a peripheral lymphoid population that is immunocompetent and expandable (22). Such patients, with peripheral but not central lymphoid reconstitutions, may require retransplantation months or years later to maintain immunologic vigor. Finally, some patients with severe combined immunodeficiency might be found, who for reasons unknown will not readily accept the conventional marrow transplant; this has been observed in certain strains of mice (23).

Furthermore, differences in histocompatibility typing and matching play important roles in cell traffic (24) and it seems possible that successes or failures of marrow takes may reflect these influences. It is already clear that the autosomal chromosome region controlling histocompatibility differences in man and animals is complex and controls not only histocompatibility determinants but also the capacities to respond to antigens and to stimulate antigenically (25, 26). Thus, many functions related to cell surface receptivity to differentiative influences many be under control of this general region of the chromosome.

Case 7 had all the clinical and immunologic parameters of combined immunodeficiency disease. The difficulty in achieving immunologic reconstitution may have been caused by the presence of residual, but undetectable, host immunity. This case emphasizes the difficulty in estimating the optimal numbers of marrow cells required for immunologic reconstitution. Whether immunologic reconstitution could have been achieved by giving 220×10^6 cells/kg intraperitoneally instead of intravenously is not known. A more detailed discussion of this fascinating patient is to be published.

Case 8, a child with severe combined immunodeficiency disease, had no HL-A identical sibling donor. The HL-A type of the child was -1, -2, -8, and -12. Fortunately, an unrelated HL-A identical and ABO compatible female donor was found. However, the donor responded to the patient's leukocytes in mixed culture. Because the child was malnourished and critically ill, it was decided to attempt a marrow graft from this unrelated but HL-A identical donor. Three transplants of small numbers of marrow cells were given. Following the third transplant, a mild GVH reaction began, which the child appeared to be tolerating well. Fourteen days after the last transplant, and before any evidence of immunologic reconstitution could be detected, an acute and fulminating Pneumocystis carinii pneumonia developed and the patient died 12 hrs later.

This case clearly illustrates that HL-A identical but unrelated and MLC-reactive donors may be used when matched siblings are not available. The severe GVH reactions that have been seen when even smaller numbers of bone marrow cells, differing by one haplotype (parent to child), are grafted were not encountered in this patient. We suggest that when an HL-A identical and/or MLC-nonreactive sibling or relative is not available, every effort should be made to locate an HL-A identical unrelated donor before using an HL-A unidentical MLC-reactive parent or sibling.

A very high percentage of patients with combined immunodeficiency disease have Pneumocystis carinii infections. Typical of such patients is an acute overwhelming fatal infection with this organism at a time when immunologic reconstitution seems to be taking place. If drugs less toxic than pentamidine, such as pyrimethamine and sulfadiazine (27), prove to be useful and safe in the elimination of Pneumocystis carinii from these children, consideration should be given to their use as therapeutic agents or even as prophylactic agents in all these children, who so frequently succumb to this organism.

The last three patients in this group received marrow that was mismatched by one haplotype. Patient LH (case 9) died 6 days after transplantation. No evidence of GVH was found at autopsy. In case 10, it was decided to attempt to modulate the

GVH reaction by using maternal plasma and cytotoxic antibodies directed toward the paternal HL-A specificity of the child. This child was nursed in a laminar flow room. After 2 weeks of intensive antibiotic therapy at a time when repeated cultures grew no bacteria from the stool, he was given maternal bone marrow intraperitoneally. In addition, maternal plasma, 5 to 10 ml/kg, was given intravenously every other day alternating with serum from an unrelated donor who was known to contain high cytotoxic antibody titers for the HL-A antigens that were inherited from the father by the child. A violent and fatal GVH reaction ensued. Blood cultures taken 48 hrs prior to death grew Pseudomonas aeruginosa, which had been cultured from the stools prior to the attempt at intestinal sterilization but not since that time. This was disappointing and probably indicates that complete gut sterilization was not achieved. High concentrations of antibiotics in the stool specimens at the times when cultures were taken may have given falsely negative results. Perhaps a more likely possibility is that bacteria surviving deep within the intestinal crypts were seeded into the blood when the intestinal mucosa became ulcerated by GVH disease (28).

In this patient, significant reduction of the intestinal bacterial flora did not reduce the severity of the GVH reaction, although it had been expected to do so from observations of some experimental animals (29, 30).

Immunologic enhancement with antibody directed against host leukocyte antigens was tried in an attempt to suppress or prevent the attack of the grafted marrow cells against the host. This has been tried in human marrow (31) and renal transplantation (32) and in a variety of experimental animals. It must be emphasized, however, that, although studies in experimental animals show that such antiserum may suppress the GVH reaction, the studies also show that antisera may accentuate the GVH disease or have no effect at all (33,34). Furthermore, the ability of the antisera to suppress the in vitro mixed leukocyte responses of donor and recipient does not allow one to accurately predict its potential for immunological enhancement in vivo. No enhancement was apparent in this patient.

The final patient, Case 11, with combined immunodeficiency, received a very small bone marrow transplant mismatched in one haplotype (10^6 total nucleated cells). No attempt at bone marrow cell separation or fractionation was made. The GVH reaction was not seen until 21 days after transplantation. The GVH disease persisted and a transient return of cellular and humoral immunity and lymphocyte counts was observed. Chromosome analysis and HL-A typing of peripheral leukocytes revealed them to be of donor origin. By 75 days after transplant, the lymphocyte responses to PHA and the serum immunoglobulins had fallen. Because, as we have shown, successful bone marrow chimeras may depend in part upon active antagonism, possibly antibody, between humoral and cellular immunity (20), a second transplant was made to try and correct the humoral deficit. In addition, malnutrition may have been important in this patient's chronic GVH reaction because, with nutritional deprivation, the humoral factor, possibly antibody, that modulates cellular immunity in vitro is markedly diminished (35) and this humoral factor may be critical in human lymphoid chimeras.

SUMMARY

Bone marrow transplantation is still in its beginning stages of development. In this review, we have focused on the use of bone marrow transplantation in the immunologic correction of combined immunodeficiency disease. From these studies, it is clear that we have achieved immunologic reconstitution in six of 11 patients with severe combined immunodeficiency disease treated in Minneapolis.

Only three of these six patients promise long term
success. Unfortunately, one child (Case 5), apparently fully reconstituted, was lost when aspiration
complicating fluid therapy for diarrhea was fatal
nearly 100 days after a successful marrow transplant
achieved immunologic reconstitution. Two children
(cases 3 and 11) died of Pneumocystis carinii and
cytomegalic inclusion virus when evidence of
immunologic reconstitution was shown. Much has been
learned from these initial efforts and in spite of
the difficulties encountered, this approach to an
otherwise uniformly fatal disease continues to hold
promise. From our experience and that of others, it
is apparent that several factors, many of which are
not well understood, may influence the outcome of
bone marrow transplantation.

Following bone marrow transplantation, the time
required for immunologic reconstitution is variable.
It may depend in part on the number of marrow cells
given, fractionation and/or separation of marrow
cells prior to their infusion, the route of administration (IP or IV), the age of the host, and other
host and donor influences as yet not well understood.
In a young patient (3 to 4 months old), small numbers
of HL-A identical sibling marrow cells can achieve
early and complete immunologic reconstitution (case
5). We presently feel that if no evidence of GVH or
immunologic reconstitution is evident by 3 to 4 weeks
following the first transplant, repeated transplantations should be made, using increasing cell dosages
at 3 to 4 week intervals until immunologic reconstitution is achieved. One patient (case 7) required
five bone marrow grafts before evidence of immunologic reconstitution was obtained. The fifth transplant, given intravenously, numbered 2×10^8 cells/
kg. A mild and characteristic skin rash was the only
clinical evidence of GVH disease. Why so many cells
were required is not clear at this time.

Early diagnosis and intensive supportive therapy
is essential if improvement in results is to be
realized. Several of our patients have died from

severe viral and Pneumocystis carinii infections (36)
while immunologic reconstitution was apparently
being achieved. We believe that the critical time of
extreme vulnerability prior to achieving immunologic
reconstitution will be more readily bridged when
effective therapy is available for these and other
pathogens. These patients should be nursed in a
protective environment with sterile isolation techniques when such facilities are available.

Bone marrow transplantation across a major histocompatibility barrier still presents important
obstacles to success. We feel that very small numbers of carefully aspirated bone marrow cells (1 x
10^6, IP) may be successful in achieving immunologic
reconstitution, either alone or with additional small
bone marrow grafts 3 to 4 weeks after the first
transplant. Judicious use of chemotherapy and/or
methods of immunodeviation may facilitate this
process and minimize the GVH disease. Adequate
nutrition may be critical in attaining this goal.

Finally, prior to transplantation, these children are usually severely malnourished. Adequate
nutrition has been clearly demonstrated to have a
profound influence on immune mechanisms. In general,
we recommend that every effort, including intravenous
hyperalimentation, be made to achieve adequate
nutrition during the time of immunologic reconstitution. The humoral antagonism that may be critical
in successful bone marrow chimeras (20) may not be
established in such malnourished children; instead,
chronic GVH disease and ultimate sepsis may ensue.

Acknowledgments

We thank Drs. P. Ferrieri, J. Matsen, and P.
L'Heureux and Mrs. J. Stemper for their numerous
microbiologic and radiologic consultations, and the
house officers and nursing staff of the University of
Minnesota Hospitals for their invaluable care and
devotion. Also, we thank Dr. C. Lopez and the Virus
Laboratory of the Minnesota State Health Department

for their extensive virological analyses, Drs. E. Gold, S. Austrian, R. Balblus, D. Tubergen, R. Anonsen, R. Papermaster, and V.H. Gordon for refer-ring their patients to us; Dr. J. Yunis for the chromosome analyses;. Dr. E. Yunis for the HL-A typing; and Drs. D. Guenther, M. Ballow and P. L'Esperance for their helpful discussions and advice. This study was supported by grants from the National Foundation March of Dimes, the John A. Hartford Foundation, Inc., and the US Public Health Service AI-08677 and HE-06314. W. D. B. is a Queen Elizabeth II Canadian Research Fellow.

REFERENCES

1. Bortin, M.M. A compendium of reported human bone marrow transplants. Transplantation 9, 571 (1970).
2. Pillow, R.P., Epstein, R.B., Buckner, C.D., Giblett, E.R., and Thomas, E.D. Treatment of bone marrow failure by isogeneic marrow infusion. N. Engl. J. Med. 275, 94 (1966).
3. Beilby, J.O.W., Cade, I.S., Jelliffe, A.M., Parkin, D.M., and Stewart, J.W. Prolonged survival of a bone-marrow graft, resulting in blood-group chimera. Brit. Med. J. 1, 96 (1960).
4. Stewart, J.W. Haemopoietic chimera. Brit. Med. J. 1, 304 (1964).
5. Mathé, G., Amiel, J.L., Schwarzenberg, L., Cattan, A., Schneider, M., De Vries, M.J., Tubiana, M., Lalanne, C., Binet, J.L., Papiernik, M., Seman, G., Matsukura, M., Mery, A.M., Schwarzmann, V., and Flaisler, A. Successful allogenic bone marrow transplantation in man: Chimerism, induced specific tolerance and pos-sible antileukaemic effects. Blood 25, 179 (1965).
6. Gatti, R.A., Meuwissen, H.J., Allen, A.D., Hong, R., and Good, R.A. Immunological reconstitution of sex-linked lymphopenic immunological defi-ciency. Lancet 2, 1366 (1968).

7. Meuwissen, H.J., Gatti, R.A., Terasaki, P.I., Hong, R., and Good, R.A. Treatment of lymphopenic hypogammaglobulinemia and bone marrow aplasia by transplantation of allogenic marrow. Crucial role of histocompatibility matching. N. Eng. J. Med. 281, 691 (1969).

8. Meuwissen, H.J., Rodney, G., McArthur, J., Pabst, H., Gatti, R., Chilgren, R., Hong, R., Frommel, D., Coifman, R., and Good, R.A. Bone marrow transplantation. Therapeutic usefulness and complication. Amer. J. Med. 51, 513 (1971).

9. Mancini, G., Vaerman, J.P., Carbonara, A.O., and Heremans, J.F. Protides Biol. Fluids, Proc. Colloq. 11, 370 (1964).

10. Fudenberg, H., Good, R.A., Goodman, H.C., Hitzig, W., Kunkel, H.G., Roitt, I.M., Rosen, F.S., Sowe, D.S., Seligmann, M., and Soothill, J.R. Primary immunodeficiencies. Pediatrics 47, 927 (1971).

11. Park, B.H., and Good, R.A. A new micromethod of evaluating lymphocyte responses to phytohemagglutinin: "Quantitative Analysis of 'T'-Cell Function." Proc. Nat. Acad. Sci. U.S. 69, 371-373 (1972).

12. Bach, F.H., and Voynow, N.K. One-way stimulation in mixed leukocyte cultures. Science 153, 545 (1966).

13. Biggar, W.D., Good, R.A., and Park, B.H. Immunologic reconstitution of a patient with combined immunodeficiency disease. J. Pediat. (1972) (in press).

14. Tung, K.S.K., Hoffman, G.C., and Lonsdale, D. Lymphoproliferative lesion in congenital thymic aplasia associated with agammaglobulinemia. Amer. J. Clin. Pathol. 52,726 (1969).

15. Park, B.H., Fikrig, S.M., and Smithwick, E.M. Infection and nitroblue-tetrazolium reduction by neutrophils. Lancet 2, 532 (1968).

16. Miller, R.G., and Phillips, R.A. Separation of cells by velocity sedimentation. J. Cell. Physiol. 73, 191 (1969).

17. Park, B.H., Biggar, W.D., and Good, R.A. Incompatible bone marrow transplantation. In preparation.
18. Good, R.A., and Cambell, B. Relationship of bone marrow plasmacytosis to the changes in serum gamma globulin in rheumatic fever. Amer. J. Med. 9, 330 (1950).
19. Park, B.H., Biggar, W.D., and Good, R.A. Paucity of thymus dependent cells in human marrow (1972) (submitted).
20. Jose, D.G., Kersey, J.H., Choi, Y.S., Biggar, W.D., Gatti, R.A., and Good, R.A. Humoral antagonism of cellular immunity in children with immune-deficiency reconstituted by bone marrow transplantation. Lancet 2, 841 (1971).
21. Fox, M. Cytological estimation of proliferating donor cells during graft-versus-host disease in F₁ hybrid mice injected with parental spleen cells. Immunology 5, 489 (1962).
22. Yunis, E.J., Hilgard, H.R., Martinez, C., and Good, R.A. Studies on immunologic reconstitution of thymectomized mice. J. Exp. Med. 121, 607 (1965).
23. Goodman, J.W., Martin, F.B., and Congdon, C.C. Histology of poor growth of parental marrow cells in F1 hybrid mice. Arch. Pathol. 89, 226 (1970).
24. Stutman, O., Yunis, E.J., and Good, R.A. Tolerance induction with thymus grafts in neonatally thymectomized mice. J. Immunol. 103, 92 (1969).
25. Yunis, E.J., Amos, D.B. Three closely linked genetic systems relevant to transplantation. Proc. Nat. Acad. Sci. U.S. 68, 3031 (1971).
26. Park, B.H., and Good, R.A. Third party mixed leukocyte culture test: A potential new method of histocompatibility testing. Proc. Nat. Acad. Sci. U.S. (in press).
27. Kirby, H.B., Kenamore, B., and Guckian, S.C. Pneumocystis carinii pneumonia treated with pyrimethamine and sulfadiazine. Ann. Intern.

Med. 75, 505 (1971).

28. Niosi, P., Matsen, J., Biggar, W.D., Park, B.H., and Good, R.A. Bacterial complications in patients with combined immunodeficiency diseases receiving bone marrow transplantation. (in preparation).

29. Keast, D. A simple index for the measurement of the runting syndrome and its use in the study of the influence of the gut flora in its production. Immunology 15, 237 (1968).

30. Jones, J.M., Wilson, R., and Bealmear, P.M. Mortality and gross pathology of secondary disease in germfree mouse radiation chimeras. Radiat. Res. 45, 577 (1971).

31. Buckley, R.H., Amos, B.A., Kremer, W.B., and Stickel, D.L. Incompatible bone-marrow transplantation: Use of immunological enhancement. N. Eng. J. Med. 285, 1035 (1971).

32. French, M.E., and Batchelor, J.R. Immunological enhancement of rat kidney grafts. Lancet 2, 1103 (1969).

33. Batchelor, J.R., and Howard, J.G. Synergic and antagonistic effects of isoantibody upon graft-versus-host disease. Transplantation 3, 161 (1965).

34. Voisin, G.A., Kinsky, R., and Maillard, J. Protection against homologous disease in hybrid mice by passive and active immunological enhancement-facilitation. Transplantation 6, 187 (1968).

35. Jose, D.G., and Good, R.A. Absence of enhancing antibody in cell-mediated immunity to tumor heterografts in protein-deficient rats. Nature (London) 231, 323 (1971).

36. Lopez, C., Biggar, W.D., Park, B.H., and Good, R.A. Virus infections in primary immunodeficiency diseases. In preparation.

TABLE 1

Case No.	Patient	Age (mo) and sex	Form of LID	Bone Marrow Donor and Marker	Number nucleated cells/kg body weight	Take of Graft	Outcome
1	DCa	5, M	Sex-linked	Sister, MLC identical CTA nonidentical; markers: PHA, MLC, DHS, karyotype, RBC type	1st TP: 7×10^7 peripheral blood IP, 7×10^7 bone marrow IP. 2nd TP: 12×10^7 bone marrow TP, incubated with ALS $1/400 \times 2$ hr at 37°C	Donor cells present (RBC, lymphocytes, sex chromosomes), gamma globulin pos., antibody pos., PHA and MLC pos	Immunologic reconstitution; good health 4 years after TP. Chimeric state and switch of blood type persist.
2.	EFe	7, F	Autosomal recessive	Sister, MLC and CTA identical; markers: PHA, DHS, gamma globulin	1st TP: 10^8 bone marrow IP. 2nd TP: 10^9 bone marrow IP	PHA pos., gamma globulin pos., antibody pos.	Immunologic reconstitution and freedom of infection 3 1/2 years after TP, tight skin and slow weight gain at present, immunologically normal
3.	CRu	13, M	Sex-linked	Sister, MLC and CTA identical; markers: PHA, gamma globulin	10^9 bone marrow IP	PHA pos., gamma E pos.	Evidence of onset of immunologic reconstitution; died of Pneumocystis carinii pneumonia, 5 weeks after TP
4.	SSi	11, M	Sex-linked	Father, MLC and CTA nonidentical; markers: RBC type, PHA	Albumin gradient fraction 3 of bone marrow: 5×10^6 IV	PHA pos., paternal RBC present	Beginning immunological reconstitution; died with GVH disease, gram-negative sepsis, 7 weeks after TP
5.	JP	4, M	Autosomal recessive	Sister, MLC and CTA identical; markers: neutrophil drumsticks	9×10^6 bone marrow IP	Drumsticks in peripheral blood rise in PHA and quantitative immunoglobulins	Moderate GVH, immunologic reconstitution, infectious diarrhea, died of aspiration pneumonia 14 weeks after TP
6.	CMa	12, M	Autosomal recessive	Brother, MLC and CTA identical; no markers	1st TP 1×10^6 bone marrow IP 2nd TP 5×10^6 bone marrow IP 3rd TP 30×10^6 bone marrow IP	None	"Congenital" GVH, PHA fluctuating; died of E coli sepsis 17 days after 3rd TP, no evidence of a take
7.	TT	10, F	Autosomal recessive	Sister, MLC identical CTA nonidentical; marker: HL-A5	1st TP 10×10^6 bone marrow IP 2nd TP 20×10^6 bone marrow IP 3rd TP 40×10^6 bone marrow IP 4th TP 113×10^6	Probably donor cells present (Loss of HL-A5). Rise in PHA and quantitative immunoglobulins, normal diptheria and tetanus antibody responses.	Mild transient GVH skin rash, good weight gain, cellular and humoral immunologic reconstition evident
8.	CMo	3, M	Autosomal recessive	Unrelated female, CTA identical, MLC nonidentical	1st TP: 7×10^5 fractionated bone marrow IP. 2nd TP: 1×10^6 unfractionated bone marrow IP. 3rd TP: 7×10^6 unfractionated bone marrow IP	None	Mild GVH 14 days after 3rd TP, severe Pneumocystis carinii pneumonia and death 30 days after 3rd TP
9.	LH	8, F	Autosomal recessive	Mother, MLC and CTA nonidentical	60×10^6 bone marrow IP incubated with ALS x 1 hr. at 37°C	None	Died 6 days after TP: parainfluenza pneumonia, no GVH
10.	BH	9, M	Autosomal recessive	Mother, MLC and CTA nonidentical	70×10^6 bone marrow IP, maternal plasma, cytotoxic antisera	None	Severe GVH; died of pseudomonas sepsis 23 days after 1st TP
11.	KR	7, F	Autosomal recessive	Father, MLC and CTA nonidentical; markers: PHA and chromosome	1st TP: 2×10^5 IP 2nd TP: 1×10^6 IP	Rise in PHA and peripheral lymphocytes, lymphocyte CTA and chromosomes all of donor origin	Severe cytomegalic inclusion virus and pseudomonas, death 104 days after 1st TP. Evidence of cellular and humoral reconstition clearly shown.

Abbreviations used in this table are:

DHS – delayed hypersensitivity; TP – transplant; MLC – mixed leukocyte culture;
CTA – lymphocytotoxic assay; PHA – phytohemagglutinin; IP – intraperitoneally;
ALS – antilymphocyte serum; GVH – graft-versus-host; IV – intravenously;
Pos. – positive; LID – lymphopenic immune deficiency

TABLE 2

HL–A Typing and Genotypes

Case No.	Recipient	Donor	Identical At HL–A	MLC
5	10–5/W28–W10 4a, 4b	10–5/W28–W10	yes	yes
			sibs	
6	2–12/x–W22 4a	2–12/x–W22 4a	yes	yes
			sibs	
7	9–W5/10–W5 HL–A12,–5 W15, W27, W17 4a	9–W15/10–W5 4a	no	yes
			sibs	
8	1, 2, 8, 12 4a, 4b	1, 2, 8, 12 4a, 4b	yes	no
		unrelated		
9	3–7/x–7 4a	3–7/2–x 4b mother	no	no
10	1–8/2–x and W22, W10, 4b	x–W5/2–x, 4b mother	no	no
11	1–W17/W32–W14 4a, 4b	1–W17/x–8 4a, 4b father	no	no

The x indicates that the HL–A specificity was not determined by the antisera available.

Patients 7 and 10 showed additional HL–A specificities not accounted for on a genetic basis.

BONE MARROW TRANSPLANTATION
FOR ACUTE LYMPHOCYTIC LEUKEMIA

Richard A. Gatti, Mark Ballow, and Robert A. Good

Department of Pediatrics
University of Minnesota Hospitals

Once it became apparent that transplantation of
bone marrow from HLA/MLC matched siblings to immunologically deficient patients was possible without an
overwhelming fatal graft-versus-host (GVH) reaction
and that correction of aregenerative pancytopenia
could also be achieved safely by this manipulation,
interest was renewed in many centers in attempting to
transplant nonleukemic bone marrow into leukemic
patients after destroying their diseased marrow
either by cytotoxic compounds, such as cyclophosphamide, or by total body irradiation with lethal exposure doses. Whereas the main thrust of our efforts in
Minnesota had been directed toward transplantation
of immunodeficiency patients, in a few isolated circumstances in which conventional approaches had been
exhausted and clinical conditions allowed testing
particular hypotheses by marrow transplantation,
attempts were made to transplant patients with
leukemia. Our early experiences are discussed briefly in the preceding chapter by Meuwissen et al. and
are published in detail elsewhere (1). Two more
recent experiences are described in this chapter.
  The first patient with acute lymphoblastic
leukemia received two transplants from an HLA/MLC
matched sibling of the opposite sex. The first
transplant was attempted immediately after a course

of cytosine arabinoside in an effort to establish a graft with minimal disruption of the patient's comfort and apparent wellbeing. Similarly, her second transplant followed 4 weeks of treatment with L-asparaginase, at a time when the patient was in complete remission.

The second patient, also suffering from acute lymphocytic leukemia, did not have a matched sibling donor. However, it had been noted during the course of matching studies that the patient's mother's serum inhibited mixed-lymphocyte culture (MLC) reactions of many individuals, including the responses of either of her parent's cells against her own (2). After 4 years of treatment with conventional cytotoxic agents, the patient relapsed again. She was given 900 rads total body irradiation, bone marrow from her father, a regimen designed after that of Storb and Thomas (3-5), and repeated intravenous infusions of maternal serum. Although a permanent graft was not established in either patient, several interesting lessons were learned. The possible reasons for the failure of the transplants to "take" are discussed.

I. Case Reports

Case 1.
S. St. was 3 years old when a diagnosis of acute lymphoblastic leukemia was established. A good remission was obtained with 6-mercaptopurine and Prednisone. Later relapses were treated with methotrexate, vincristine and cyclophosphamide. Histocompatibility studies revealed that an older brother was HL-A identical and also presumptive-haplotype identical. Mixed-lymphocyte cultures were mutually unresponsive. Several potential markers were present, including male/female karyotypes and Rh typing (donor, rhrh; recipient, RhRh). The donor was blood group O; the recipient, group A.

In 1970, cytosine arabinoside therapy was instituted. On the basis of several preliminary reports suggesting various immunosuppressive effects of this agent, including diminished antibody responses to certain antigens, we decided to attempt a marrow transplant immediately after the patient's last course of cytosine arabinoside, at a time when the patient was in remission and extremely leukopenic. Under light general anesthesia, 2.7×10^9 nucleated cells were withdrawn from the patient's 8-year-old brother and administered intraperitoneally to the patient (the patient weighed 25 kg). Both patient and donor were discharged from the hospital the following day and followed as outpatients.

Two weeks following transplantation, 3% group O erythrocytes were present in the peripheral blood. The bone marrow contained 12% blasts. The donor-type erythrocyte population was increased slightly 3 weeks after transplant; however, by 5 weeks posttransplantation, 40% blasts were present in the bone marrow and chemotherapy with Vincristine and Prednisone was restarted.

Despite the severe leukopenia, the patient's delayed hypersensitivity skin tests and in vitro lymphocyte responses to stimulation with phytohemagglutinin (PHA) remained within normal ranges throughout this entire period. Two months later, the patient's serum was negative for lymphocytotoxic antibodies against her brother's cells and against a panel of 18 different HL-A specificities. Subsequent MLC studies continued to show mutual unresponsiveness.

In November, 1971, the patient was again in relapse with 80% lymphoblasts in her marrow. L-asparaginase therapy was initiated with 2000 units intramuscularly three times weekly for 4 weeks, at the end of which time she was in complete remission. One week later, she received an additional five daily doses of 2000 units each followed by intraperitoneal administration of 5.8×10^9 nucleated bone marrow cells form her brother (patient's weight was 26 kg). The following week, another five daily doses of L-asparaginase (2000 units each) were given.

Weekly differential agglutination studies failed

to reveal any donor Rh type erythrocytes. Bone marrow studies performed 30 days after this second transplant showed 15% donor-type karyotypes. Shortly thereafter, immature cells appeared in the peripheral blood. A repeat bone marrow examination at 40 days posttransplantation no longer revealed metaphases with male karyotypes and this marrow contained 60% lymphoblasts. There were no clinical signs of a graft-versus-host reaction following transplantation. In vitro lymphocyte responses to PHA were severely depressed for several weeks after transplantation. Skin tests were also negative to mumps and to Candida during this period. However, two months later both PHA responses and skin tests had returned to normal. Immunoglobulin levels during this time showed only a transient decrease in IgG.

The patient was then treated with Prednisone and methotrexate. (The latter agent had been discontinued early in her course of treatment when she developed a progressive anemia, leukopenia, hepatomegaly with elevated liver enzymes, and a chronic cough with roentgenograms suggestive of pulmonary fibrosis. At this time, hepatic fibrosis was documented by liver biopsy. All findings subsided when methotrexate was discontinued.) Two weeks later, she again developed signs of methotrexate toxicity. Four months following her second transplant, the patient died with overwhelming sepsis from Salmonella. Postmortem examination revealed Candida organisms in many tissues, including lungs, lymph nodes, and intestinal wall. Leukemia cells were seen both in hematopoietic organs and in the kidney. Several large ulcerations were noted in the gastrointestinal tract.

Case 2.

M. Ho., a 10-year-old white female with lymphatic leukemia, was admitted in September, 1971, for bone marrow transplantation. She had been treated for more than 3 years with conventional chemotherapeutic agents and was no longer deriving benefit from any of these agents. Her peripheral leukocyte count had been less than 1000/mm3 during the 6 weeks prior to transplantation. The bone marrow was markedly hypo-cellular and contained almost 100% lymphoblasts.

Histocompatibility studies in search of a matched sibling donor revealed that none was avail-able. The patient was mutually responsive with all siblings in MLC. In the course of these studies, it was discovered that the mother's serum markedly inhibited MLC reactions of many related and unrelated individuals, including the response of her husband's cells against the patient. The inhibitory factor was associated with the immunoglobulin-containing fraction of her serum in numerous studies. The inhibition did not appear to be related to HL-A types (2). In preliminary studies, no adverse effects were noted when this maternal serum was administered to the patient intradermally, intramus-cularly, or intravenously. Blood groupings were: patient, O; mother, A; father, O. The father was therefore selected as the marrow donor. One week prior to transplantation a precipitous drop in the patient's platelet count necessitated the administra-tion of platelets on short notice. The only immedi-ately available donor with compatible blood groups was the child's father. Three platelet packs were given.

The patient was placed on a soft, then a liquid diet for several days before admission in order to minimize the side effects of total body irradiation on the gastrointestinal tract. She was then admitted to a sterile laminar flow room (SciMed, Inc.) where all hospital care was administered under conditions of protective isolation. No attempt was made to sterilize the patient's gastrointestinal tract. Food however, was prepared under sterile conditions and was sterilized before being served. Following 950 rads total body irradiation on September 20, 1971, 9×10^9 nucleated bone marrow cells from the father in a volume of 125 ml were given to the patient intravenously after passing the marrow through a 100u blood administration filter (patient's weight, 33 kg).

441

Methotrexate was given intravenously on days 1
(15 mg/m^2), 3 (10 mg/m^2 thereafter), 5, 7, 11, and 14
in order to minimize an expected GVH reaction.
Hyperimmune Pseudomonas gamma globulin (for experimental uses only; supplied by Parke-Davis) was alter-
nated with doses of regular gamma globulin every few
days. Because the patient had been on hydrocortisone
immediately prior to transplantation, this was continued during the immediate posttransplantation (PT)
period.

The patient developed a typical postirradiation
febrile pattern over the first few days; vital signs
and blood chemistry studies remained stable. On
day 1 PT, a generalized rash appeared rather suddenly
that resembled the rash often seen with Pseudomonas
sepsis. Consequently, Carbenicillin (2 gm. q. 3 hr,
intravenously) and Gentamycin (40 mg. q 4 hr, intravenously) were started. Blood cultures were being
drawn routinely twice daily. When cultures failed to
substantiate sepsis and the rash did not become worse
over the next 48 hours, these antibiotics were discontinued. During this period, the patient received
numerous units of leukocytes and platelets. All
units were oxygenated and then irradiated with 3000
rads prior to administration. Many of these units
were collected with the aid of a cell separator
(American Instrument Co.). The patient's WBC never
rose above 1500 cells/mm^3. Oral mycostatin (2
million units q. 6 hr) was administered to minimize
overgrowth of known Candida organisms in the mouth,
stool, and urine.

High fever continued without apparent cause
until, on the ninth PT day, blood cultures grew
coagulase-positive Staphylococcus aureus. Nafcillin
(1 gm. q. 4-6 hr, intravenously) and Vancomycin
(0.5 gm. q. 6 hr per os) were added to her therapy
and several more units of leukocytes obtained by cell
separator removal were administered. The cultures
cleared; however, her fever continued. Roentgenograms
of the chest began to show signs of infiltration a
around day 9 PT. These improved somewhat when the

patient was forced to move about her room more
actively and to exercise with blow bottles. On day
12, a severe tachypnea, a slight cough, and a progression of the areas of infiltration on lung films
films prompted the initiation of Pentamidine isethionate (130 mg/day, intramuscualrly) despite repeatedly
negative sputum specimens for Pneumocystis carinii.
Marked improvement of breathing, chest films, and
temperature followed over the next 48 hours. The
patient did not, however, become afebrile.

A bone marrow aspiration at this point showed
very few cells of any kind. Several of these were
interpreted as possibly being "leukemic". There was
no evidence of engraftment. At this point, a second
marrow transplant from the same donor was attempted.
Several days later, too soon to be related to a GVH
reaction, a recurring high temperature prompted
initiation of Gentamycin. The following day, a
fusiform bacillus grew from blood cultures. Amphotericin B was also added to treat a persistent oral
and esophageal candidiasis that was creating great
discomfort for the patient. The patient died the next
morning, 5 days after the second transplant, following an episode of tachycardia and hypotension. Blood
cultures drawn just before death· grew Clostridium
perfringens and Fusobacterium gonidaformans. These
same organisms were grown from many tissues obtained
at postmortem. Postmortem examination revealed
450 ml of bloody fluid in the abdomen. Gaseous blebs
were found in almost all tissues. No evidence of
leukemia or ongoing hematopoiesis was found in bone
marrow or other tissues. The gastric mucosa was
eroded by foci of Candida infection. Lymphoid
elements were markedly depleted in bowel and lymph
nodes, although a few well-defined follicles were
found in the spleen.

DISCUSSION

Despite the renewal of interest in bone marrow
transplantation since 1968, successful engraftment is

still limited to only one of every two patients
transplanted for leukemia. Of the 50 well-documented
patients with this disease who have received transplants of allogeneic bone marrow since 1968, only two
are surviving without evidence of their leukemia (6,
7). The experience described by Fialkow et al. (8)
provides another reservation with regard to the
potential role of bone marrow transplantation in the
treatment of leukemia. These investigators observed
the recurrence of leukemia, following total body
irradiation and marrow transplantation, in donor-type
cells. A second very similar case has recently been
observed by this same group of investigators (9).
Such experiences further reduce expectations of
success and make it increasingly difficult to justify
the heroic efforts involved in marrow transplant
attempts for leukemia.

By contrast, new advances in supportive medicine,
such as laminar flow rooms, cell separators, and an
ever-increasing armamentarium of antibiotics, now
allow some patients to survive for many weeks following lethal doses of irradiation, thus giving the
patient and the transplant team an increasing chance
of establishing a marrow graft. In addition, on the
horizon are agents with antiviral activities that
have potential usefulness in reducing sepsis associated with GVH reactions and possibly in preventing
transmission of the leukemia to the donor cells after
transplantation. Finally, one must consider that a
patient with end-stage acute lymphocytic leukemia
usually still has a normal physiology with the
exception of the leukemic process. Theoretically,
at least, reversal of this process would result in a
totally intact individual. All of these factors must
be carefully considered many times during the long-
term clinical care of such patients. The importance
of these considerations in determining the outcome of
each transplant cannot be overstressed. Because of
the meager successes of marrow transplantation in
leukemia, most investigators have waited too long to
obtain complete remissions in their patients prior to

transplantation. This further lowers the chances of successful management by regimens including marrow transplantation.

Both of the patients reported here were stable and afebrile at the time of their transplants. Case 1 had received two blood transfusions prior to transplantation. The failure of engraftment following the second transplant attempt in this patient may have been related to presensitization by the first transplant. On the other hand, Graw et al. (10) recently reported engraftment of eight of nine leukemia patients who received multiple blood transfusions prior to bone marrow transplantation. This evidence stands in direct contrast to the results of studies in dogs (11) showing a marked reduction in the incidence of engraftment following presensitization with blood transfusions. It was also possible that the cytosine arabinoside that our patient was receiving just prior to her first transplant suppressed antibody formation to donor antigens (12-15). Further, it seems clear in retrospect that despite a severe leukopenia in this patient at the time of the first transplant, her immunologic capacities remained intact. By contrast, despite the depressed skin test reactions and PHA responses at the time of the second transplant, engraftment of the allogeneic, histocompatible marrow was not achieved. There is, of course, the additional possibility that the L-aspariginase, besides depressing cell-mediated immune functions (14,15), may have prevented engraftment of donor cells.

A recent survey prepared from the records of the Bone Marrow Transplant Registry (16) suggests that the chances of engraftment are greater among HL-A identical donor-recipient pairs (56%) than among nonidentical pairs (43%). This observatjion is even more striking among immunodeficiency patients who have received bone marrow transplants (82% versus 36%, respectively). On the other hand, Mathe and others (17) have long argued that a GVH reaction may actually be an important positive factor in combating

445

the leukemic process. In this regard, although the data of the Registry must be considered with a number of reservations and the groups are not large enough to produce statistically significant numbers, when GVH disease is absent, the leukemia recurrence rate is 67% (20/30); when it is present, 22% (4/18) relapse. The median survival time is not significantly different between the two groups (16).

The use of methotrexate to minimize the GVH reaction is based primarily on studies of allogeneic marrow grafting in dogs (5). Although some amelioration of GVH reactions appears to have been achieved in humans given nonidentical marrow and methotrexate immunosuppression, the results are difficult to evaluate (3,6,18,19). It seems clear, however, that in a situation such as that of our second patient, where only a one-haplotype-identical MLC mismatched donor was available, a GVH reaction following total body irradiation with lethal doses would almost certainly have resulted in fatal consequences unless some means were taken to reduce the severity of the GVH reaction (20). The inhibitory in vitro effect of the maternal serum on MLC reactions between donor and recipient was not, in this instance, clinically useful. Although an inhibitor of the MLC reaction was available from the mother's serum, we chose to use the methotrexate regimen as well because we could not assume that this inhibitory influence in vitro could be translated into effective prevention of GVH in vivo. This serum was not cytotoxic to lymphocytes from many sources under a variety of laboratory conditions (2); however, it is possible that it may actually have prevented the engraftment of patenral marrow cells either by a direct in vivo cytotoxic effect or by altering cell traffic pattenrs. As in the first patient, we were confronted with a history of blood transfusions prior to transplantation. In this case, the last transfusion of platelets had been given only 1 week before transplantation and the platelet donor was the father. Although the numbers of nucleated marrow cells that each of our patients received were not high, they were compatible with engraftment in similar situations by other investigators (2,5).

SUMMARY

Two children with acute lymphocytic leukemia were treated with bone marrow transplantation. In the first case, no attempt was made to further depress host cell-mediated immunity beyond that which occurred following chemotherapy with cytosine arabinoside for her first transplant and L-asparaginase for her second transplant. The sibling donor was HL-A/MLC compatible. Transient engraftment was noted following the second attempt. In the second patient, a matched sibling donor was not available. Following total body irradiation with 950 rads, the father's bone marrow was administered. To minimize the expected GVH reaction, serum from the patient's mother, which was known to markedly inhibit MLC reactions between father and patient, was administered along with methotrexate. Neither a GVH reaction nor engraftment was achieved. The role of bone marrow transplantation in the treatment of leukemia is considered.

ACKNOWLEDGMENTS

We wish to thank Dr. Edmond Yunis for his continuing advice and assistance in the performance of HL-A typing on family members of bone marrow transplant recipients. We also wish to thank Dr. Jeff McCullough and his co-workers for the continuing supply of leukocyte packs for transfusion that they provided with the aid of a cell separator.

This work was supported by grants from The National Foundation-March of Dimes, the John A. Hartford Foundation, Inc., and the U.S. Publich Health Service (AI-08677 and HE-06314). R.A.G. is a recipient of a U.S. Public Health Service Research Career Development Award.

REFERENCES

1. Meuwissen, H. J., Rodey, G., McArthur, J., Pabst, H., Gatti, R. A., Chilgren, R., Hong, R., Frommel, D., Coifman, R., and Good, R. A. Am. J. Med. 51, 513 (1971).
2. Gatti, R. A., Yunis, E. J., and Good, R. A.: Clin. Exp. Immunol. (1973) (in press).
3. Buckner, C. D., Epstein, R. B., Rudolph, R. H., Clift, R. A., Storb, R., and Thomas, E. D. Blood 35, 741 (1970).
4. Lochte, H. L., Levy, A. S., Guenther, D. M., Thomas, E. D., and Ferrebee, J. W. Nature 196, 1110 (1962).
5. Storb, R., Epstein, R. B., Graham, T. C., and Thomas, E. C. Transplantation 9, 240 (1970).
6. Thomas, E. D., Buckner, C. D., Rudolph, R. H., Fefer, A., Storb, R., Neiman, P. E., Bragant, J. I., Chard, R. L., Clift, R. A., Epstein, R. B., Fialkow, P. J., Funk, D. D., Giblett, E. R., Lerner, K. G., Reynolds, F. A., and Slichter, S. Blood 28, 267 (1971).
7. "ACS/NIH Organ Transplant Registry", 2nd rep. 1972.
8. Fialkow, P. J., Thomas, E. D., Bryant, J. I., and Neiman, P. E. Lancet 1, 251 (1971).
9. Thomas, E. D., Bryant, J. I., Buckner, C. D., Clift, R. A., Fefer, A., Johnson, F. L., Neiman, P., Ramberg, R. E., and Storb, R. Lancet 1, 1310 (1972).
10. Graw, R. G., Yankee, R. A., Rogentine, G. N., Leventhal, B. G., Herzig, G. P., Halterman, R. H., Merritt, C. B., McGinniss, M. H., Krueger, G. R., Whang-Peng, J., Carolla, R. L., Guillion, D. S., Lippman, M. E., Gralnick, H. R., Berard, C. W., Terasaki, P. I., and Henderson, E. S. New Eng. J. Med. (1973) (in press).

11. Storb, R., Epstein, R. B., Rudolf, R. H., and Thomas, E. D. J. Immunol. 105, 627 (1970).

12. Gray, G. D., Mickelson, M. M., and Crim, J. A. Transplantation 6, 805 (1968).

13. Gray, G. D., Perper, R. J., Mickelson, M. M., Crim, J. A., and Zukowski, C. F. Transplantation 7, 183 (1969)

14. Mitchell, M., Wade, M., Bertino, J., and Calabresi, P. Proc. Amer. Assn. Cancer Res. 9, 50 (1968).

15. Harris, J. E., and Hersh, E. M. Cancer Res. 28, 2432 (1968).

16. Bortin, M. M., Rimm, A. A., Santos, G. W., and Thomas, E. D. "ACS/NIH Organ Transplant Registry. 2nd Rep. 1972.

17. Mathe, G., Amiel, J. L., Schwarzenberg, L., Cattan, A., Schneider, M., de Vries, M. J., Tubiana, M., Lalanne, C., Binet, J. J., Papiernik, M., Semen, G., MAtsukura, M., Mery, A. M., Schwarzmann, V., and Flaisler, A. Blood 25, 179 (1965).

18. Santos, G. W., Burke, P. J., Sensenbrenner, L., and Owens, A. H. Excerpta Med. Int. Congr. Ser. 197, 24 (1969).

19. Mathe, G., Amiel, J. L., Schwarzenberg, L., Choay, J., Troland, P., Schneider, M., Hayat, M., Schlumberger, J. R., and Jasmin, C. Brit. Med. J. 2, 131 (1970).

20. Gatti, R. A., Kersey, J. H., Yunis, E. J., and Good, R. A. Progr. Clin. Pathol. (1973) (in press).

TRANSPLANTATION: A CRITICAL APPRAISAL

L.J. Greenberg, E.J. Yunis, D.B. Amos
and A. Rosenberg

Department of Laboratory Medicine
University of Minnesota
Minneapolis, Minnesota

Department of Microbiology
Duke University Medical Center
Durham, North Carolina

No other area of medical science has profited
more from international collaboration at workshops
and conferences than transplantation. We hope that
the lectures and discussions in this volume have also
added to our mutual understanding of this complex and
rapidly growing field. In this summary chapter we
shall try to provide the reader with an appraisal of
the current state of the art of human transplantation. We shall utilize material from this lecture
series, from the more recent studies of others, and
from personal experience.

THE HISTORICAL BASIS FOR HUMAN TRANSPLANTATION

The impetus for transplantation in man derived
primarily from three biological landmarks: the work
of Gorer (1-4) and Snell(5,6) on the elucidation of
the H-2 system in mice and its relationship to tissue
transplantation; the studies of Medawar (7,8), which
established the immunologic basis of allograft rejection; and the observation by Amos(9) that serum
obtained after allogeneic skin graft rejection would
agglutinate donor leukocytes. This discovery by
Amos (9) that leukocytes shared H-2 transplantation

antigens with other tissues provided the basis for
the serological analysis of histocompatibility antigens in man.

THE HL-A SYSTEM

Since these early studies, we have seen ever
increasing efforts by scientists all over the world
to define the essential parameters for successful
human organ transplantation. These efforts have led
to the elucidation of the HL-A histocompatibility
system in man. In its present state of development,
this system is said to be composed of two series of
segregant specificities known as LA (first), which
has at least 13 allelomorphic antigens, and 4
(second), which has at present 27 antigens (10-17).
The antigens of the HL-A system have been defined
serologically with the aid of both mono- and polyspecific complement fixing antisera in a lymphocytotoxicity assay. Any assessment of the role of HL-A
in organ transplantation is entirely dependent upon
the accuracy of the assignment of antigenic specificities. It is relevant to discuss how these assign-
ments are currently derived. An HL-A antigen is
usually defined by the identical reactions of two or
more sera with cells from families or with a cell
panel from at least 50 unrelated donors. When new
antibodies are found that are even more restricted in
their reactivity than the original type specific
sera, the antigen is often redefined on the basis of
those new sera. Of course, as Walford points out, it
is possible to redefine the definition of antigens to
an absurdity (18). Some HL-A antisera react with
cells that manifest a specific HL-A antigen and with
other cells that seemingly lack the antigen. When
such reactions are found to coincide with a second
specificity common to all or most of the additional
cells, one of two assumptions is usually made.
Either the more broadly reacting antiserum is said to
contain two antibodies, or else it is said to contain
an antibody that cross-reacts with two antigens.

452

CROSS-REACTIVITY AND ANTIGEN FREQUENCY

The nature of the cross-reactivity between specificities is still under investigation; it relates to the complex relationship between antibody specificity and antigen structure. Cellular antigens may include several determinants with varying degrees of immunogenicity. Variants that can be serologically distinguished can still share large areas of similar molecular topography.

Whereas the immunochemist can distinguish antigen-antibody reactions on the basis of polypeptide structure, serology per se does not permit such a definitive genetic analysis of the immune system nor does it relate directly to the property of immunogenetics. The difficulties derive in part from the complex nature of antigens (immunogenicity involves the primary, tertiary, and carrier structure of the participating molecules) and in part from the fact that immune cells of the responder can form many different binding configurations with antigen molecules, resulting in a rather heterogenous response. Consequently, many factors, such as antibody affinity, gene dosage, cross-reactivity, antigen density, accessibility of antigenic sites, and zeta potential differences on cell membranes, must be considered in the response against cellular antigens. Competitive and synergistic interactions between antibody and immunocyte and genetic factors controlling both types of response are also highly relevant and complex.

When faced with the problem of documenting HL-A specificities, the question of which reaction is homotypic and which is cross-reactive is frequently debated. It is generally accepted that the allelic HL-A specificities are defined by "short" antisera that react with low frequency within a population. There is a tendency of HL-A reactivity to get "shorter" and "shorter," as can be illustrated by the splitting of 4c (19,20). The ancestral antigen was 4a, from which 4c was separated. The 4c antigen was thought to be present only when 4a was also present, but 4a could be found without 4c. Then, 4c was subdivided into three components, W5, W18, and HL-A5, each controlled by a different allele (19). Recently, W18 was subdivided into two allelic specificities (21). These alleles could have evolved by stepwise mutations from some ancestral precursor types of alleles of the system. These precursor components corresponding to primitive antigenic specificities may be shared by all the antigens of the family and therefore have higher frequencies in the population, whereas antigenic determinants of more recent mutations are more restricted.

Ceppellini has called "supertypic" the factors shared by more than one allelic variant of the antigen (22). Obviously, it is possible to arrange the alleles with very restrictive frequency as mutually exclusive genetic factors among the offspring of heterozygous parents. However, some "compound" sera of broad reactivity, including those that react freely with two or more HL-A specificities, such as HL-A3 and HL-A11, or HL-A2 and W28, or the subspecificities of HL-A9, HL-A10 and W19, appear to be monospecific by the criterion of absorption.

Amos and Yunis (23) studied such a situation with a subject BC, whose serum was used to determine specificity Ao14. This serum reacted with cells that carried HL-A3 specificity (positive) and also with cells generally considered to be HL-A3 negative. By employing different immunization cycles, they were able to define three classes of cells serologically. Early antibody primarily detected class I individuals, represented by "classical" HL-A3, and to a lesser degree class II cells, which were either HL-A11 or a variant form of that antigen. The late antibody response was characterized by lymphocytotoxic reactions to class I and class II cells and also by weak reactions of class III cells. The definition of class III was more complex and was correlated with HL-A1 and other reactions not defined by known HL-A specificities. Absorptions using cells

from donors of each BC class indicated that BC sera
were operationally monospecific. Class II and III
cells were not as efficient in absorbing the antibody as were class I cells. Eluates recovered following absorption with platelets from either class I,
II, or III donors demonstrated specificity similar to
that observed with the unabsorbed serum.

Amos and Yunis (23) explain the data in the
following way: (1) the differences between classes
may be caused by a complex cross-reactivity between
antigens, antibodies, or both; (2) a marked antigen
strength effect of the HL-A3. Alternatively, the
Ao14 gene may be arranged in the HL-A system in a
manner similar to the G gene of the Rh gene complex,
which is in genetic disequilibrium with the C and D
genes. Anti-CD sera are generally assumed to contain
anti G plus anti-D and anti-C. The G antigen is not
a compound specificity, because red cells from one
Rh-negative donor react with anti-G sera. The G
effect can explain the apparent cross-reactivity and
the antigen strength related to HL-A3 cells if we
assume that BC serum contains highly cross-reactive
antibodies to both Ao14 and HL-A3. Therefore, HL-A3-
Ao14 cells are class I, HL-A11-Ao14 are class II, and
HL-A1-Ao14 are class III. HL-A11 and HL-A1 in the
cis position may depress Ao14 as the antigen C
depresses antigen D in the cis position. Of course,
this does not explain the observed positive correlation between certain antigens of the first and second
series referred to as linkage disequilibrium.

Monospecificity by absorption is not necessarily
the same as monospecificity by elution. By differential elution with a pH gradient Dorf et al. (24) were
able to show that serum BC, although completely
absorbable by cells of the different classes, could
be fractionated into a variety of antibodies of over-
lapping specificity, apparently a universe of antibody molecules.

At the risk of hypothesizing ad nauseum, we
would like to introduce another thought on the subject of HL-A polymorphism. One mechanism by which a

species can increase and differentiate its gene complement during evolution is by gene duplication followed by independent mutational changes in the resulting gene copies (25). Numerous examples of such duplications appear in the literature (26-28). We may rationalize HL-A specificities 1,3 and 11 by a duplication-mutation mechanism in which HL-A11 is the product of a more ancestral gene and HL-A1 and A3, the more recent mutated duplicates. Under this hypothesis, specificities 1,11 and 3,11 segregate together, detection of HL-A11 being obscured by the serologic cross-reactivity of the more recently mutated duplicates. The situation may be analogous to that seen in the immune response to haptenated proteins. Because of the immunodominance of the hapten, a population of antibodies molecules is elicited that is strongly directed against the hapten. During the course of evolution, continued mutation and duplication of the HL-A11 gene may have given rise to more immunologically restricted gene products. In the present case HL-A3 is the most immunologically restrictive.

ISOLATION AND CHARACTERIZATION
OF MEMBRANE CONSTITUENTS

An understanding of the molecular mechanisms controlling the synthesis of membrane antigens and the immune response can no doubt provide valuable guidelines for tissue transplantation. However, owing to inherent difficulties in this area, progress is being made along selected lines limited to very specific goals, such as isolation and chemical characterization of cell surface antigens, studies on the migration of antigens of antibody-treated cells, and chemical definition of specificity in hapten antibody complex formation. We shall not discuss hapten antibody complex formation in this summary. Any isolation procedure aimed at defining a biological activity is critically dependent on the specificity of the assay employed. In the quest for

456

the isolation of HL-A antigens, we must rely on the
specificity of the serum available. In essence, the
concept used in serology is more properly termed
"selectivity." A satisfactory serum is one that
reacts at some chosen concentration level with one
antigen and not with others. Therefore, a similar
degree of selectivity can be obtained with a number
of different sera. However, in the procedure of
purification of the antigen, the degree of purity of
homogeneity must be expressed quantitatively as
units of activity per mass of material isolated and
purified. In a classical enzyme isolation procedure,
we strive toward maximum activity per milligram of
material isolated. It is very difficult to produce
a truly quantitative definition of activity if the
biological assay requires intact cells and a detection system that related to an event different from
the combination of antibody and antigen, as in the
case of the lymphocytotoxicity test. The competitive
assay, where purified antigen fractions are used to
block the normal test cell, is a viable alternative
for continuous activity measurements. However, the
question of activity standardization still remains a
problem because it is not possible to standardize
either cells or antibodies.

A totally different approach to the problem is
presented in the chapter by Popp et al. (29). These
authors, recognizing the difficulties in such
activity measurements, approach the problem by side
stepping the activity issue and concentrating their
efforts on the identification of recurring amino acid
sequences from tryptic peptides of the plasma membrane. They describe their efforts to correlate
recurring sequences with the genetic pattern of the
mice employed for the studies. Although it has been
possible to separate and identify 52 peptide chains
present in red cell membrane constituents by isoelectric focusing in 8 M urea (30), it must be
remembered that the antigenic determinants of globular proteins in many instances depend on the secondary and tertiary structure of the protein. The best

example of this type of dependency is found in the INV system of the immunoglobulins (31).

GRID HYPOTHESIS

In a sense, the assumptions by Popp and his collaborators about the correspondence of sequences and antigenic sites is on the other end of the spectrum of membrane interactions envisioned by the so-called grid model of Boyse and Old (32). This model of the cell membrane envisions the different membrane determinants and receptors as forming patterns, the positions and sequence of positions of which recur over a considerable distance. Three independent determinants, ABC, can for example, create BCA and CBA in a unidimensional grid and a large number of patterns in two- or three-dimensional grids. The main experimental support for this concept comes from blocking studies (32) and from work utilizing fluorescein-labeled antibody, which reveals recurring patterns on the cell surface (33).

The validity of the blocking test, however, as a measure of the proximity of any pair of antigens was recently challenged by the work of Davis (34). Employing a ferritin-conjugated alloantibody, Davis (34) demonstrated that the spatial arrangement of the membrane components that possessed H-2 isoantigens was markedly altered by the attachment of a second antibody directed toward mouse gamma globulin or ferritin. He further pointed out that other membrane antigens might also be affected in a similar manner.

Furthermore, the variability of the membrane response with temperature (35) and the whole concept of capping (36) is more compatible with a more flexible membrane model (37). In such a model, the membrane has the latent capability of forming several patterns of structural response to different molecules that bind to it. If we assume a surface density of determinants of $4-8 \times 10^3/\mu^2$, as in the case of concanavalin receptors (38), the area covered by the 35 Å head of IgG alone would come to

458

the range of 1% of the surface; or considering the
whole IgG, the change in surface contact for the cell
would fall in the 10% maximum range. Such changes
are energetically significant on any type of structure, regardless of whether or not they occur at
sites of metabolic regulation. If we also assume
that minimizing the total free energy of the membrane
leads to different patterns or structures on the membrane surface, then we can ask what percentage of the
sites must be covered for a new pattern or structure
to appear. This can be accompanied by another variation of the same question. How many binding sites
per cell must be available so that a structural
rearrangement can take place? A very reasonable
mechanism for such changes is a cooperative rearrangement represented by a simple Ising model (39).
In such cases, the binding shows a sigmoid curve,
and the onset of the membrane changes has a threshold
value. Although the concept of threshold reactivity
has been well documented by many pharmacological and
neurophysiological studies both in vivo and in vitro,
quantitative evaluation of threshold histocompatibility parameters is lacking. Although we know that
lymphocyte reactivity in mixed culture and to various
mitogens has a threshold, the application of this
information to transplantation has not been ade-
quately explored. With respect to HL-A typing, the
phenomena of CNAP (cytotoxic negative absorption
positive) and CNIP (cytotoxic negative immunogenicity
positive)(40) may reflect antigen densities that are
beneath the threshold for complement-mediated cell
lysis but the practical application of these phenomena for organ transplantation has not been determined.

CLINICAL ASPECTS OF TRANSPLANTATION

Skin Grafts

The first attempts to correlate histocompatibility, as defined by leukocyte agglutination, with

459

primary skin graft survival (41-44) were disappointing and inconclusive. The differences between survival times of grafts from compatible and incompatible donors were too small to evaluate. In an effort
to clarify this situation, graft survival was
examined as a second-set phenomenon (45). It was
felt that moderate preimmunization would amplify the
differences between compatible and incompatible
donors. The results of this study indicated that 16
compatible grafts were rejected as a first set
phenomenon, whereas 14 out of 17 incompatible grafts
were rejected in an accelerated manner. These data
were interpreted to mean that the Hu-1 (now called
HL-A) leukocyte antigens were transplantation antigens and, when matched between donor and recipient,
resulted in prolonged graft survival. A number of
points in this study, however, must be emphasized.
To begin with, moderate immunization was employed,
because when hyperimmunization was used, most of the
grafts, whether compatible or incompatible, were
rejected in an accelerated fashion, very often as
white grafts. Under conditions of moderate immunization, as for example by sequential and widely
spaced injections and/or skin grafts, recipients
$R_1R_2R_3$ developed humoral antibodies, some of which
were specific for donor leukocyte antigens. These
subjects demonstrated a preference for compatible
grafts. In the case of recipients $R_4R_5R_6$ however, no
specific agglutinating antibodies were detectable.
Furthermore, after the highest preimmunizing dose of
leukocytes, grafts designated as incompatible survived longer than did the compatible ones. It is
rather difficult to accept in toto the conclusions of
the authors (45) that these leukocyte antigens exert
a major role in graft survival or rejection.

Kidney Grafts

With the advent of tissue typing, it was hoped
that the results of kidney transplantation could be
dramatically improved. However, the picture that

emerged was disappointing and often bizarre (46,47).
Incompatibility was not necessarily associated with
rapid graft rejection. For example, in one small
early series, an unrelated and almost certainly
incompatible kidney survived for longer than 11 of
13 grafts from close relatives. Attempts to correlate graft survival with phenotypic similarity for
HL-A antigens were only partially successful (46).
Although many of the failures can possibly be attributed to inadequate and inaccurate typing, difficulty
is still being experienced in predicting compatibility. It seems probable that the rare phenotypically
identical donor-recipient pairs show a very high
survival rate but one distinguished serologist has
commented privately that success of a transplant
depends more upon where it was carried out than on
the tissue typing results. Although this was of
course a cynical and exaggerated comment, one reflection of the difficulty involved in donor selection
is the paucity of published reports confirming the
correlation. Large collaborative schemes in which
both clinicians and serologists combine to improve
and standardize their respective practices are still
required to clarify the relationship. In part, the
difficulty is caused by immunogenetic factors affecting the recipient. This may explain the occasional
reported example of prolonged survival of blood
group A or B incompatible kidneys, because the A and
B antigens appear to be as potent in most instances
as HL-A (47).

HL-A Typing by Lymphocytotoxicity
Testing and Homograft Prognosis

As our ability to define the HL-A system has
improved, renewed efforts to correlate HL-A typing
and homograft reactions have been attempted (48-54).
The general conclusions are still that graft survival
is lowest between unrelated pairs, intermediate
between parent-child combinations, and highest for
HL-A identical siblings. However, as might be

expected, the best results have been between
identical twin transplants (55–57) and dizygotic twin
transplants (58), whereas in the remainder of the
published reports there is an ever increasing number
of examples that cannot be rationalized on the basis
of HL–A matching (48,59–62). By way of example, a
clinical evaluation of 29 renal transplants were compared with respect to leukocyte typing and graft
function (59). Eleven transplants were classified as
a good match and good function, whereas 13 grafts
were designated poor matches but had good function.
The same authors (59) found that in over 100 transplants graft survival was practically the same with
related or cadaver donors, 73% versus 68% survival,
respectively.

Of course, we may still argue that the problem
is not one of donor–recipient matching but that graft
rejection is related to prior immunization of recipients. This immunization may result from multiple
transfusions during dialysis or from prior experience
with a variety of cross-reactive bacterial, viral, or
fungal antigens, all of which could bring about
accelerated graft rejection. This argument is
weakened by the moderate success that has been
achieved in patients with multiple transplants (56).
In fact, an analysis of the data on second transplants suggests that they may function better than
the primary graft (56). Hume et al. (56) feel that
this may be because of the protective function of
humoral antibodies resulting from the first transplant. Alternatively, there may have been a degree
of exclusion of the most immunogenetically imcompat-
ible antigens for the particular recipients involved.

MLC Testing and Homograft Prognosis

Another means of assessing donor–recipient
interactions is the mixed-leukocyte culture (MLC)
(63–65). This test, which is thought to be the in
vitro counterpart of the graft-versus-host reaction,
can detect antigenic disparity between lymphocytes

but does not define the antigens that are involved. Although it was first thought that MLC reactions measured histocompatibility, when one tried to relate MLC with homograft reactions, only a cloudy picture emerged. To begin with, MLC tests between HL-A identical siblings as a rule do not result in stimulation (66,67) although there are some reports of MLC-positive HL-A identical pairs (66-68). In the case of nonidentical pairs, the MLC test has always been positive (69). However, Terasaki et al. (70) have recently reported that a patient with combined immunodeficiency disease, having 12 HL-A specificities expressed phenotypically, did not react in MLC to his genotypically HL-A identical sibling, who had three detectable specificities. Although there is no clear-cut correlation between MLC tests and graft survival, a negative MLC or a low level of stimulation in related pairs is associated with some instances of prolonged graft survival (71,72). With respect to unrelated subjects, Koch et al. (73) compared skin graft rejection in HL-A identical pairs, including some that were stimulatory and some that were nonstimulatory in MLC, to a nonidentical stimulatory pair. There was very little difference in rejection times.

BONE MARROW GRAFTS

Early attempts to transplant bone marrow in man and outbred animals were also seriously hampered by incompatibilities between donor and recipient, manifested as graft rejection or graft versus host disease (GVH). In addition, prolonged immunodeficiency of the patient preceding and accompanying marrow grafting further complicated the clinical picture. Significant advances in our ability to define histocompatibility parameters through HL-A tissue typing and MLC testing, coupled with judicious immunosuppressive therapy, provided new hope for clinical marrow grafting. The most success was in patients with severe combined immunodeficiency and

aplastic anemia (74-77) when transplanted with marrow from HL-A identical siblings. However, even
under optimum conditions, i.e., marrow grafts from
HL-A identical siblings that did not react with
recipient lymphocytes in MLC, marrow transplantation
was associated with fatal GVH disease (79-82).
Thomas et al. (78-83), employing HL-A identical siblings that were nonreactive in MLC, reported successful marrow grafts between opposite sexes. In one
case (83), a female patient in remission from lymphoblastic leukemia was treated with chemotherapeutic agents, given total body radiation, and transplanted with marrow from an HL-A matched brother.
Although treatment with methotrexate suppressed GVH
disease and facilitated engraftment, leukemia
recurred after 135 days in which more than 50% of the
blast cells were donor type malignantly transformed.
In a recent report by Dupont et al. (84), however,
a patient with severe combined immunodeficiency was
successfully transplanted with marrow from a nonidentical HL-A, MLC-negative donor. Although this
observation emphasizes the importance of MLC in
graft prognosis, much more data are needed on
marrow grafting to properly assess the situation.

HISTOCOMPATIBILITY NETWORK

From the foregoing discussion, which attempts to
interpret the state of the art today, one is forced
to conclude that although HL-A typing and MLC testing
are generally adequate yardsticks of histocompatibility under optimum conditions, they are inadequate
predictors of allograft behavior between unrelated
subjects.

Well then, where should we look for the answers?
To begin with, we should probably diversify and also
intensify our attempts to identify the antigenic
factors involved. Although our other skills, including clinical management, appear to be generally
adequate for the support of the postoperative HL-A
identical or identical twin pairs, greater care is

indicated for the recipient of an incompatible kidney where the greater amounts of immunosuppression required to prevent rejection can intensify all the problems of management. Preparation of the kidney, including an evaluation of the role and methods of elimination of passenger lymphocytes and selection and care of the pretransplant patients, are also important. Included in this category are an evaluation of frozen or other leukocyte-poor blood for transfusion or the administration of antigen prior to transplantation and the avoidance of endstage and chronically debilitated dialysis patients wherever possible. Many of these measures are common sense but few if any are standard practice between transplant teams. The continuing dialog between serologists in the form of histocompatibility testing workshops has, unfortunately, no clinical counterpart.

In the laboratory, improved tests for histocompatibility antigens are urgently needed. In the mouse, the animal from which most of the basic information about transplantation antigens has been derived, 30 or more histocompatibility systems are demonstrable (85). In man, only ABO and HL-A antigens have been described on lymphocytes, platelets, and fibroblasts. However, even in the mouse, most of the H antigens can only be demonstrated through transplantation studies.

Some idea of the potential relevance of non-HL-A antigens comes from an analysis of the rejection times of grafts between HL-A identical siblings. Rejection times range from 14 days or less to 80 days or more. The expression of non-HL-A antigens may differ greatly from tissue to tissue; certainly this is true for the mouse, where it has been suggested that tissue distribution may be a useful method of distinguishing between antigenic systems. However, if the same difference exists between HL-A and non-HL-A factors of man as is known for H-2 and non-H-2 factors of mouse, adequate immunosuppressive procedures should be capable of rendering non-HL-A

factors relatively trivial in clinical transplantation and the main emphasis must continue to center
on HL–A and HL–A associated (linked) attributes.

In this context Yunis and Amos (86) have presented evidence that suggests that allograft rejection is dependent on immunization against the products of two and possibly three separate, but closely
linked, genetic systems: HL–A, MLC, and hypersensitivity delayed reaction (HDR). Their evidence for
an HDR locus is mainly circumstantial and is based on
studies both in the mouse and man. These authors
(87) have reinterpreted the work of Snell et al. (88,
89) relating to the strong association between H–2
phenotype and tumor susceptibility. They point out
that the best correlation occurs when the mouse
strains challenged belong to the same ancestral
stock. The most clearcut example is in the case of
the H–2k group, represented by CBA or C3H, C57Br/a
or C57Br/cd, and ST (87). With regard to CBA and
C3H, descendants of Strong's C family are both 100%
susceptible to C3H tumors whereas the other strains
are almost 100% resistant. Br/a and Br/cd are both
almost 100% susceptible to a BR/a tumor whereas the
other strains are resistant. Amos and Yunis (87)
feel that these data are consistent with the hypothesis of allelic HDR genes in different mice,
separate from H–2. Although the concept of an HDR
locus is certainly compatible with the consensus of
opinion implicating delayed hypersensitivity as the
major immunologic mechanism underlying rejection of
homografts (90–93), the circumstantial evidence
derived from the mouse data is open to question. To
begin with, is the H–2 phenotype-tumor susceptibility
correlation really good presumptive evidence for all
normal tissue graft behavior? Second, is there
sufficient bona fide documentation of the ancestral
histories of all strains of mice? And finally,
should we not verify the original H–2 designations
with present-day reagents and assays?

With respect to the evidence for HDR in man,
Amos and Yunis (87) cite the work of Koch et al.

(73), who compares skin graft rejection times between
HL-A identical unrelated subjects, both stimulatory
and nonstimulatory in MLC, with rejection of skin
from a stimulatory nonidentical. There is essentially no difference in rejection times. Although
the findings of Koch et al. (73) can be interpreted
in terms of an additional locus, such as HDR, they
very clearly strengthen the concept of separate
loci for HL-A and MLC.

Further evidence for a separate MLC locus comes
from the recent work of Dupont et al. (84), who
report several instances in which the MLC response is
negative in spite of HL-A disparities. These nega-
MLC responses are not associated with any particular
HL-A haplotype or with the presence of lymphocytotoxic or blocking antibodies. These very interesting
and provocative studies must be considered when one
attempts to describe the architecture of the human
histocompatibility network. Amos et al.(94) suggests the designation HL-1 for the histocompatibility
complex comprising HL-A, MLR-S, and HDR.

IMMUNOSUPPRESSION

No volume dealing with organ transplantation is
complete without a consideration of the influence of
immunosuppressive therapy, for without such therapy,
there are very few successful transplants. We shall
not attempt to trace the development of all types of
immunosuppressive therapy but rather shall focus
briefly on regimens that are in vogue today.
Although a combination of corticosteroids, azathioprine, and antilymphocyte serum (ALS) is most
frequently employed, the most promising agent is ALS.
Its full potential in man has not yet been realized
because of the difficulty of standardizing the product and of establishing meaningful dose-response
parameters. The great power of ALS to inhibit
cellular immunity in mice accounts for its striking
ability to prolong the survival of allografts. However, the effect is not antigen specific and

depresses the whole immune system. As a consequence, the patient is not only vulnerable to bacterial, viral, and fungal infections but also suffers a breakdown in immunological surveillance mechanisms, which may explain why severely immunosuppressed patients have developed malignancies. This lack of specificity is the greatest obstacle in immunosuppressive therapy and frequently one must consider the advantages of treatment and the disadvantages incurred by immunologic crippling. The whole area of drug action is presently in a state of ferment. With the realization that at least two populations of lymphocytes exist, the so-called T and B cells, both of which may include a variety of subpopulations, and that macrophages also play a major role in certain immunologic interactions, new methods for selectively breaking a particular form of immune response become possible. Furthermore, the proliferative changes that precede the manifestation of graft rejection require the participation of a wide variety of metabolic pathways potentially susceptible to blockade. The finding by Berke et al. (95) that the lymphoid cells at the anatomical site of graft rejection are uniquely effective and represent an extraordinary enrichment of effector cells at their site of action appears to offer a new approach to the study of selective drug action.

Although the areas of investigation covered in this book may ultimately provide the magic formula for tissue transplantation, transplantation is not an end in itself. For even when immunosuppression, donor selection by histocompatibility, and tolerance are understood, applied transplantation is expensive, impractical for society, and painfully traumatic for the family.

REFERENCES

1. Gorer, P.A., J. Pathol. Bacteriol. 44, 691 (1937).
2. Gorer, P.A., J. Pathol. Bacteriol. 47, 231

(1938).

3. Gorer, P.A., J. Pathol. Bacteriol. 54, 51 (1942).
4. Gorer, P.A., Lyman, S., and Snell, G.D., Proc. Roy. Soc., Ser. B 135, 449 (1948).
5. Snell, G.D., J. Nat. Cancer Inst. 11, 1299 (1951).
6. Snell, G.D. In "Conceptual Advances in Immunology and Oncology," p. 323. Harper (Hoeber), New York, 1963.
7. Medawar, P.B., J. Anat. 78, 176 (1944).
8. Medawar, P.B., Brit. J. Exp. Pathol. 27, 15 (1946).
9. Amos, D.B., Brit. J. Exp. Pathol. 34, 455 (1953).
10. Dausset, J., Acta Haematol. 20, 156 (1958).
11. van Rood, J.J., Thesis, Leiden, 1962.
12. Walford, R.L., Gallagher, R., and Troup, G.M., Transplantation 3, 387 (1965).
13. Terasaki, P.I. and McClelland, J.D., Nature (London) 204, 998 (1964).
14. Payne, R., Tripp, M., Weigle, J., Bodmer, W., and Bodmer, J., Cold Spring Harbor Symp. Quant. Biol. 29, 785 (1964).
15. Dausset, J., Ivanyi, P., and Ivanyi, D. In "Histocompatibility Testing 1965" (D.B. Amos and J.J. van Rood, eds.) p. 51. Munksgaard, Copenhagen, 1965.
16. Bodmer, W., Bodmer, J., Adler, S., Payne, R., and Bialek, J. Ann. N.Y. Acad. Sci. 129, 473 (1966).
17. Ceppellini, R., Curtoni, E.S., Mattiuz, P.L., Miggiano, V., Scudeller, G., and Serra, A., In "Histocompatibility Testing 1967" (E.S. Curtoni, P.L. Mattiuz, and R.M. Tosi, eds.), p. 149. Munksgaard, Copenhagen, 1967.
18. Walford, R.L., personal communication (1971).
19. Payne, R., Tripp, M., Weigle, J., Bodmer, W., and Bodmer, J., Cold Spring Harbor Symp. Quant. Biol. 29, 285 (1964).
20. Bodmer, W.F. and Payne, R., In "Histocompatibility Testing 1965" (D.B. Amos and J.J. van

Rood, eds.), p. 141. Munksgaard, Copenhagen, 1965.

21. Thorsby, E., Kissmeyer-Nielsen, F., and Svejgaard, A., In "Histocompatibility Testing 1970" (P.I. Terasaki, ed.), p. 137. Munksgaard, Copenhagen, 1970.

22. Ceppellini, R. In "Progress in Immunology" (D.B. Amos, ed.), p. 973. Academic Press, New York, 1972.

23. Amos, D.B. and Yunis, E.J., Science 165, 300 (1969).

24. Dorf, M.E., Eguro, S.Y., and Amos, D.B. Transplantation (1972)(in press).

25. E.B. Lewis, Cold Spring Harbor Symp. Quant. Biol. 16, 159 (1951).

26. Ingram, V.M., Nature (London) 189, 704 (1961).

27. Baglioni, C., Proc. Nat. Acad. Sci. U.S. 48, 1880 (1962).

28. Balin, E., Hereditas 58, 1 (1967).

29. Popp, R.A., Francis, M.W., and Popp, D.M. In "Tissue Typing and Organ Transplantation" (E.J. Yunis and D.B. Amos, eds.) Academic Press, New York, 1972.

30. Litman, G., Merz, D., and Good, R.A. (Personal communication).

31. Grubb, R. In "The Genetic Marker of Human Immunoglobulins", p. 152. Springer-Verlag, Berlin and New York, 1970.

32. Boyse, E.A., Old, L.J., and Stockert, E., Proc. Nat. Acad. Sci. U.S. 60, 886 (1968).

33. Cerrotini, J.C. and Brunner, K.T., Immunology 13, 395 (1967).

34. Davis, W.C., Science 175, 1006 (1972).

35. Taylor, R.B., Duffus, W.P.H., Raff, M.C., and de Petris, S., Nature (London), 233, 225 (1971).

36. Raff, M.C., Steinberg, M., and Taylor, R.B., Nature (London) 225, 553 (1970).

37. Singer, S.J. and Nicolson, G.L., Science 175, 720 (1972).

38. Inbar, M. and Sachs, L., Nature (London), 223, 710 (1969).

39. Wannier, G.H. In "Elements of Solid State Theory", Chapter 4. Cambridge Univ. Press, London and New York, 1959.
40. Yunis, E.J., Ward, F.E., and Amos, D.B. In "Histocompatibility Testing 1970" (P.I. Terasaki, ed.), p. 351. Munksgaard, Copenhagen, 1970.
41. Colombani, J., Colombani, M., and Dausset, J. Ann. N.Y. Acad. Sci. 120, 307 (1964).
42. Dausset, J., Colombani, J., Feingold, N., and Rapaport, F.T., Nouv. Rev. Fr. Hematol. 5, 17 1965.
43. van Rood, J.J., van Leeuwen, A., Eernisse, J.G., Frederics, E., and Bosch, J.L., Ann. N.Y. Acad. Sci. 120, 285 (1964).
44. Dausset, J. and Colombani, J., Proc. Congr. Int. Soc. Blood Transfusions., 8th, 1962.
45. Dausset, J., Rapaport, F.T., Ivanyi, P., and Colombani, J., In "Histocompatibility Testing 1965" (D.B. Amos and J.J. van Rood, eds.), p. 63. Munksgaard, Copenhagen, 1965.
46. Terasaki, P.I., Marchioro, T.L., and Starzl, T.E., Nat. Acad. Sci. - Nat. Res. Counc., Publ. 1229, 83 (1965).
47. Starzl, T.E., Marchioro, T.L., Hermann, G., Brittain, R.S., and Waddell, W.R., Surgery 55, 195 (1964).
48. Amos, D.B., Hattler, B.G., MacQueen, J.M., Cohen, I., and Seigler, H.F. In "Advances in Transplantation" (J. Dausset, J. Hamburger, and G. Mathé, eds.), p. 202. Williams and Wilkins, Baltimore, 1967.
49. Ceppellini, R., In "Human Transplantation" (J. Dausset and F.T. Rapaport, eds.), p. 21. Grune & Stratton, New York, 1968.
50. Dausset, J., Rapaport, F.T., Legrand, L., Colombani, J., and Marcelli, B.A., In "Histocompatibility Testing 1970" (P.I. Terasaki, ed.), p. 381. Munksgaard, Copenhagen, 1970.
51. Mickey, M.R., Kreisler, M., Albert, E.D., Tanaka, N., Linscott, S., and Terasaki, P.I.,

Tissue Antigens 1, 57 (1971).

52. van Rood, J.J. In "Progress in Immunology" (D.B. Amos, ed.), p. 1027. Academic Press, New York, 1972.

53. Amos, D.B. and Yunis, E.J. In "Tissue Typing and Organ Transplantation" (E.J. Yunis and D.B. Amos, eds.). Academic Press, New York, 1972.

54. Simmons, R.L., Kjellstrand, C.M., and Najarian, J. In "Tissue Typing and Organ Transplantation" (E.J. Yunis and D.B. Amos, eds.). Academic Press, New York, 1972.

55. Ginn, H.E., Jr., Unger, A.M., Hume, D.M., and Schilling, J.A. J. Clin. Lab. Med. 56, 1 (1960).

56. Hume, D.M., Magee, J.H., Kaufman, H.J., Jr., Rittenbury, M.S., and Prout, G.R., Jr., Ann. Surg. 158, 608 (1963).

57. Murray, J.E. and Harrison, J.H., Amer. J. Surg. 105, 205 (1963).

58. Merrill, J.P., Murray, J.E., Harrison, J.H., Friedman, E.A., Dealy, J.B., and Dammin, G.J., New Engl. J. Med. 262, 1251 (1960).

59. Hume, D.M. In "Human Transplantation" (J. Dausset and F.T. Rapaport, eds.), p. 151. Grune & Stratton, New York, 1968.

60. van Rood, J.J., van Leeuwen, A., Pearce, R., and van der Doas, J.A., Transplant. Proc. 1, 372 (1969).

61. Sengar, D.P., Mickey, M.R., and Terasaki, P.I., Transplantation 7, 246 (1969).

62. Terasaki, P.I. and Mickey, M.R., Transplant. Proc. 3, 1057 (1971).

63. Bain, B., Lowenstein, L. and MacLean, L.D., Nat. Acad. Sci. - Nat. Res. Counc., Publ. 1229 121 (1965).

64. Hirschhorn, K., Firschein, L.L., and Bach, F.H., Nat. Acad. Sci. - Nat.Res. Counc. Publ. 1229, 131,(1965).

65. Bach, F.H., Science 156, 1196 (1968).

66. Amos, D.B. and Bach, F.H., J. Exp. Med. 128, 623 (1968).

67. Bach, F.H., Albertini, R.J., Amos, D.B., Ceppellini, R., Mattiuz, P.L., and Miggiano, V. L., _Transplant. Proc._ 1, 339 (1969).

68. Yunis, E.J., Plate, J.M., Ward, F.E., Seigler, H.F., and Amos, D.B., _Transplant. Proc._ 3, 118 (1971).

69. Sorensen, S.F. and Nielsen, L.S., _Acta Pathol. Microbiol. Scand._ 78B, 719 (1970).

70. Terasaki, P.I., Miyajima, T., Sengar, D.P.S., and Stiehm, E.R., _Transplantation_ 13, 250 (1972).

71. Bach, J.F., Debray-Sachs, M., Crosier, J., Kreis, H., and Dormont, J., _Clin. Exp. Immunol._ 6, 821 (1970).

72. Jeannet, M., _Helv. Med. Acta_ 35, 168 (1970).

73. Koch, C.T., Frederiks, E., Eijsvoogel, V.P., and van Rood, J.J., _Lancet_ 2, 1334 (1971).

74. Buckley, R.H., _In_ "Progress in Immunology" (D.B. Amos, ed.), p. 1061. Academic Press, New York, 1972.

75. De Koning, J., Dooren, L.J., van Bekkum, D.W., van Rood, J.J., Dicke, K.A., and Radl, J., _Lancet_ 1, 1223 (1969).

76. Gatti, R.A., Meuwissen, H.J., Allen, H.D., Hong, R., and Good, R.A., _Lancet_ 2, 1366 (1968).

77. Thomas, E.D., Rudolph, R.H., Fefer, A., Storb, R., Slichter, S., and Buckner, C.D., _Exp. Haematol._ 21, 16 (1971).

78. Thomas, E.D., Buckner, C.D., Storb, R., Neiman, P.E., Fefer, A., Clift, R.A., Slichter, S.J., Funk, D.D., Bryant, J.I., and Lerner, K.E., _Lancet_ 1, 284 (1972).

79. Bortin, M.M., Saltzstein, E.C., Waisbren, B.A., Kay, S.A., Hong, R., and Bach, F.H., _Transplantation_ 11, 573 (1971).

80. Graw, R.G., Herzig, G.P., Rogentine, G.N., Yankee, R.A., Leventhal, B.G., Whang-Peng, J.J., Halterman, R.H., Kruger, G., Berard, C., and Henderson, E.S., _Lancet_ 2, 1053 (1970).

81. Levey, R.H., Klemperer, M.R., Gelfand, E.W., Sanderson, A.R., Batchelor, J.R., Berkel, A.I.,

and Rosen, F.S., Lancet 2, 571 (1971).

82. Meuwissen, H.J., Bach, F., Hong, R., and Good, R.A., J. Pediat. 72, 177 (1968).

83. Thomas, E.D., Bryant, J.I., Buckner, C.D., Clift, R.A., Fefer, A., Johnson, F.L., Neiman, P., and Ramberg, R.E., Lancet 1, 1310 (1972).

84. Dupont, B., Anderson, V., Hansen, G.S., and Svejgaard, A., Transplantation (1972)(in press).

85. Haughton, G., Folia Biol. (Prague) 15, 239 (1969).

86. Yunis, E.J. and Amos, D.B., Proc. Nat. Acad. Sci. U.S. 68, 3031 (1971).

87. Amos, D.B. and Yunis, E.J., Cell. Immunol. 2, 517 (1971).

88. Snell, G.D., Smith, P., Gabrielson, F., J. Nat. Cancer Inst. 14, 457 (1953).

89. Snell, G.D., Russell, E., Fekete, E., and Smith, P., J. Nat. Cancer Inst. 14, 485 (1953).

90. Brent, L., Progr. Allergy 5, 271 (1958).

91. Lawrence, H.S., Physiol. Rev. 39, 811 (1959).

92. Lawrence, H.S., Annu. Rev. Med. 11, 207 (1960).

93. Lawrence, H.S., In "Human Transplantation" (J. Dausset and F.T. Rapaport, eds.), p. 11. Grune & Stratton, New York, 1968.

94. Amos, D.B., Seigler, H.F., Simmons, R.L., and E.J. Yunis, Transplantation (1972)(Submitted for publication).

95. Berke, G., Sullivan, K.A., and Amos, B., J. Exp. Med. 135, 1334 (1972).

SUBJECT INDEX

A

Actinomycin C, as prophylactic immuno-
  suppressant, 202
  for rejection therapy 216-217
Acute lymphocytic leukemia, bone marrow
  transplantation for, 437-449
Anemia, after renal transplantation 239
Antibiotics, for posttransplant infections,
  223
Antibodies
  human, in leukocytes, 1-7
  MLC reactivity inhibition as test for, 115
Antigens, human, in leukocytes, 1-7
Antilymphocyte globulin (ALG), use
  following kidney transplantation,
  198-200, 467-468
Anuria, after kidney transplantation,
  203-205
Arterial anastomosis, in kidney transplantation, 194-195
Azathioprine, use following kidney
  transplantation, 200
  toxicity from, 235

B

Bleeding, gastrointestinal, from renal
  immunosuppression, 234-235
Bone marrow transplantation, 463-464
  for acute lymphocytic leukemia,
  437-449
  in immunodeficiency disease, 413-449
  method for, 414
  MLC test in, 81-82
Brain death, criteria of, in renal transplant
  donors, 180-182

C

Cadaver donors, for kidney transplants,
  m 180-184
Calcium metabolism, disorders in, from
  renal immunosuppression, 236-238
Cataracts, from renal immunosuppression,
  235
Children, renal transplantation in, 192-193
  248-249
Creatinine clearance test, following renal
  transplantation, 197
Cushing's disease, from renal immunosuppression, 233-234
Cyclophosphamide, as prophylactic
  immunosuppressant, 202

D

Diabetes
  renal transplants in, 168-169, 247-248
  steroid type, from renal immunosuppression, 234
Dialysis (*see also under* Kidney transplantation)
  application of, 135-141
  renal transplantation compared to,
  143-157
Dipyridamole, as prophylactic immunosuppressant, 202

E

Erythremia, after renal transplantation, 239
Eurotransplant, kidney transplants in,
  matching in, 51, 65

475

F

Fungal infections, in immunosuppressed patients, 221

G

Genetics, of HL-A antigens, 13-47
Glomerulonephritis, renal transplants for, 167, 168
Granulocytes, effects on mixed-lymphocyte reactivity, 108

H

H-2 antigens, HL-A antigens compared to, 19
Hemodialysis, *see* Dialysis
Hemolytic uremic syndrome, renal transplants for, 169
Heparin, as prophylactic immunosuppressant, 202
Hepatitis, in posttransplant patients, 230
Herpes infections, in posttransplant patients, 230
Histadyl, as prophylactic immunosuppressant, 202
Histocompatibility
  of lymphocytes HL-typing use in, 75-77
  matching of, in donor selection, 117-133
    importance in kidney transplants, 242-244
  tests, in cadaver donors, 182-184
HL-A system and tests
  H-2 antigens compared to, 19
  in cadaver donors, 182-184
  genetics of, 13-47, 49
  control aspects, 79-81
  in histocompatibility and donor selection, 120-121
  in human transplantation, 452
  hypothesis for, 47
  leukocyte histocompatibility testing using, 75-77
  studies and uses of, 1-11
  use in kidney transplant prognosis, 49-69
HL-A transplantation antigens
  assay of, 384-387

distribution of 381-384
purification of, 387-388
solubilization and characterization of, 381-412
  by autolysis, 388-390
  by papain, 390-394
  by potassium chloride, 396-397
  by sonication, 394-396
Hypertension, from renal immunosuppression, 236

I

I^{131} hippuran renogram test, following renal transplantation, 197
Immunodeficiency disease, bone marrow transplantation for, 413-449
Immunosuppression, 467-468
  following kidney transplants, 198-202, 219-239, 266-269
Infections
  following renal transplantation, 220
  differential diagnosis, 229-230
  diagnosis, 224
  neurologic complications, 228
  prevention, 222-224
  pulmonary type, 224-228
  treatment, 223, 231-232
Irradiation, of kidney graft, 202
Isoniazid, as prophylactic immunosuppressant, 202

K

Kidney
  antigens of, 285-287
  antibodies to 297-299
  availability of, 287-288
  lymphocyte response, 292-293
  processing of, 289-292
Kidney transplantation, 165-283, 460-463
  of allografts
    biology of, 285-327
    pathology of, 329-355
  antibiotic therapy following, 198
  antilymphocyte globulin use following, 198-200
  azathioprine use following, 200

cadaver donors for, 180-184
  brain death criteria in, 180-182
  infection and, 222-223
  preparation prior to surgery of, 182-184
complications of, 202-219, 334-335
  anuria or oliguria, 203-205
  hyperacute rejection, 207-208, 333-334
  infection, 215-216
  rejection, 210-217, 267, 315-319
    morphology, 329-333
  renal failure, 202-203
    from recurrent disease, 217-219
  technical type, 205-207
  treatment of, 216-217
  tubulur necrosis, 208-210
dialysis prior to, 135-141, 171-173, 190
  preparation for, 173-175
  surgery and, 175-176
dialysis vs., 143-157
in high-risk patients, 150, 151
  prognosis, 244-246
histocompatibility importance in, 242-244
in HL-A identical patients, 336-337
HL-A typing for, 49-69, 461-463
immunosuppressive therapy following,
    198-202, 266-267, 269
  complications of, 219-239
  Cushing's disease from, 233-234
  malignancy from, 232-233
irradiation of graft following, 202
living donors for
  ethical problems of, 178-179
  medical evaluation of, 177, 264-265
  selection and evaluation of, 176-179
mortality causes, 153-154, 270-271
multiple, 249-250, 277-278
organ harvest for, 184-187
  from cadaver donor, 187
  in related living donors, 184-186
posttransplant care, 196-202
  laboratory tests, 197-198
prednisone use following, 201
preparation for, 173-175
prior to renal transplantation, 135-141,
    171-173
recipient in, 187-190
  nephrectomy in, 187-190
  preparation, 187-190

selection of, 166-176, 262
  criteria, 166-171
  workup for, 262-263
rehabilitation in, 250
renal disease effects on, 274
results of, 239-250, 279
  in abnormal urinary tracts, 246-247
  in ideal vs. high-risk patients, 244-246
  in children, 248-249
  in diabetics, 247-248
technical problems during, 194-195
technique of, 190-195
  in anephric patient, 193-194
  in children, 192-193

L

Laboratory tests, following renal
  transplantation, 197-198
Leucoagglutination, in discovery of H-2
  antigens, 13
Leukemia, acute lymphocytic type, bone
  marrow transplantation for, 437-449
Leukocytes
  antigens and antibodies in, 1-7
  mixed culture test using, see Mixed
    leukocyte culture test
Leukopenia, infection in immunosuppression and, 223
Lungs
  infections of, in post transplant
    patients, 224-228
  "transplant lung" disease of, 229
Lupus erythematosus, renal transplants
  for, 169
Lymphocytes
  in vitro transformation of, 72-73
  response to kidney antigens, 292-293
  stimulation of, in histocompatibility
    matching and donor selection,
    121-126
Lysozyme, urinary, following renal
  transplantation, 197-198

M

Malignancy, from renal immunosuppression, 232-233, 281-283

Methylprednisone, use following kidney
transplantation, 201
Mixed-lymphocyte culture (MLC) test
and reactivity
after allografting, 110-111
in bone marrow transplantation, 81-82
cellular contributions to, 96-100
clinical uses of, 93-115
cultures for, 73-75
genetic control aspects of, 79-81
in histocompatibility matching, 78-79
with donor selection, 121
inhibition of, as test for antibody, 115
use in transplantation, 71-91
Musculoskeletal disorders, after renal
transplantation, 238-239

N

Nephrectomy, prior to transplantation,
187-190
Nervous system, fungal infections of, in
posttransplant patient, 228

O

Oliguria, after kidney transplantation,
203-205

P

Pancreatitis, after renal transplantation, 239
Papain, solubilization of HL-A trans-
plantation antigens by, 390-394
Perfusion, of kidneys, prior to transplanta-
tion, 183-184
Prednisone, use following kidney trans-
plantation, 201
Pulmonary embolisms, in posttransplant
patient, 229
Pyelonephritis, renal transplants for, 167

R

Rejection, after kidney transplantation
clinical patterns of, 315-319

differential diagnosis of, 211-215, 337
hyperacute, 207-208
infection with, 215-216
lymphocyte participation, 293-297
morphology of, 329-333
pathology of, 307-314
Renal failure
after kidney transplantation, 202-203
due to recurrent disease, 217-219

S

Skin, grafts of, 459-460
Sonication, solubilization of HL-A antigens
by, 394-396
Splenectomy, prior to kidney transplantation, 188
Steroid diabetes, from renal immunosuppression, 234

T

Thrombosis, from renal immunosuppression, 205, 235-236
Thymectomy, prior to kidney transplantation, 188
Tissue typing, in human transplantation,
surgical aspects, 159-163
Transformation, of lymphocytes, in vitro,
72-73
Transplant fever, etiology of, 229-230
Transplant lung, description and etiology
of, 229
Transplantation antigens
chemical tags for, 357-380
HL-A type, 381-412
isolation and chemistry of, 359-367
Transplants and transplantation
of bone marrow, see Bone marrow
transplantation
clinical aspects of, 459-467
critical appraisal of, 451-474
cross-reactivity and antigen frequency
in, 453-456
grid hypothesis in, 458-459
histocompatibility and donor selection in,
117-133
historical basis for, 451-452, 464-467

HL-A system in, 452
immunity of, genetic control of, 79-81
isolation and characterization of
   membrane constituents in, 456-458
of kidneys, 165-283
  dialysis vs., 143-157
  HL-A typing in, 49-69
mixed leukocyte culture test in, 71-91
of skin, 459-460
tissue typing in, 159-163

immunosuppressive therapy in,
   467-468
Tumors, of kidney, transplants for,
   168-169

V

Venous anastomosis, in kidney transplantation, 194